FAMILY HOMŒOPATHY.

BY

JOHN ELLIS, M. D'.,

LATE PROFESSOR OF THE THEORY AND PRACTICE OF MEDICINE IN THE NEW YORK MEDICAL COLLEGE FOR WOMEN; FORMERLY PROFESSOR OF THE THEORY AND PRACTICE OF MEDICINE IN THE WESTERN HOMŒOPATHIC MEDICAL COLLEGE OF CLEVELAND, OHIO; AND OF THE NEW YORK HOMŒOPATHIC MEDICAL COLLEGE; AUTHOR OF THE "AVOIDABLE CAUSES OF DISEASES," "MARRIAGE," ETC.

TENTH EDITION.

DETROIT, MICH:

E. R. ELLIS, M. D., Secretary of, and Professor of SURGERY in the DETROIT HOMŒOPATHIC COLLEGE,

AND

J. YOUNGHUSBAND, M. D., LL. D., President of, and Professor of THEORY AND PRACTICE in the DETROIT HOMŒOPATHIC COLLEGE.

1872.

PREFACE.

On presenting a treatise on domestic medicine to the homœopathic portion of the community, while there are so many works already in existence, it is proper that the author should state some of the motives which have induced him to write it.

First: He has done it in compliance with the often expressed wish of many of his patrons, for a work of the character of the one he here presents, and at the request of some of the leading pharmaceutists of our country. His aim has been to present in a compact form, as good a description of the symptoms of the various diseases, as possible in a small compass, and to give the prominent indications for the use of a limited number of our most important remedies, with specific and somewhat positive directions as to the stage of the disease in which they should be used, and the length of time during which they should generally be continued; thus simplifying the practice, and leaving as little as possible to the discretion of the prescriber. He is satisfied that the success of even a physician does not always depend upon the number of remedies with which he is acquainted, but upon his understanding how to make the best possible use of such as he does administer, and this is more manifestly true in the case of lay practitioners. If a large number of remedies, and numerous indications for their use are given, the domestic prescriber is often confused, and finds it impossible to decide between the merits of the different remedies; and if no directions are given as to the period of time a remedy should be continued, a frequent change often prevents any good effects being derived from the treatment. The author has purposely avoided the alphabetical arrangement in noticing the remedies indicated for the various diseases. The first one on the list has been placed there, either because it is generally required at the commencement of the disease, or is more frequently required than those which follow. The reader will please bear in mind that this is a domestic work, and has not been written to instruct physicians in regard to the proper treatment of diseases, but to guide those comparatively unacquainted with medical lore; therefore the aim has been to make it as simple and useful as possible. If the author had written this work for the profession he certainly would have recommended earnestly the high dilutions; and that a frequent repetition of doses and the alternation of remedies should be avoided as far as practicable.

Second: One of the leading motives which has induced the author to write this volume has been to have an opportunity to call the attention of the homœopathic portion of the community to another work, which he has written, denominated, "The Avoidable Causes of Disease, Insanity, and Deformity," published by Messrs. Mason Brothers, 5 and 7 Mercer street, New York; a work which, in the opinion of the author, is of far more importance, and of much greater value to every man, woman, and child, than any work on domestic medicine can possibly be. That is a work to be read while well, so as to be able to shun the causes of disease; and if sick it should be read so as to understand the conditions required for a restoration to health. The most skilful application of remedies often fails to relieve, for the want of the very information contained in that volume; and, although the work was written for general circulation, yet the author has no hesitation in expressing the opinion that even physicians can obtain as much practical information from its pages, which will enable them to treat successfully, especially chronic diseases, as they can find in any other single volume which has ever been written. Knowing, then, the value which the author sets upon that work, the reader of this will pardon the frequent reference to the "Avoidable Causes of Disease," in the following pages.

NEW YORK, *June*, 1864.

INTRODUCTION.

LAW OF CURE.

HOMŒOPATHY differs from all other systems of medical practice, in being based upon a law of nature; and it is, therefore, strictly a scientific system. "Like is cured by like," is the fundamental law—that is, a remedy will cure symptoms when they arise from some other cause, similar to those which it will itself cause if it is taken during health. The allopathic materia medica, or knowledge of the action of remedies, is derived from the empirical administration of poisons to the sick, their use in domestic practice, their being taken through accident or design, and the giving of them to brutes; and allopathists are guided simply by past experience in administering them to the sick, with no fixed rule or law to guide them. The homœopathic materia medica is the result of carefully proving remedies on the healthy, or the giving of them during health, and accurately noting down the symptoms which they cause; and when given to the sick, they are administered in accordance with the law of cure named above. Homœopathic remedies, then, act in the direction of the disease, and simply excite a reaction which overcomes the diseased action. It follows, as a necessary consequence, that if remedies are given which will excite symptoms similar to those which already exist, they must be given in small doses, or they will most certainly aggravate the symptoms seriously, and experience has shown that this is unnecessary, hence the small doses of homœopathy.

SIZE OF THE DOSE.

The size of the doses which are administered by homœopathists is simply the result of experience; every physician aims to give such doses as he finds most efficacious. The selection of the right remedy is of far more importance, as a general rule, than the size of the dose, provided the latter is not so great as to cause any serious aggravation of the symptoms. Yet, in some cases, the right dose is very important. According to the author's experience, many of the happiest cures ever effected are the result of using the high dilutions, but it requires accurate knowledge and great skill to select the right remedy, and to decide on the frequency of the repetition of the dose, when the high dilutions are used. The low dilutions are generally used in domestic practice, and the author is by no means satisfied that they should not be, for they can be repeated, with a prospect of success, and without injury, more frequently than the high dilutions, and there is less objection to alternating two remedies, when the low dilutions are used, which is generally satisfactory to the patient and friends. The action of the low dilutions is more transient than that of the high, and when they are used, a second remedy will often be required long before the first can safely be dispensed with, therefore, if the low dilutions are used, it is difficult for the physician even to avoid alternating remedies to a greater or less extent.

The directions in this volume in regard to the repetition of doses and alternating remedies, in the treatment of the various diseases, have been given upon the supposition that the low dilutions are to be used. If the thirtieth, or higher dilutions are used, they should not, generally, be repeated in acute diseases more frequently than once in from six to twelve, or twenty-four hours; in chronic cases, once or twice a week—never more frequently than once a day at most; generally it is better not to repeat so long as the patient continues to improve.

MEDICINAL AGGRAVATIONS.

If the symptoms are worse after taking one or more doses of the remedy, especially if they grow suddenly worse within half an hour of taking the medicine, omit the remedy; and if the aggravation has been caused by the remedy, it will generally soon cease, but if it should not cease, select another remedy, and give one dose, and repeat it at long intervals. A remedy which has caused an aggravation may be repeated when the relief which follows the aggravation has ceased, but it should be given at longer intervals, or be made much weaker by being diluted with a large quantity of water.

If relief to the symptoms follows the use of a remedy, continue it, but lengthen the intervals between the doses. If the patient ceases to improve, select another remedy, but do not change the remedies while there is any manifest improvement.

DOSE AND ADMINISTRATION OF REMEDIES.

In acute diseases, and in other cases where a prompt action of the remedy is desired, it is generally best to give the medicine dissolved in water. If the remedy is in the form of globules, dissolve twelve of them in half a glass of cold water; if it is in the form of a tincture, drop one drop into a glassful of water; if it is in the form of powder, put half as much as will lie on a three-cent piece into half a glass of water—in either case stir the solution well, and give to an adult two teaspoonfuls or one tablespoonful for a dose; to a child, one teaspoonful for a dose. Powders may also be given dry on the tongue, giving for a dose as much as will lie on the point of a penknife blade. In chronic cases, or in acute cases which are not very urgent, the remedy may be given either dry on the tongue or dissolved in cold water. If it is in globules, give four to an adult or two to a child; if in powder, give as much as will lie on the end of a penknife blade to an adult, or half as much to a child; if it is in the form of a tincture, drop one drop on a lump of sugar, or into a spoonful of water, and give the whole of it to an adult, or one fourth of it to a child, if only a single dose is to be given, but if several doses will probably be required, dissolve the same quantity of the tincture in ten spoonfuls of water, and give as directed in acute cases, to an adult two spoonfuls, or to a child one teaspoonful. Never use the same glass or spoon for two remedies without carefully washing it.

DIET.

Patients under homœopathic treatment should avoid high-seasoned dishes and all condiments, with the exception of salt and sugar, which should be used only sparingly. Smoked meats and fish, all strong-scented and pungent vegetables, pastry of all kinds, and confectionery, should be shunned. He should avoid all alcoholic and fermented drinks, tobacco, and opium, except when he has been long addicted to their use, in which case he should use them very sparingly, or, what is better, gradually discontinue their use. It is generally better that he should drink neither tea nor coffee, or certainly nothing more than black tea.

More specific directions in regard to diet will be found in connection with the treatment of the various diseases.

LIST OF REMEDIES RECOMMENDED IN THIS WORK.

ABBREVIATIONS, FULL NAMES, AND COMMON NAMES.

1. Aconite—Aconitum napellus—Monk's Hood.
2. Aconite—tincture, or globules saturated with the tincture.
3. Apis mel.—Apis mellifica—poison of the Honey Bee.
4. Arnica—Arnica montana—Leopard's Bane.
5. Arsenicum—Arsenicum album—Arsenic.
6. Belladonna—Deadly Nightshade.
7. Bryonia—Bryonia alba—White Bry
8. Calcarea carb. or Calcarea carbonica—Carbonate of lime.
9. Cannabis or Cannabis sativa—Hemp.
10. Cantharis—Cantharides—Spanish Fly.
11. Carbo veg. or Carbo vegetabilis—Charcoal.
12. Chamomilla—Chamomile.
13. China—China officinalis—Cinchona—Peruvian Bark.
14. Cina—Wormseed.
15. Coffea—Coffea cruda—Coffee.
16. Colocynth—Colocynthis—Bitter Cucumber.
17. Cuprum—Cuprum met. or metalicum—Copper.
18. Drosera—Round-leaved Sun-dew.
19. Dulcamara—Bitter Sweet.
20. Gelsemium semp.—Gelsemium sempervirens—Yellow Jessamine.
21. Helleborus—Helleborus niger—Black Hellebore.
22. Hepar sulph. or Hepar sulphuris—Sulphuret of Lime.
23. Hyoscyamus or Hyoscyamus niger—Henbane.
24. Ignatia or Ignatia amara—St. Ignatius' Bean.
25. Ipecac or Ipecacuanha.
26. Lachesis—Poison of the Lance-headed Serpent.
27. Lycopodium—Wolf's Claw.
28. Mercurius prot.—Mercurius protiod.—Protiodide of Mercury.
29. Mercurius viv.—Mercurius vivus (Mercurius sol. may be used in its place)—Mercury.
30. Mercurius cor.—Mercurius corrosivus—Corrosive Sublimate.
31. Natrum mur.—Natrum muriaticum—Muriate of Soda.

32. Nitric acid—Nitri acidum.
33. Nux vom.—Nux vomica.
34. Opium.
35. Phosphorus.
36. Pulsatilla—Pasque Flower.
37. Platina.
38. Rhus tox.—Rhus toxicodendron—Poison Oak.
39. Rheum—Rhubarb.
40. Sabina—Savine.
41. Secale cor.—Secale cornutum—Ergot of Rye.
42. Silicea—Silex.
43. Spongia—Burnt Sponge.
44. Stannum—Tin.
45. Stramonium—Thorn Apple.
46. Sulphur.
47. Tartar emetic—Tartarus emeticus—Stibium.
48. Veratrum—Veratrum album—White Hellebore.

TINCTURES FOR EXTERNAL AND INTERNAL USE.

1. Arnica—Arnica montana—Leopard's Bane.
2. Calendula—Calendula officinalis—Marigold.
3. Urtica urens.
4. Camphor or Camphora in tincture or globules.

The reader will please bear in mind that the above list of abbreviations and variations of the names of the remedies, contains simply those which are in this book, and not all that are sometimes used in putting up domestic cases. For instance, *Aconite, Acon., Aconitum nap., Aconitum napellus*, all denote the same remedy, and so in other cases. If the first three or four letters are right on your label, and there is no second name on the label, you have the right remedy. If there is a second name, the first two or three letters should correspond with those of the remedy named in the book, if in the book there is any second name ; but if there is no second name to the remedy in the book, you have the right remedy, for when there are two remedies with the same first name, the first three letters of the second name are always given.

DOMESTIC HOMŒOPATHIC PRACTICE.

CHAPTER I.

FEVERS.

No class of diseases has attracted more attention, or has been the subject of more speculation, than febrile diseases. As this is a practical work, I do not intend to spend either much time or space in considering such speculations ; but a few remarks on some of the theories which have prevailed seem necessary, to counteract certain pernicious methods of treatment which are prevalent, having such theories for their foundation. Among the most pernicious of the various theories which have prevailed will be found the one which ascribes fevers to the fluids of the body, especially to the bile, the phlegm, and blood—to a superabundance of these fluids, or to their depraved state.

The "black bile" was a bug-bear with Hippocrates, the father of allopathy, and his descendants have been bilious ever since ; and if we can judge from the common expression so frequently sounding in our ears, "I am bilious," they have not labored in vain in their efforts to convince the community that an excess of bile is the cause of a large share of their ills, especially fevers. "You are bilious," says the doctor, by which the patient understands that his stomach is filled with bile ; and what is more simple, or apparently natural, than to cure this state of things by an emetic or cathartic. If an emetic is given, the first effort of vomiting may not reach the bile, simply because the stomach contains none; but by the efforts of vomiting, and the irritation caused by the emetic, the inverted action which has been established in the stomach extends to the upper portion of the intestines, below the entrance of the gall duct, and the bile, which should flow down through the bowels to aid in the process of digestion, passes up into the stomach, and is thrown up; and the more the patient vomits the more bile he discharges, until he is astonished to think he was not sick before, from being so bilious. So the poor patient is humbugged into the belief that he is bilious, through his own senses; the doctor makes a convert to his sagacity and method of practice, but he fails to show his poor deluded victim how the throwing off of the small quantity of bile which is secreted for an hour or two during the operation of the emetic, is to furnish any permanent relief, or prevent its continued secretion; but as, after the action of the emetic is over, the bile pursues its usual course, and does not trouble the patient more than heretofore, he is satisfied with the wonderful skill of his doctor. Even if there is an excess of bile secreted, the fault is with the liver, and remedies should be given to correct its deranged action; simply evacuating the stomach and bowels by emetics and cathartics amounts to little, except to do injury. Although priding themselves in a "combined experience of three thousand years," only a few of the most intelligent physicians of the dominant school are beginning to make the discovery that blood-letting exercises little or no control over febrile or inflammatory diseases, except for injury—often exhausting the vital energies, and destroying the power of resistance which is so much needed at the critical stage of the disease.

Hoffman and Cullen introduced the nervous theories of fever. Hoffman taught that the chill is caused by a spasm of the capillary, or most minute blood-vessels, and that the heat and excitement which follow are but the reaction of the system to overcome this spasm. But there would seem to be much greater evidence of a collapse of the minute blood-vessels than of spasm. The nervous theories, in a great measure, overthrew the theories founded upon the blood and secretions, but, as we have seen, did not destroy the methods of practice founded upon them, for the latter continue to this day. Having said this much in regard to the theories of the past, I shall allow all theories to rest in the grave with their authors, for they are of no practical value. The homœopathist has a practical law to guide him in the selection of his remedies, and so strong is my confidence in the superiority of the system for the treatment of all febrile diseases, that I would rather trust an intelligent layman, with simply a good domestic work and case of medicines to treat me, than to risk the treatment of the best allopathic physician in the world, in any febrile disease.

We have what physicians call idiopathic fevers; by which are meant diseases which are essentially and primarily febrile diseases, and do not depend upon local disease. Among the fevers of this class we have ephemeral fevers, typhus and typhoid fevers, intermittent, remittent, and yellow fevers. During the course of such diseases, local congestions, and even inflammation, may supervene; but these local affections are secondary—rather the consequence of the fever than the cause of it. We have also symptomatic fevers, or fevers which are caused by local inflammation or local disease. Such fevers sometimes assume a typhoid or an intermittent form during their course, or become complicated with the latter affections, especially when they occur in localities where, or during seasons when, typhoid or intermittent fevers are prevailing. Then we have eruptive fevers.

EPHEMERAL FEVER.

This consists of a single paroxysm of fever, commencing generally with chills, pains in the head, back, and limbs, followed by fever, attended by the latter symptoms, and terminating, in the course of twenty-four or forty-eight hours, in a profuse perspiration, or some other critical discharge, such as a profuse flow of urine, or a diarrhœa. This is a very common disease, especially during the prevalence of other febrile and eruptive diseases. It is not improbable but that the causes which produce such fevers, acting on constitutions partially protected against them, or which are not very susceptible, may produce simply this ephemeral fever ; as it is more common, as has just been noticed, during the prevalence of other febrile affections. It is not always easy to distinguish this disease from the commencement of other febrile diseases, except by its duration, and this is of no great moment, as we always select our remedy by the symptoms which exist, and not by the name of the disease. It may also be caused by exposure, sudden changes of temperature, errors of diet, mental emotions, &c.

Treatment.—*Aconite*, if the skin is hot and dry, the pulse full and hard, and the face flushed, is the proper remedy. It may be given in solution every hour until perspiration ensues.

Dose, see page 7.

Bryonia: If typhoid or typhus fever is prevailing, or if the pains in the head are dull, and the hands and feet disposed to be cool, *Bryonia* may be given instead of *Aconite*, or it may follow the latter remedy at the end of twelve hours, and be repeated once in four hours.

Belladonna may be selected instead of *Bryonia*, and given once in two hours, if the pains in the head are sharp and cutting, the eyes red, with sensitiveness to light and noise ; and if there is delirium.

A warm bath, when it is convenient, or simply bathing the feet in warm water, if great care is used against exposure afterward, will be useful. A glass of cold water, or even of hot water, milk, and sugar, and covering up warm in bed, will often afford considerable relief, by aiding the *Aconite* in promoting perspiration.

TYPHUS FEVER.

Very little is known in regard to the cause of this disease. It occurs most frequently in situations where persons are crowded together, especially when there is added to this, unwholesome food and vitiated and confined air, as aboard ships, in crowded hospitals, prisons, camps, and large cities. But this disease not unfrequently occurs in country places, and even in mountainous regions, and also among those who are well housed and fed, and who pay the utmost regard to cleanliness. It is supposed to be, to a limited extent, contagious, and it often depends upon an epidemic influence. This disease prevails more frequently during the autumn and winter, but it may occur during any season of the year.

Symptoms.—Often loss of appetite, weariness, sleepiness, and dull headache. precede the attack. Sometimes the disease begins abruptly by a chill, followed by symptoms of fever. There is dull pain in the head, and perhaps in the back and limbs—the mental faculties soon become torpid and dull—the pulse, if at first full, soon becomes feeble and frequent, often beating from 100 to 110, 120, or even, in the course of the disease, as frequently as 140 or 150 in a minute. The extremities soon become cool, and even cold, but the body and head hot, the face flushed, and of a purple tint. The tongue at first may be coated white, but it soon becomes brown and dry. The urine is small in quantity and reddish The bowels are generally costive. These symptoms continue, with a gradual increase, until about the end of six or seven days from the commencement of the chills and fever, when other symptoms are superadded. The tongue becomes encrusted with a brown or black coating, and is generally dry. There oozes from the gums and mucous membrane of the mouth dark bloody mucus, which dries and accumulates on the teeth, lips, gums, and even on the soft palate, in some cases. Such crusts are called sordes. The pulse becomes frequent and feeble, the body hot and dry, the extremities cold, a peculiar offensive odor often exhales from the body, and there is twitching of the tendons, or cords, in the extremities. The patient slides down in bed involuntarily, becomes very feeble, lies on his back, picks at the bedclothes, or at imaginary objects; muttering delirium ensues, or even stupor or coma, more or less profound. Occasionally the lungs become congested, and there is oppression in breathing and cough. Sometimes there are involuntary evacuations from the bowels, retention of urine, hemorrhage from the bowels, or from the nostrils, effusion of blood beneath the skin, causing dark spots like bruises. There is frequently an eruption on the neck and body, and sometimes on the limbs, varying in size from a pin's head to the fourth of an inch in diameter, varying in color from red to purple, violet, or even black. A fine rash, of transparent vesicles, from the size of a mustard-seed to that of a pin's head, frequently makes its appearance at this stage of the disease. There is almost always more or less deafness. There is often a very great tendency to excoriation, ulceration, and mortification of the parts of the back and hips, on which the patient lies, caused by pressure, when the utmost care is not used to prevent it. The average duration of this fever is about fourteen days, but it may abate by the seventh or ninth, or continue until the twenty-first day.

Favorable Symptoms.—The tongue gradually begins to clean at the tip and edges, the pulse becomes less frequent and fuller, the skin over the body becomes cooler and less dry, the extremities warmer, a gentle uniform perspiration may ensue, the delirium, stupor, and deafness, subside, the patient takes more interest in the things around him, and begins to feel some appetite, and steadily recovers.

Unfavorable Symptoms.—A very frequent or an irregular pulse, or slow and scarcely perceptible pulse. The extremities become cold and clammy, or the whole surface becomes covered with a cold clammy sweat. The countenance assumes a death-like aspect, and the patient gradually sinks and dies. Sometimes death is preceded by convulsions, and often by profound coma or insensibility.

Treatment.—To prevent this disease, pure air and cleanliness are very essential; all decaying vegetables should be carefully removed from the cellar; stagnant water should be drained from the cellar, and from beneath the house; the sink should be kept clean, dish washings and vegetable substances should not be thrown about the doors, and in gutters, to decompose and vitiate the air. If the disease is prevailing, and individuals have been exposed to patients sick with it, or to the same causes which have produced it in those already suffering, *Rhus tox.* and *Bryonia* may be taken alternately, forty-eight hours apart, as preventives.

Dose, see page 7.

Bryonia: During the first stage of the disease, before the stage of prostration or collapse arrives, *Bryonia* is generally the most important remedy, especially when there is dull pain in the head, with mental and physical torpor, great heat over the body and temples, with cold extremities, coated tongue, light colored or brown, and dry, and when there is great soreness over the body.

If the disease commences with a full pulse, and warm extremities, great benefit will result from giving *Aconite* once in two hours, for twelve or twenty-four hours, or until the extremities are cool, before giving *Bryonia*.

It should be remembered that we can rarely if ever "break up" either this disease or typhoid fever. It is the opinion of many writers that this can never be done; it is quite certain that it generally runs its course, and all we can expect is to lessen its severity, and bring it to a favorable termination. If we would derive the full benefit which remedies are capable of exerting in this and other diseases which have a somewhat specific duration, we must avoid changing our remedies often. *Bryonia*, when indicated in this disease, should generally be continued once in two or three hours, until the sixth or seventh day, or even longer if the patient seems to be doing well. The patient may be regarded as doing well, so long as he is not getting materially worse. If there are sharp pains in the head, with sensitiveness to noise and light, with or without delirium, early in the disease, *Belladonna* may be given instead of *Bryonia* once in two hours, until such symptoms are relieved.

Nux vomica: This remedy may be given in the first stage of the disease, when there is pain in the top and back of the head, when the skin and eyes are yellow, and the tongue yellow or dry, when there is pain, soreness, or fullness and weight in the right side beneath the short ribs, in the region of the liver, and constipation. This remedy will rarely be required for more than two or three days, when it should be followed by *Bryonia*. *Nux vomica* may be given during any stage of the disease, if the above symptoms occur.

Rhus tox.: As the disease approaches the stage of collapse, or great prostration, and the extremities become colder, the pulse weaker, and sordes begin to appear on the teeth and gums, and the tongue becomes dry and dark, *Rhus tox.* should take the place of *Bryonia*, and be given once in two hours. *Rhus tox.* may be given early in the disease, if the prostration is very great, but in the stage of prostration it is our main remedy, especially when there are muttering delirium, sliding down in bed, cold perspiration, or the dark spots on the skin, and the eruptions named in the description of the symptoms; also, if the bowels should become loose with dark offensive passages, and the breath very offensive.

Arsenicum: If, notwithstanding the use of *Bryonia* and *Rhus tox.*, the tendency to decomposition and dissolution increases until the pulse becomes very small, or irregular, and the surface cold and clammy, *Arsenicum* should be given either alone or alternately with *Rhus*, one hour apart. This remedy is especially indicated, if there are profuse, watery, or offensive discharges from the bowels, with or without burning thirst.

Carbo veg.: If *Arsenicum* fails to check the tendency to dissolution, and the pulse becomes scarcely perceptible, or irregular, the skin even over the body cool and clammy, this remedy may be given instead of *Arsenicum* every hour.

Camphor: If, during the course of the disease, especially about the seventh or fourteenth day, very great prostration of strength suddenly ensues, the pulse becomes small and irregular, the surface cold and clammy, give one drop of the common tincture or spirits of *Camphor*, in a little sugar and water, every fifteen minutes, until the symptoms of excessive prostration are relieved, provided they are relieved within two hours. If at the end of that time reaction does not ensue, give *Arsenicum* and *Carbo veg.* alternately, one hour apart.

Gelsemium semp.: This is a new remedy, which has been used to a greater or less extent by many physicians, in this and typhoid fever. At the commencement of the fever it sometimes does very well, but at present the particular indications for its use are not sufficiently understood. It may be given at the commencement of the attack, when the veins of the head are congested or full, with dull headache, delirium, or wavering of sight, and be repeated every hour until free perspiration ensues. If no change in the symptoms results within from twenty-four to forty-eight hours, select another remedy. Some physicians give drop doses of the tincture, others prefer the dilutions or globules. Either will answer.

There are other remedies which may be required for the successful treatment of certain cases of typhus fever, especially for the various complications which may arise, such as congestion of the lungs, diarrhœa, vomiting, hemorrhage from the bowels or nose, and bed sores, but as these complications quite as frequently occur in the course of typhoid fever, and as the indications are similar, the reader is referred to the treatment of that disease in such cases; also for suggestions as to diet, &c.

TYPHOID FEVER.

It is the opinion of many physicians and writers, that this is but a milder and modified form of typhus fever, and that it arises from the same cause. There is the same tendency to decomposition of the blood and solids of the body as witnessed in genuine typhus; and in cases which tend to a fatal termination, in the last stage, the symptoms are generally the same as in the latter disease. Typhoid fever generally commences more gradually, is slower in its progress, and longer in its duration than typhus fever. In typhus fever the bowels are generally constipated, whereas in typhoid fever there is predisposition to diarrhœa and soreness in the bowels on the right side of the lower half of the abdomen. Diarrhœa and soreness of the bowels are not always present, especially under homœopathic treatment, for I have seen well-marked cases of typhoid fever run their course without the occurrence of such symptoms. In fact, under our treatment, when they do occur, they are rarely very troublesome, when they have neither been developed nor aggravated by cathartic remedies. Diarrhœa may precede the febrile symptoms, it may commence with them, or it may commence during the middle or later stages of the disease. The average duration of typhoid fever is twenty-one days, but it may terminate in fourteen days, or linger for four or five weeks, but rarely for so long a period under homœopathic treatment.

Symptoms.—The disease sometimes commences abruptly by a chill, followed by symptoms of fever; but it often comes on insidiously, and increases gradually, so that it is difficult to fix the exact point of the commencement of the disease. The patient complains of weariness, uneasiness, soreness of the limbs, slight headache, torpor of the mental faculties, and indisposition to muscular action; there is heat of the body and temples, with a tendency to cool extremities. The disease may be so slight as scarcely to require the patient to take to his bed during its course, or it may be very severe, with severe headache, great mental and physical torpor, deafness, delirium, cold extremities, burning heat of body, frequent and small pulse, and, during the latter stages of the disease, dry tongue, sordes on the teeth, offensive breath, and twitching of the tendons. Between the mild and severe cases described above, we may have every degree of severity in different cases. We have the same tendency to hemorrhage from the nose and bowels, effusions of blood in and beneath the skin, and bed sores, as in typhus fever. There is frequently a troublesome cough, caused by a slow inflammation of the air-passages, or bronchia, and also obstinate vomiting caused by irritation or inflammation of the stomach. The tendency to diarrhœa and abdominal tenderness has already been noticed. For the symptoms which denote a fatal tendency, consult the section on typhus fever.

Treatment.—To prevent the disease in the case of individuals exposed, *Rhus tox.* and *Bryonia* may be given two days apart, as suggested for the prevention of typhus fever, and the same care in regard to cleanliness and ventilation is essential.

Bryonia: This remedy is about as important for the treatment of this disease as in the treatment of typhus fever, especially during the first ten or twelve days of the disease, and when the bowels are constipated. The reader may consult the indications for this remedy, *Rhus tox.*, *Arsenicum*, *Carbo veg.*, and *Gelsemium semp.*., under the head of typhus fever. In slight cases where there are no local complications, no other remedy may be required during the first stage of the disease but *Bryonia.*

Dose of this and other remedies, see page 7.

Rhus tox. may take the place of *Bryonia* during the latter stages of the disease, provided there is great prostration, with sordes or crusts on the teeth, and twitching of the tendons. If *Rhus tox.* does not check the tendency to a typhus state and dissolution, *Arsenicum* must be given every hour, and finally *Carbo veg.*—if *Arsenicum* fails—in desperate cases.

Gelsemium semp. will often do well at the commencement of the disease when there is great fullness about the head, severe headache or delirium, with or without derangements of sight. Also, if in the course of the disease head symptoms occur, which are not relieved by other remedies, give *Gelsemium* every hour. The above are all the remedies generally required in uncomplicated cases, where there is neither local congestion nor inflammation, but in a majority of cases there are symptoms which require other remedies.

Pulsatilla : This remedy, either alone or alternately with *Bryonia,* will often be useful when typhoid fever commences with a diarrhœa, or when this symptom occurs early in the disease, if there is a bitter taste, whitish tongue, or watery, bilious, or even mucous evacuations from the bowels. Later in the disease, if the stomach is acid, if there are nausea and vomiting, with diarrhœa, it may still be of service.

China is often of service during the forming stage of the disease, when there is a painless, watery diarrhœa, with rumbling in the bowels, paleness of the face, and ringing in the ears.

Arsenicum : This remedy should be given at any stage of the disease when there are watery, slimy, whitish, greenish, or more particularly brownish evacuations from the bowels. If the passages from the bowels become bloody or slimy, or if there is straining with the discharges, *Mercurius viv.* may be given instead of *Arsenicum.* For dark mahogany-colored passages, *Nitric acid* is the remedy.

If nausea and vomiting occur, with tenderness of the stomach on pressure over it, *Ipecac* may be given ; and if at the end of twelve hours these symptoms are not relieved, give *Veratrum*. *Arsenicum* should follow *Veratrum* at the end of twenty-four hours, if the symptoms are not relieved. If the nausea and vomiting are very obstinate, and not relieved by remedies, and everything the patient takes is immediately thrown up, let him take nothing into the mouth, except the proper medicine, dissolved in a few drops only of water, and give an injection of thin rice water, arrow root, or corn starch, night and morning—about a teacupful. This will relieve the thirst, sustain the strength, and not aggravate the stomach symptoms. This course can be continued until the stomach will tolerate nourishment, when the above liquids may be cautiously administered by the mouth, at first only a teaspoonful at a time.

When there is a troublesome cough and bronchial irritation, which are not relieved by *Bryonia* or *Rhus tox*, *Belladonna* is generally the most important remedy, and may be given alternately with one of these remedies. If *Belladonna* fails to relieve, *Sulphur* should take its place at the end of twenty-four hours. *Phosphorus* will be useful when there is great oppression of the chest, with cough with or without expectoration.

For great oppression of the brain, when the patient lies in an unconscious state, or with muttering delirium, if *Bryonia* and *Rhus tox.* do not relieve, give *Arnica* once in two hours. If *Arnica* fails to relieve the above symptoms within twelve hours, give *Belladonna*. If there are great stupor and drowsiness, which other remedies fail to relieve, give *Opium*.

If the above remedies fail to relieve severe pain in the head, delirium, or oppression of the brain, wet a large towel in cold water, and wrap it around the entire head and face above the eyes, and cover the wet towel entirely with four or five thicknesses of dry flannel; pin the flannel snugly around the head, so that it will keep its place and exclude the cold air. Wet the towel once in two or three hours, until there is some improvement, then only once in six hours.

For bleeding from the nose, if it occurs in typhus or typhoid fever at the commencement of the fever, give *Aconite* alternately with *Bryonia*. If it occurs during the fever before the stage of prostration, give *Pulsatilla* every hour, and if it fails to relieve, give *Calcarea carb.* If during the latter stage of the disease, give *Arnica* every hour, and follow it with *Carbo veg.*, if necessary. If the remedies do not soon stop the bleeding, consult the article on hemorrhage from the nose, especially the mechanical measures there described.

For hemorrhage or bleeding from the bowels, give *Pulsatilla*, followed by *China*, if the patient becomes very weak and faint. Apply cloths wrung from cold water over the bowels, and change them often until the bleeding stops.

Cathartic remedies should never be given during the treatment of either typhoid or typhus fevers, for I have in several instances, especially in typhoid fever, seen an irritation of the stomach and bowels caused by their use, which no subsequent treatment could cure. Many die from this cause. If the bowels are costive, give nothing more, in addition to the remedies named, than a free injection of tepid water once in two or three days. I have often had patients go one, two, or even three weeks, without a passage, and do well. Still injections, as directed above, will do no harm.

To prevent bed sores, carefully watch the back and hips, and if there are any red, dark, or excoriated spots on the skin, wash them in a solution containing a teaspoonful of *Arnica tincture* to a teacupful of water, once a day, and apply over the parts strips of the common adhesive plaster of the shops. Remove them every day, and wash in the *Arnica* wash. If this does not relieve the parts, all pressure should be taken off the red or excoriated points by the means of cushions and pillows.

General Directions.—The sick-room should be well ventilated by the admission of fresh air, instead of being fumigated by burning substances. The light of the sun should be freely admitted, all day, into the sick-room, to purify the atmosphere, and cheer the patient. The patient should be freely sponged over the entire surface of the body with tepid water at least once a day, and the bed and the patient's linen should be often changed.

Diet.—In cases of typhus fever, and even of typhoid fever, where there is no irritation of the mucous membrane of the stomach and bowels, manifested by nausea, vomiting, diarrhœa, pain and tenderness on pressure over the stomach and bowels, the patient, from the commencement of the disease, may be encouraged to eat regularly, but moderately, of boiled rice, tapioca, sago, and roasted potato, or of dry toast or cracker, with a small quantity of baked apple. The moderate use of such articles will sustain the patient's strength, and keep up the secretion of gastric juice, so that the patient will be able to take other nourishment much earlier than he could otherwise do with safety. If he has continued to take the above articles from the commencement, when the stage of collapse or great prostration ensues, if the prostration is very great, as it generally is in malignant typhus, the patient, if able, may be allowed to chew a little beefsteak and swallow the juice. Or the juice of the beef may be obtained by cutting or slicing the beef thin, putting it into a bottle, and setting it into boiling water for an hour or two. When the prostration is not very great, as is generally the case in typhoid fever where there is no irritation of the stomach and bowels, it is better, perhaps, not to resort to animal nourishment until the fever has entirely abated. But in all cases where there are nausea and vomiting or diarrhœa, with tenderness on pressure over the right side of the lower part of the abdomen, no nourishment should be taken but liquids, such as rice water, arrow root, toast water, the thin part of oat meal or corn meal gruel, and weak black tea. Nor should food in substance or animal food be given in such cases until after the fever has entirely passed off, and been gone for three or four days, and the patient has a good appetite. And even then it is necessary to use the utmost care in changing to a more substantial and stimulating diet. At first, for a day or two, the rice water, arrow root, or gruel, should be made thicker simply; then, after a day or two more, be made into a thin pudding; and then, after a few days more, dry toast may be given three times a day—never more frequently; after a day or two more, the patient may be allowed to chew beefsteak, and swallow the juice, and after having done this for two days he may swallow the meat. Be thus careful and relapses will rarely follow; but if the patient is allowed to take food in substance, or animal food, especially broth, as soon as he begins to desire it, a relapse will often follow, and death not unfrequently. Nothing is lost by being thus careful, for the patient will gain strength steadily, in fact, rapidly, on rice water, gruel, &c. I have often known relapses follow, and in several instances death, when animal broths, toast or rice, and other solid articles of food, have been given too soon. In all febrile diseases, if the patient has been several days or weeks without solid food, or without animal food, it is necessary to return to its use with great care, as directed above; for little or no gastric juice is secreted in such cases, and the food, if taken, will not be digested, but will decompose and irritate the stomach and bowels. The patient may be allowed, in addition to the above liquids, to drink cold water, molasses and water, or warm water, milk, and sugar, freely during the course of these fevers when there is no irritation of the stomach and bowels, which is aggravated by their use. A roasted apple put into a bowl of water makes a pleasant drink; also steep a few dried apples in water and drink the liquid. As far as possible have around the patient only those who are needed to take care of him.

INTERMITTENT FEVER,

(FEVER AND AGUE.)

This disease is supposed to be caused by poisonous exhalations arising from decomposing vegetable substances. It rarely occurs north of fifty-six degrees of north latitude; for although there may be sufficient heat, the seasons are too short. The nearer we approach the equator the more violent do these fevers become, and the more constantly do they prevail; whereas, in temperate climates they do not usually prevail until the latter part of summer and autumn. If individuals are attacked with intermittent fever in the winter or spring, it is generally from the disease, or rather its cause, being latent in the system, and then developed by some exciting cause, such as over-exertion, over-eating, or exposure. Persons do not take this fever from residing in sections of country where it prevails during the winter, spring, and latter part of the fall, after severe frosts have come. Heat and moisture are essential for the development of its cause, but too much wet weather may prevent the generation of the poison in certain localities by covering up decomposing vegetable matter; therefore, in very wet seasons, the lower grounds are usually most healthy, and higher grounds which are ordinarily exempt from disease become sickly. It is inferred that decomposing vegetable substances are necessary for the production of the poison which causes this fever, from the fact that in no situations are intermittent fevers so prevalent as along the banks of rivers, and in the deltas of tropical streams, which, in their periods of flood, deposit large quantities of vegetable substances, which, upon the subsidence of the waters, are exposed to the heat of the sun; also, when grounds are overflowed and then allowed to dry up, as in the case of mill-ponds, where the water is drawn off, exposing moist, dead vegetation. These fevers are very prevalent in new countries, but it often happens that they do not prevail to any considerable extent among new settlers, until they have cleared up the forests so as to expose a large extent of soil to the sun.

Varieties of Intermittent Fever.—By an intermittent fever, we understand a febrile disease in which there are paroxysms of fever, with an intermission between them, during which the patient is free from fever. When the paroxysms occur once in twenty-four hours the fever is called a quotidian. When they occur once in forty-eight hours it is called a tertian. When they occur once in seventy-two hours it is called a quartan. We sometimes have what are called double types. In the double quartan the patient has a fever two days and skips one day. In the double tertian the patient has a fever every day, as in a quotidian; but it is known from the latter by the fact that the paroxysm either occurs at a different hour every other day, or is more severe, or not as regular in all its stages, on alternate days. We may have intermittent fever without or with very slight chills or sweat; we may have a severe paroxysm of fever followed by profuse perspiration without being preceded by chills. A very slight fever may be followed by a profuse sweat. A paroxysm of intermittent fever may consist principally of chills without being followed by much fever or perspiration; or we may have a chill followed by heat and perspiration—regular ague and fever.

Symptoms.—Each paroxysm of an intermittent fever, when regular and fully developed, consists of three stages, namely: a cold, hot, and sweating stage, which usually succeed each other in the order named. Sometimes the chill comes on suddenly, without premonitory symptoms; but it is often preceded by a feeling of languor, weariness, stretching and yawning, impaired appetite, with slight fever and pain in the back and limbs. There are sometimes slight paroxysms of such symptoms for two or three days before regular paroxysms commence.

The cold stage is usually ushered in by yawning, stretching, pains in the head, back, and limbs, and by feelings of chilliness in the limbs, which soon extend over the whole body, sometimes seeming to run in streaks, especially up and down the back. Shivering or trembling soon ensues, and even shaking; the teeth chatter, the surface is pale and contracted, the hands are shrunken, and the ends of the fingers often purplish. The breathing is irregular and hurried, and there is oppression of the chest, with a disposition to sigh. Nausea and vomiting frequently occur during this stage. The pulse is small, sometimes very frequent, sometimes slow and irregular. There may be very great thirst or very little, also severe pains in the head, back, and limbs, irritability of temper, delirium, and in children, convulsions. The cold stage generally lasts about one hour, but it sometimes continues but for a few minutes, whereas in other instances it lasts for three or four hours, or even for a longer period.

The hot stage generally follows the cold gradually, chills alternating for a time with flashes of heat. Gradually the whole surface becomes warm, but for a time the least exposure of the surface of the body causes chilly sensations. At length the heat prevails, the skin is distended with blood, the eyes sparkle, the mouth is hot and dry, the tongue furred, and there is often, but not always, great thirst. Nausea and vomiting are occasionally present, the breathing is rapid, the pulse is generally frequent, full, and strong, the skin dry, the urine scanty and high colored. There is almost always violent pain in the forehead and temples, with throbbing and feeling of distension, and severe pain in the back. There is sometimes delirium, and, in cases of children, frequently convulsions. Sometimes a rash, like nettle resh, makes its appearance and vanishes with the fever. The duration of the hot stage varies from one to twelve, or even twenty-four hours, before it begins to abate.

The sweating stage follows gradually, the perspiration commencing on the face, neck, and breast, and extending over the whole body. It may be scanty, profuse, or very copious. When the perspiration commences, the febrile symptoms begin to abate, and gradually pass off, and the pains in the back and head cease, the skin becomes cool, and the pulse less frequent, the mouth moist, and the urine, which had been scanty during the fever, becomes free, and often deposits a sediment on cooling.

The whole duration of the paroxysm varies greatly. The average duration of the paroxysms in the quotidian variety is perhaps eight or ten hours; in the tertian, six or eight hours; in the quartan, five or six hours. Sometimes they are much longer, instead of shorter, in the tertian and quartan than in the quotidian. The paroxysms may last in some cases but two or three hours, in other cases for eighteen hours, and in tertian and quartan fevers from thirty to fifty hours. The paroxysms generally shorten as the disease becomes of longer continuance. Young children rarely shake, but the hands, feet, nose, and ears, become cold, and perhaps blue; even such symptoms may be absent.

During the intermission the patient is free from fever, but feels languid, with slight uneasiness in the head, back, and stomach. The appetite is poor, the countenance is pale and sallow; but the above symptoms generally abate, as the disease continues, if the patient improves.

The first attack of intermittent fever is usually the worst the patient ever has, and subsequent attacks are milder, and more easily controlled by homœopathic treatment.

In sections of the country where intermittent fevers prevail, various affections, such as neuralgia, rheumatism, hysterics, hiccough, diarrhœa, and even epilepsy, occasionally occur in a regular intermittent form, but without chills and fever, evidently caused by the poison which gives rise to intermittent fever. These diseases, when they become thus paroxysmal, are regarded as masked cases of ague, or intermittent fever, and require the same class of remedies as regular intermittents; at least such remedies should be given alternately with the remedy appropriate for the disease which has assumed a paroxysmal character.

Preventive Treatment of Intermittent Fever.—Persons residing in sections where these fevers prevail, from the beginning of summer to late in the fall, should avoid the early morning air; also the late evening and night air, as far as practicable; admit the solar rays freely all day into their sleeping rooms, for sunlight is the great purifier of the atmosphere; and avoid building their houses in the neighborhood of marshes, mill-dams, &c., especially on the side, where they will be compelled to breathe the atmosphere from such localities, as the wind ordinarily blows. Higher grounds in such a direction will generally be more unhealthy than lower grounds on the opposite side of the marsh, pond, or stream. During the months of July, August, September, and October, take *China* and *Arsenicum* alternately, one week apart.

Treatment of Intermittent Fever.—Little difficulty will generally be found in curing old cases of ague promptly, by the use of homœopathic remedies, in ordinary doses, even though they may have been treated allopathically and empirically, for months and years. Sometimes, under such circumstances, a single dose of the proper remedy will accomplish a permanent cure. But it will be found far more difficult to cure promptly recent cases, where the patient has never had the disease before. In such cases, if we use the ordinary dilutions, it will generally require from two to four weeks to get entirely rid of the fever, but after such a treatment the disease is *cured*, and relapses are rare; whereas, if the paroxysms are suppressed, by quinine and other remedies, relapses generally occur again and again for about two seasons, and sometimes for a longer period. I expect this work to fall into the hands of many individuals in the Western country, especially in the section where the author has long resided, who have not access to a homœopathic physician, and I shall endeavor to give them such information as will prevent them, under any circumstances, from being tempted to resort to the empirical treatment of allopathy and nostrum venders. Calomel, blue pills, and cathartics, are of no use in any form of miasmatic disease, and, where used, they often endanger the future health, and even lives of patients. I well know that patients who have the ague for the first time are not always satisfied to wait for a permanent cure by the homœopathic dilutions; they are generally a little better satisfied to wait the treatment after having suppressed the disease repeatedly by large doses, without curing it. I well know that patients may be travelling, or away from home, or have important business to attend to, when it may be desirable to stop the paroxysms at once. This disease may occur for the first time during the latter months of pregnancy, or soon after childbirth, when, in my opinion, the paroxysms should be stopped. Or it may assume a dangerous character, when it must be checked at once to save life with any certainty. This last class of cases is so important, that I have thought best to consider it separately, under the head of congestive or pernicious fever. The article on this form of the disease will be found after the section on remittent or bilious fever. For the above reasons I shall tell the reader how to cure the disease with the ordinary dilutions by a persevering treatment; how, in case the patient becomes impatient, to hurry up the cure with very small doses of quinine; and finally, how to stop it at once by the use of large doses of quinine, with the greatest certainty and safety practicable.

In all cases where dangerous symptoms occur during the course of intermittent or remittent fevers, the reader should consult carefully the section on congestive or pernicious fevers. Among dangerous symptoms which may occur will be found the following: Great drowsiness, stupor, difficulty of speaking, loss of consciousness, much delirium, or convulsions. Again: A long-continued chill, with great paleness or blueness, followed by slight fever, excessive and long-continued perspiration, great faintness and oppression, with weak and irregular pulse, sinking at the pit of the stomach, or profuse vomiting and diarrhœa. If one or more of the above symptoms occur, do not fail to consult the section on congestive fevers.

Aconite: If the paroxysms of an intermittent fever are very severe, the skin hot and dry, the pulse full, with violent pain in the head, *Aconite* may be given every hour until perspiration ensues, commencing about one hour before the chill is expected.

Dose of this, or any of the following remedies, except *Quinine*, see page 7.

Ipecac: In recent cases, especially if there is any nausea or vomiting during the paroxysm, or feeling of fullness and oppression in the chest, with great thirst during the fever, *Ipecac* should be given once in three or four hours, when the patient is awake, during the intermission, and *Aconite* as directed during the fever. This remedy (*Ipecac*), in such cases, should be continued for five or six days at least. It will also be useful, at the commencement of the treatment, when symptoms like the above occur, in old cases of ague.

Nux vom.: This remedy is perhaps more frequently required at the commencement of the treatment of recent cases of ague than any other, excepting *Ipecac.* It is indicated if there are bilious symptoms, yellow skin and eyes, bitter taste, fullness or pain in the region of the liver or stomach, nausea and vomiting, or constipation, thirst during the chill, but moderate thirst during the fever and sweat, and thirst after the sweat. It may be given alone once in two or three hours; or, if nausea is a prominent symptom, it may be given alternately with *Ipecac,* two hours apart. *Nux vom.* is also very frequently required in old cases of intermittent fever, and in such cases it is especially indicated when the above symptoms pertaining to thirst are present, also when there are derangements of the stomach or liver.

Pulsatilla: This remedy will be found useful, either in recent attacks or long-continued cases, when there is watery or bilious diarrhœa, with or without sick stomach and acid vomiting; and if the paroxysms occur in the afternoon or evening, and if the patient be of a mild disposition, or a woman, these will be still further indications for this remedy.

In recent cases of ague the above are generally the most important remedies for the first eight or ten days of the treatment, after which either *Arsenicum* or *China* will often be required, either to take their place, or, if derangements of the stomach and liver still linger, to be given alternately with the *Nux vom.*, two hours apart. In such cases *Arsenicum* will generally be required, and, if necessary, to be followed by *China*, at the end of a week or ten days more.

Arsenicum: After the bilious and stomach symptoms have been relieved by the above remedies, and the disease somewhat modified by their use, as it will be, no remedy is as frequently required as this, and no one will more frequently cure old cases of ague than the one we are considering. The following are the chief indications for *Arsenicum:* Very little thirst during the fever; chill and heat set in about the same time, or alternate with each other; burning heat, as if boiling water were flowing through the veins; watery diarrhœa, distress in the region of the heart, great debility; and when all the stages are not well marked, as, for instance, if there is little or no chill, or chill and fever but little or no sweat. This remedy is useful when there is with this disease a tendency to dropsy. *Arsenicum* may be given once in two hours during the intermission.

China: This remedy will be of service where *Quinine* has not been administered recently, when there is a sallowness of the skin, a well-marked chill or shake, fever and sweat, with thirst before and during the chill, and during the sweat, but not much thirst during the fever; and especially if the patient is hungry during the fever and intermission; soreness, tenderness, and enlargement in the region of the spleen, or beneath the left short ribs, is a particular indication for the use of this remedy. *China* may be given once in three hours during the intermission.

In all new cases of regular ague; or of attacks occurring in individuals who have not had the disease for several years, which practically amounts to nearly the same thing, too much should not be expected of the remedies in a short time. Select the proper remedy or remedies, and persevere in their administration, and do not change oftener than has been directed above, nor as often, if the patient is doing well.

In addition to the above, there are several other remedies which may be required in obstinate cases of recent ague, and also in old cases which have been dosed with *Quinine*, *Fowler's solution*, *Cholagogue*, patent pills, &c., &c.; or which have continued a long time without treatment.

Ignatia: This remedy will be found useful when the chills are moderated by external heat, pale face, or alternately pale and red—thirst during the chill only; and in the case of children, if either the cold or hot stage is attended with convulsions. *Ignatia* may be given once in two hours during the chill, fever, sweat, and intermission.

Natrum mur.: This is one of our best remedies for the treatment of old cases of ague where the disease has been frequently suppressed, especially if there is thirst during the chill and fever, with dry tongue, pains in the bones, yellowish complexion, and great debility. Success with this remedy will be more certain if, in addition to the above symptoms, the paroxysms occur in the morning, or fore part of the day, and the fever has but a single type. I have rarely found *Natrum mur.* of any service in recent cases; but late in the fall, after patients have had the disease during the summer, it often acts like a charm. Six globules may be taken dry on the tongue, or dissolved in water, night and morning only.

Corbo veg.: This is a valuable remedy in old cases of the disease, especially where patients have had the ague frequently for years, and when there are rheumatic pains in the teeth and limbs before or during the fever, and when paroxysms occur in the evening or at night, and terminate with a profuse perspiration. A dose may be given night and morning.

Arnica: In old cases of ague, where the following symptoms exist, a drop of the tincture of this remedy, dropped on the tongue at the commencement of the chills will sometimes stop the chills, and cure the disease at once. Pains in the bones before the paroxysm, constant disposition to change position, each one being found uncomfortable during the fever, loathing of meat during the intermission, loss of appetite, and yellowish complexion.

Bryonia: When the paroxysms have been composed almost entirely of chills, followed by little or no fever or sweat, this remedy has rarely failed to afford prompt relief from all the symptoms.

Quinine: It is better, as a general rule, to avoid *Quinine* entirely, excepting when dangerous symptoms occur; but it sometimes happens, in recent cases of ague, that after three or four weeks' treatment the paroxysms, although lighter, still persist; the countenance becomes very pale, and the spleen swollen and tender, with perhaps bleeding from the nose; and the patient and friends become alarmed and impatient, and it seems desirable to hurry up the cure. In such cases give to an adult one grain, or to a child one half a grain of *Quinine* four hours before the paroxysm is expected, and the same quantity at the termination of the paroxysm; continue this treatment until they cease; then give one dose only a day, for a few days.

The first decimal trituration of *Quinine* will do even better than the above if you have it, or can readily get it; commencing five hours before you expect the paroxysms, give one grain of this trituration every hour until the patient has taken four or five doses, and continue this treatment until the patient is cured. It will be well to continue other remedies once a day for two or three weeks, especially *Nux vom.* or *Arsenicum.*

By pursuing the course here directed, you will generally get a permanent cure, if you do not commence with the *Quinine* sooner than I have named. Such small doses of *Quinine* will have little or no influence over recent cases of ague at their commencement, except to aggravate the symptoms and do harm.

If the patient is not willing to wait to be cured by the homœopathic dilutions, or, if for any reason it is thought advisable to stop the paroxysms at once, this can be done by the proper use of *Quinine* with far more safety than by the use of any other remedy known. It will require, for an adult, about eighteen or twenty grains of *Qnınine* to stop the paroxysms. One half should be given about ten hours before the chill is expected, and the other half at the end of six hours from the time of taking the first dose. In a majority of cases, no chill or fever will follow, but sometimes a short paroxysm will follow, which may either be delayed or commence earlier than usual. It is well to give six or eight grains of *Quinine* six hours before the next paroxysm would occur if the disease had continued. But to stop the paroxysms is not to cure the disease ; but after the paroxysms have been thus suppressed, the disease can often be permanently cured, without any return, if the following directions are carefully followed. The disposition of the paroxysms to return is much stronger every seventh day, for several weeks, than on other days ; therefore, let the patient take eight grains of *Quinine* once a week, about thirty-six hours before the same day and hour of the week when the last chill occurred, and continue to do this punctually for at least four weeks. Also take a dose of *Arsenicum* morning and noon, and *Nux vom.* before tea and at bedtime, and continue them for at least four or five weeks. Carefully avoid over-exertion, over-eating, and exposure, and the disease will not generally return again the same season, but the next May, June, or July, there will be danger of a return. To prevent this, the patient may take five grains of *Quinine* once a week for a few weeks; and the *Arsenicum* and *Nux vom.* should again be taken for several weeks. In the first attack a cure can often be effected in this way, but if the disease has heen broken up with *Quinine*, even once or twice only, and allowed to return, it will rarely succeed, and in such cases to give *Quinine*, except it may be in minute doses after at least two or three weeks of previous treatment with the ordinary dilutions of other remedies, will be but to prolong the duration of the disease indefinitely.

If *Quinine* is to be used to stop the paroxysms, I much prefer the full doses I have named, and few of them, to giving it in small doses often repeated. About so much is required to break up the disease, and if it is given in full doses in the intermission, as I have directed, its administration is almost always followed by a profuse perspiration, and relief to all local congestions and general symptoms; whereas, if it is given in one, two, or three grain doses, often repeated, it excites the circulation and nervous system, and increases local congestions, and is very apt to increase the following paroxysm.

If *Quinine* is to be given to children to break up the paroxysms, it will require about as many grains as the child is years old, to accomplish this object. The dose should be divided and given as directed for adults. It may be given to children by the mouth, or by injection in a little starch. Adults generally prefer *Quinine* in the form of pills. The pills can be made by moistening the *Quinine* with a thick solution of *Gum Arabic.*

In conclusion, I desire to say, distinctly, that the use of *Quinine* is rarely necessary, or for the best, in the treatment of intermittent fever, as it generally prevails in our country. Under the use of the ordinary dilutions of our medicines, the disease will gradually abate, the paroxysms become less severe and delayed, and the patient will feel better during the intermissions, and he will be radically cured. In old cases, or where the patient has frequently had the disease before, he will generally be cured promptly by our remedies, often without the return of another paroxysm; and generally the patient will be relieved in a few days.

TYPHOID INTERMITTENTS.

It not unfrequently happens, during the fall of the year, that persons residing in sections of country where both intermittent and typhoid fevers are prevailing, are attacked by a fever partaking the character of both, and furnishing corresponding symptoms. In this form of the disease patients rarely have a regular shake, and the sweating stage is generally somewhat deficient. The patient has a regular paroxysm of fever every day, or every other day, at about the same hour, with perhaps at first very few symptoms of fever between the paroxysms, excepting a frequent pulse; but as the disease continues, and the paroxysms grow less severe, the tongue becomes dry, the body constantly hot, the extremities cool, and sordes, or dried mucus crusts, collect on the teeth in severe cases, and the disease continues the usual course of typhoid fever, but generally rather tedious, lasting three or four weeks.

Treatment.—*Bryonia*, *Ipecac*, and *Arsenicum*, are the chief remedies for the early stage of the disease; *Bryonia* and *Ipecac*, if there are nausea and vomiting, or fullness and uneasiness in the chest and stomach. *Arsenicum* should take the place of *Ipecac* in a few days, and be given alternately with *Bryonia*, especially if there is any disposition to diarrhœa; and even if there is not, this is generally the most important remedy for the successful treatment of this disease, and may be continued alternately with *Bryonia* until the stage of prostration, when, if the teeth become covered with sordes, or dark crusts, the breath offensive, and the extremities cold, it may be given alternately with *Rhus tox.* For suggestions as to diet, in this and intermittent fevers, consult the paragraph on that subject at the end of the section on remittent fevers.

REMITTENT OR BILIOUS FEVER.

The disease denominated, in the Western country, chill fever, is usually but a light form of this disease; in other instances it is only an intermittent fever. Remittent fever prevails in all parts of the United States where intermittent fevers originate, and it is but a severer form of the same disease, arising from the same cause. It usually prevails during August, September, and October: but it may occur at any season of the year. As remittent fever is but a modification of the same disease as intermittent fever, we find every shade of the disease, from the slightest intermittent to the severest remittent, and likewise one running or passing into the other. Remittent fever is subject to the same types as intermittent, but the quotidian is the most frequent, the paroxysms occurring at about the same hour every day. The paroxysms may consist of chills, fever, and sweat, or the chills may be slight or absent, and the sweat may be trifling.

Symptoms.—The premonitory symptoms are similar to those of intermittent fever—languor, drowsiness, aching pains in the head, back, and limbs, followed, sooner or later, by slight chills, alternating with flashes of heat. The chills may be quite severe, or entirely absent. The flashes of heat increase until the fever is fully developed, when the pains in the head, back, and limbs, become very severe. The pains in the back and limbs are often so severe as to resemble those of inflammatory rheumatism, but they may be distinguished from the latter by the absence of pain on motion. The pains in the head, back, and limbs, are generally much more severe in this disease than in typhoid or typhus fever, and the patient suffers intensely, and is alive to his sufferings. Sometimes during the fever the patient becomes chilly on the slightest exposure of the body, as when raising the bedclothes. The skin is hot and dry, the surface reddened and expanded, the respiration hurried, and the pulse frequent and full. The eyes soon become yellow, the tongue coated with a white or brownish fur. Sometimes there are nausea and bilious vomiting, and a sense of weight and fullness is often felt at the pit of the stomach, and to the right of it, or in the region of the liver. The urine is scanty and high colored, and there is generally a loss of appetite. Sometimes there is great thirst, in other instances very little. The patient is restless and wakeful, but seldom delirious. The above symptoms continue without abatement for from twelve to twenty hours, and in some instances for thirty-six hours, after which they begin to abate, with the appearance of moisture about the neck and face. This gradually increases, until the body is covered with a gentle perspiration, and the patient is much relieved, and perhaps able to sleep. The headache, thirst, and nausea are much relieved, but not gone, and the pulse is nearly natural. This is the remission; it is not always as complete as described above; there may be less perspiration, and more heat and headache. The remission generally occurs in the morning. The remission is exceedingly variable in duration, sometimes lasting not more than two or three hours, and in other cases twelve or even twenty-four hours, when the paroxysms occur only every other day. When the remission is over, another paroxysm of fever commences, which may, or may not, commence with a chill and end with a perspiration, but frequently without either. Another remission follows the paroxysm, and thus the paroxysms and remissions alternate. Sometimes the paroxysms grow less severe and shorter, and the remissions longer and more distinct until the disease becomes an intermittent whereas in other cases the paroxysms become longer and more severe, and the remissions less distinct and shorter, until the disease reaches its height, when the skin generally becomes yellow, and there is often more or less pain and tenderness in the region of the stomach. The bowels are usually constipated, but occasionally there is diarrhœa. Sometimes the disease assumes a typhoid character, with dry and dark tongue, sordes, or crusts on the teeth, and cool extremities.

The usual duration of this fever, under the ordinary homœopathic treatment, is from one to two weeks; if complicated with typhoid fever, about three weeks The disease terminates, usually, either at the end of one of the paroxysms, which ends in a free perspiration, a bilious diarrhœa, a profuse flow of urine, or it becomes intermittent. In some instances it abates gradually, without any marked crisis. The first signs of a favorable change are a return of moisture to the tongue, with a disposition to clear off about the tip and edges, a less frequent pulse, a cooler and moister skin, especially when uniform over the whole body. Copious dark passages from the bowels sometimes occur, and are regarded as favorable. Unfavorable symptoms: Very small or irregular pulse; cold extremities, with a cold, clammy sweat extending over the limbs and body, with increasing frequency of pulse; eructations of dark or bilious matters from the stomach; reddish watery evacuations from the bowels, discharged involuntarily; sunken features, or muttering delirium or stupor.

In all severe attacks where dangerous symptoms occur, especially during the first two or three paroxysms, the reader should consult carefully the next section on congestive or pernicious fevers.

Treatment of Remittent Fevers.—Emetics and cathartics should be carefully avoided, for by their use a simple remittent fever is often changed into a dangerous gastric or pernicious fever. A simple copious injection of tepid water may be used once in three or four days; but even this is generally unnecessary, unless the bowels feel full and uncomfortable. During febrile diseases the patient eats but little, and takes no exercise, and we cannot expect him to have passages from the bowels regularly as in health; nor is it desirable that he should have.

Aconite: This is one of the most important remedies at the commencement of this disease, especially when the skin is hot and dry, the pulse full, and there is violent pain in the head, back, and limbs, red eyes, faintness on rising up, shooting pains in the chest, with oppression, and short and anxious respiration, palpitation of the heart, and red and scanty urine. Give this remedy every hour.

Dose of this. or any other remedy named, see page 7.

Belladonna: It is generally best to give either *Belladonna* or *Bryonia* after giving three or four doses of *Aconite*, during severe paroxysms of this disease. *Belladonna* should be selected when there are sharp cutting or throbbing pains in the head, especially over the eyes, with intolerance of light, restlessness, sleeplessness, or delirium; and in children when there are starting and jerking, or convulsions; repeat the dose every hour.

Bryonia: This remedy should be selected in preference to *Belladonna*, and be given after *Aconite* during the paroxysms, when the pains in the head are dull, or throbbing, with intense pains in the back and limbs, sensation of load or weight at the stomach, pain and soreness in the region of the liver, or beneath the right short ribs, yellow skin, cough and oppression of the chest, and offensive breath and bitter taste, with a dry tongue. If *Belladonna* is indicated at the commencement, it should generally give way to *Bryonia* at the end of three or four days.

If the above remedies are faithfully given during the paroxysms, they will rarely fail to render the latter lighter, and the remissions more distinct in the course of a few days. They need not be continued during the remission when the remissions become distinct, but one of the following remedies may be given once in two hours.

Ipecac when there are nausea and vomiting, painful pressure and fullness at the pit of the stomach. with aversion to all food, and a yellow complexion. *Ipecac* need not be continued longer than during two or three remissions.

Nux vomica may be given instead of *Ipecac*, or follow that remedy during the remissions, when there are marked bilious symptoms, such as yellow skin and eyes, swelling and tenderness, with pain in the region of the liver; cramp-like pains in the stomach, with sensitiveness on pressure and bitter taste, with or without bilious vomiting; also where there is a sensation as if the brain were bruised, and humming in the ears, or pain in the back portion or top of the head.

Arsenicum: If *Nux vomica* does not relieve the stomach symptoms in the course of a few days, especially if nausea and vomiting continue, with great thirst, and soreness of the stomach on the slightest pressure, *Arsenicum* should take the place of *Nux vomica.* This remedy will be still further indicated if in connection with such symptoms the extremities begin to become cool, and the pulse more frequent and less full, and the remissions less distinct. When such symptoms exist *Aconite* will not be needed, but *Arsenicum* may be given alternately with *Bryonia* one hour apart, during both the remission and the fever. If at the end of twenty-four or forty-eight hours the nausea, vomiting, thirst, burning and tenderness of the stomach, are not relieved, *Veratrum* should be given instead of *Bryonia*, alternately with *Arsenicum*, one hour apart, and be continued until such symptoms are relieved. In a case like the above the reader will do well to read what is said in regard to the treatment of similar symptoms, when they occur in the course of typhus and typhoid fevers.

But it rarely happens that such aggravated symptoms arise when the patient has been treated from the commencement with Homœopathic remedies. Generally when *Aconite*, *Belladonna*, *Bryonia*, *Ipecac*, and *Nux vomica*, or such of these remedies as are indicated have been given as directed, after a week or ten days, the paroxysms become lighter, and the stomach symptoms and bilious derangement are somewhat relieved. The disease may even approach an intermittent form by the remissions becoming more distinct. When the severity of the disease has been thus relieved, *Nux vomica* may be given once in two hours during the fever, and *Arsenicum* may be given during the intermission once in two hours, and be continued until the febrile paroxysms cease.

China: This remedy may be required in lingering cases, and when given two or three times a day, it will generally aid in restoring the appetite and strength after the fever has abated.

Quinine: This remedy exercises the same control over remittent fever that it does over intermittent. It will rarely fail to break up the paroxysms at once in any case where there is a distinct remission, if given in a sufficient quantity during the remission. If for any of the reasons named for breaking up the ague, it is thought best to stop this disease, *Aconite*, *Belladonna*, or *Bryonia*, should be given as directed above, until the close of the second paroxysm, in order to be certain as to the character of the disease; then as soon as the skin becomes moist, and the pain in the back and head is relieved in a measure, give ten grains of *Quinine*, if the patient is an adult, and after waiting six hours, give ten grains more; at the end of twenty-four hours give eight or ten grains more, especially if any fever follows the first two doses; after which treat the case precisely as directed in the treatment of intermittent fever when full doses of *Quinine* are used. If the disease returns, it will generally be as an intermittent, and rarely as a remittent; but it should not be permitted to return.

General Measures.—Frequent sponging the body with warm water, or a warm bath, often affords great relief. When it is not convenient to give a bath, the patient may be set on a stool in a tub, a sheet wrung from warm water may be wrapped around him, and then warm water may be poured over the sheet for ten or fifteen minutes, or even longer if the patient is not faint. This measure will not generally answer during the latter stages of the disease, as the patient will not bear the erect position without feeling faint or exhausted. I generally prefer hot water to cold, and think it has a better influence over the febrile excitement; and also, its use is more likely to relieve the severe pains in the back and limbs than the application of cold water. For local congestions, or pain and soreness of the liver, spleen, stomach, or even of the head, a towel may be wrung from cold water and applied over the part, and four or five thicknesses of dry flannel placed over the wet cloth so as to cover it entirely; then bind a dry cloth around the body or head and over the flannel, so as to confine the whole and exclude the cold air. The wet cloth when first applied is cold, but it soon becomes warm, and even hot from the reaction which it excites. The towel requires to be wet only once in six or eight hours, and on that account this cold compress is far less troublesome than warm applications, and as a general rule it is much more efficacious. The patient should occupy a light room into which the sun shines during the day, and an abundant supply of fresh air should be admitted.

Diet, &c.—Both in this disease and in intermittent fever, if there is no irritation of the stomach or bowels manifested by vomiting, diarrhœa, pain or soreness on pressure, the patient may be allowed to eat moderately of rice, toast, cracker or other light food three times a day, and to drink corn or oat-meal gruel, toast-water, milk-and-water, and cold water. But if there are symptoms of irritation or inflammation of the stomach or bowels the same care is required in regard to diet as in typhoid fever when it is attended by a similar irritation. For directions in such cases consult the paragraph on diet in the section on typhoid fever. When either this disease or intermittent fever has been broken up by the use of *Quinine* within a few days after the attack, the patient can return to a nourishing and substantial diet much sooner than when the disease has continued for a longer time, as the digestive organs do not become so debilitated in such cases.

CONGESTIVE, SINKING, OR PERNICIOUS FEVER.

Thus far I have been treating of intermittent and remittent fevers as they usually occur, but in this section the attention of the reader will be called to much more dangerous forms of these fevers, which are occasionally met with, and which require to be promptly and properly treated to rescue the patient from death in a majority of cases. Although I would not recommend any layman to treat such formidable cases, or in fact any severe attack of disease when a *homœopathic* physician can be obtained, yet it is very important that all who nurse or attend the sick should understand what symptoms denote a dangerous attack of intermittent or remittent fever. I feel constrained to notice this disease and its proper homœopathic treatment distinctly, in a domestic work, from the fact that a large and increasing number of the citizens and travellers in the Western country, who have no convenient access to a physician of our school, rely upon a domestic book and case in preference to sending for an allopathic physician, except in surgical or obstetrical cases. It is very important that all such have a work upon which they can rely with safety in our febrile diseases. I have known within the circle of my acquaintance not less than three patients lose their lives, as I have every reason to think, for the want of the very information contained in this section.

This disease may be intermittent or remittent, but its most common type is *tertian*, in which the paroxysms occur once in two days; they may return every day. There are two varieties of the disease, one in which the poison seems to spend its force on, or at least seems chiefly to affect, the brain; in the other the organs of circulation, respiration, secretion, and digestion.

Symptoms and Treatment where the Brain is involved.—Symptoms of this form of the disease may manifest themselves during the first, or any subsequent paroxysm of an intermittent or remittent fever. The paroxysms of chills and fever, one or both, are attended with a greater or less degree of stupor; generally the first symptom noticed is simply drowsiness, coming on with or during the paroxysm, and disappearing with it. The patient is forgetful, does not remember what he has done, desired, or said; he often stammers, and uses one word for another, and even stops when speaking in the middle of a sentence. This dullness may gradually increase until it is with difficulty that the patient can be made to attempt to answer questions, and he fails to complete his sentences if he attempts. At length he passes into a state of profound stupor, from which he cannot be aroused. There are sometimes snoring and blowing out of the lips during respiration, as in apoplexy. Sometimes there is rigidity of the muscles about the jaws, and swallowing is difficult or impossible; occasionally convulsions ensue. The pulse is often full, not very frequent, and sometimes even slower than natural; but as the disease progresses, if it is towards a fatal termination, it becomes small, irregular, and perhaps frequent. In some cases severe symptoms occur during the first paroxysm, but more frequently simple drowsiness occurs in the first, with a degree of slowness and hesitation of speech, and the state of stupor is not fully developed until the second paroxysm. If the paroxysm does not end fatally after continuing from two or three to twenty-four hours, some perspiration takes place; sensation gradually returns, and the patient becomes conscious, or at least partially so, for there generally remains during the intermission or remission, some dullness of hearing and of the mental faculties, with more or less drowsiness. The length of the remission will depend on the type of the fever, and will vary from a few hours to thirty-six hours, when another paroxysm will follow if the disease is not arrested by remedies, and the second or third paroxysm generally proves fatal, when uninfluenced by treatment.

Treatment when the Brain is the chief Organ affected.—*Nux vom.* is the most important remedy for the paroxysm, when there is drowsiness, forgetfulness, confusion of ideas, or stupor, and when the bowels are constipated. Repeat the dose every hour.

Dose of this or any of the following remedies, see page 7.

Opium: If the stupor is very profound, the pulse small and irregular, with snoring respiration, this remedy may be given instead of *Nux vom.* during the paroxysm, if the latter remedy fails to relieve the stupor.

Bryonia: Next to *Nux vom.* this remedy is more frequently required than any other, especially if there are in addition to the head symptoms, dryness of the tongue and lips, yellowness of the eyes and skin, and if there is fullness in the region of the liver and stomach. When it is indicated it should be given every hour during the paroxysm, but *Nux vom.* may be given every hour during the remission. But it will not do to rely upon these or any of our other remedies in the dilutions, for if we do, more than one half of those suffering from a severe attack of this disease will be very sure to die.

During the paroxysm warm applications should be made to the feet, such as warm dry flannel, hot bricks or stones wrapped in flannel, or bottles of hot water, taking care not to burn the patient's feet if he is unconscious. The head should be slightly elevated, and the temples, forehead, and top of the head, frequently sponged with a cloth wet in warm water; or what is generally more efficacious, a large towel may be wrung from cold water and spread over the entire head, and four or five thicknesses of dry flannel over the wet cloth, and pinned so as to keep it in place, and exclude the cold air. The cloth may be wet every hour until consciousness returns, or the symptoms of drowsiness are relieved.

Quinine: The prompt use of this remedy is our main dependance; and it will rarely disappoint our expectations. In *all* cases of this fever, as soon as the paroxysm begins to abate, or the skin becomes moist, and the drowsiness and forgetfulness are in a measure relieved, ten grains of *Quinine,* if the patient is an adult, *must* be given, and repeated once at the end of six hours. Twenty-four hours from the last dose ten grains more must be given; after this the patient should be treated exactly as directed for the prevention of a return of intermittent fever when it has been broken up with *Quinine. Nux vom.* if there is a sensation of weight or load at the pit of the stomach, may be continued while the patient is taking *Quinine.* If it fails to relieve give *Bryonia.*

It is not necessary that the patient should become unconscious during the paroxysm, in order to require that *Quinine* should be given to insure his safety, for if there is simply unusual drowsiness, forgetfulness, confusion of ideas, and hesitation in speaking, or symptoms of convulsions, especially when the patient is an adult, we shall have good reason to fear that he will die during the next paroxysm, if we do not give *Quinine* and prevent it.

Symptoms when the Organs of Circulation and Respiration, or the Heart, Lungs, and Digestive Organs, are chiefly involved.—The first paroxysm of chills and fever which the patient has may manifest the dangerous character of the disease, or dangerous symptoms may not occur until the patient has had one or two, or even several paroxysms. The appearance of the patient is peculiar, the features are shrunken, and the face and extremities of a livid paleness; the skin contracted and the fingers shrivelled; the eyes sunk in their sockets, though clear and bright; the extremities, and sometimes the whole body, are chillingly cold, and perhaps moistened with a cold clammy perspiration, or the body may be hot while the extremities and face are in a cold or clammy state. There is often sighing respiration, and sometimes inspiration requires a double effort for its accomplishment. There is generally hurried or irregular breathing, want of breath, and a desire to be fanned and to have the windows open The pulse is small, very frequent, often from 120 to 160 in a minute ; it may be fluttering, irregular, intermittent or even absent at the wrist ; the heart may beat hard or very feebly ; the tongue may be natural, pale and cold, or dry ; there may be a feeling of weight at the pit of the stomach, tenderness on pressure, and intense internal heat, with unquenchable thirst, even when the extremities and surface of the body are cold. Vomiting is a very frequent symptom ; sometimes there are excessive nausea and retching ; the bowels may be costive, but frequently the reverse, with copious watery or bloody evacuations. Instead of vomiting or diarrhœa there may be great faintness on the least exertion. Frequently there is great restlessness or uneasiness ; occasionally there are cramps in the calves of the legs, and in the upper extremities; sometimes the patient is able to walk about when the pulse is absent at the wrist. Some of the symptoms resemble those of Asiatic Cholera. All of the above symptoms are rarely present in any one case. Sometimes a paroxysm of intermittent or remittent fever runs its usual course, but ends in an exhausting perspiration.

The febrile reaction is generally slight; sometimes very little fever follows the coldness and prostration, but generally in the first paroxysm, after the symptoms described have continued for three or four hours, the skin becomes gradually warmer and the pulse fuller, and some fever follows; or the skin may lose its clammy feel, and the ghastly expression disappear, the vomiting and purging cease without perceptible fever. In some cases there are only slight attempts at reaction, the paroxysm continuing on for from one to three days, when, if not relieved, the patient dies. In such cases the coldness increases, the respiration becomes slower, with increased sighing, with a gradual failure of the pulse, and at last of the mental faculties; the patient usually dies tranquilly in such cases.

During the intermission or remission, the patient may feel very comfortable and be able to be up and around, with a natural pulse and surface, and some return of appetite. If the disease is a remittent, there are more or less symptoms of the paroxysm remaining during the remission, such as a frequent pulse, uneasiness at the stomach, general languor, or distress. Generally if the disease is not arrested by treatment, the same train of symptoms set in at the end of twenty-four or forty-eight hours from the commencement of the first attack, and with increased severity. The second paroxysm often proves fatal, and the third generally does, but not always, even without treatment, for sometimes the paroxysms grow lighter instead of harder, and the disease ends in an ordinary remittent or intermittent.

Not a few cases of simple intermittent or remittent fever are converted into a pernicious sinking fever by the use of emetics and cathartics, and so frequently have such results followed, that many of the most successful allopathic physicians at the West shun their use entirely in the treatment of patients suffering from these fevers. The free use of stimulants and stimulating doses of *Quinine*, by increasing the paroxysms of fever, or by over-exciting the organism during the remission, may cause fatal prostration, and I am satisfied from my observation that many patients die from this cause. Unnatural stimulation, if continued steadily for days, must be followed by corresponding or unnatural depression. Stimulants should never be used in the treatment of ordinary intermittent or remittent fevers, and if they are ever useful in sinking fevers, as they may be sometimes, it is only when they are given simply during the great prostration of the paroxysm, and carefully avoided during the fever and intermission or remission.

Treatment when the Organs of Circulation, Respiration, and Digestion, are chiefly involved.—Give one drop of the tincture of *Camphor* every five minutes, in a little sugar-and-water, and if, at the end of an hour, the alarming symptoms are not relieved, select another remedy.

Veratrum: This is one of the most important remedies for the treatment of the form of the disease we are now considering, during the paroxysm, especially when there are great nausea and vomiting, or profuse, watery, or bloody evacuations from the bowels; also when there are great coldness and lividness of the surface, thirst, cramps in the extremities, and cold clammy perspiration. This remedy, when the above symptoms exist, should generally be given every half hour, and if relief does not soon follow, *Arsenicum* may be alternated with it, at intervals of half an hour.

Dose of this or either of the following remedies, see p. 7.

If the patient vomits up the medicine immediately on taking it, dissolve it in less water, and give but a part of a teaspoonful at a time.

Arsenicum: This is a very important remedy, not only during the paroxysm, but also during the intermission, and should generally be continued until the severity of the disease is overcome, especially when the stomach and bowels are the chief organs affected—when there are vomiting, great thirst, profuse watery or bloody evacuations from the bowels, and a cold surface, or a cold clammy perspiration; also when there is very feeble or irregular pulse with great oppression of the chest. *Arsenicum* may be repeated every half-hour or hour; if there is much vomiting, it should be given alternately with *Veratrum* or *Ipecac.*

Ipecac: This remedy should be given when there are nausea and vomiting, which *Veratrum* does not relieve. It may take the place of the latter remedy at the commencement of the treatment, when with the nausea and vomiting, there is great oppression of the chest with sighing respiration. It may be given every half-hour or hour.

Bryonia: This remedy will be found useful in cases where there is little or no vomiting or diarrhœa, but great chilliness and coldness, oppression of the chest, with a frequent disposition to draw in a long breath, or sigh; it should be given alternately with either *Arsenicum* or *China,* in such cases; generally with the former. *Bryonia* is also one of the most important remedies during the reaction or fever; also in all cases where the fever does not terminate fatally, or in recovery, within the first few days, but tends, as it frequently does, to assume a typhoid character, with a dry tongue, crusts on the teeth, and offensive breath. It may be given once in one or two hours.

China: If we were to risk the treatment of this disease without the use of *Quinine*—which I think we should never do—*China* would become the most important remedy when there is great faintness on the slightest movement, small and fluttering pulse, or intermittent pulse, without nausea, vomiting, or diarrhœa, but with great oppression of the chest, with a desire to be fanned, and for fresh air.

Quinine: This is the chief remedy upon which we must depend, to prevent a return of the paroxysm or lessen its severity, nor need we be very particular about waiting for a remission before giving *Quinine* in this form of the disease, for we have not to fear excessive reaction or febrile excitement, for the danger is that we shall not be able to get up any reaction and that the patient will die during the stage of prostration. I am satisfied that we have no remedy equal to this to sustain the vital energies during desperate paroxysms of this disease. Then in all cases where there are great faintness and prostration of strength, small fluttering or irregular pulse, death-like coldness of the surface, the skin perhaps bathed in a cold perspiration, oppression of the chest and want of breath, if the remedies named above do not soon cause an improvement, ten grains of *Quinine* should be given at once, and after waiting six hours, teu grains more should be given; and at the end of twenty-four hours ten grains more should be given. If there are great nausea and vomiting but no diarrhœa the *Quinine* may be given by injection, stirred up in two tablespoonfuls of thin starch. If there are both vomiting and diarrhœa, the stomach will often tolerate and be settled by ten grains of *Quinine*, if it is made into pills and taken at once; but if it should be thrown up, *Arsenicum* and *Veratrum* should be given alternately until the paroxysm is over and the stomach in a measure settled, when the *Quinine* must be given, as directed above. If it has not been thought necessary to give *Quinine* during the prostration of the paroxysm, it should always be given, as directed above, as soon as the paroxysm is fairly over and the patient feels relieved, so as to prevent a return of the dangerous symptoms. We should never risk, in an adult, less than two ten-grain doses the first twenty-four hours, and in severe cases in robust individuals, give two doses of twelve grains each.

It is not necessary that all of the symptoms named should be present in any case to justify, and absolutely require, the use of *Quinine* in order to insure the safety of the patient. If one or more of the following symptoms are present it will not be safe to risk another paroxysm: An unusual paleness or lividness of the face during the paroxysm, absence of chills when the extremities are very cold; a want of uniform heat during the fever; excessive vomiting and purging with great prostration during the paroxysm; a gone and sinking sensation at the pit of the stomach, and disposition to faintness; a very frequent, feeble, or irregular pulse; also if there is a prolongation of the cold stage, and this is very severe and followed by less fever than might have been anticipated. If any of the above symptoms are prominent *Quinine* should be given.

After the paroxysms have been broken up by *Quinine*, the patient should be treated as directed under the head of intermittent fever when *Quinine* has been used, If the disease returns it will generally be as a simple intermittent or remittent, without dangerous symptoms. In all cases where *Quinine* is used the other homœopathic remedies should be selected as directed above, and given regularly during the interval between the doses of *Quinine*, when the patient is awake. Neither in this nor in any other febrile affection, where there is no unusual disposition to sleepiness or stupor, should the patient be awakened for the purpose of giving him medicine; for undisturbed rest is very important.

It sometimes happens, in the western country, that this disease is complicated with typhus or typhoid fever; in such a case *Quinine* should be given when there are distinct and well-marked paroxysms, but it will only break up the paroxysms, after which the typhus or typhoid fever will run its course, and should be treated as directed under the head of that disease; excepting that eight or ten grains of *Quinine* should be given every seventh day, counting the day on which the last paroxysm occurred, for at least three weeks.

When in the case of children, the paroxysms of intermittent fever cause convulsions, it perhaps is generally best to stop the paroxysms by the use of *Quinine*, as their frequent return may establish a tendency to convulsions, which it is desirable to avoid.

Quinine is most readily given to young children by injection, suspended in a tablespoonful of thin starch. To a child from six months to one year old, one grain may be thus given and repeated at the end of six or eight hours, and again at the end of twenty-four hours, and after that every seventh day, giving at the same time, as directed under the head of intermittent fever, such remedies as are indicated, for several weeks. One half grain of *Quinine* may be added to the doses directed above for every year of the child's age over one year, whether it is given by injection or by the mouth.

General Measures.—When there are great coldness of the extremities and prostration of strength, warm applications may be made to the cold parts and the patient should be kept quiet in bed. If there is a cold clammy perspiration on the limbs it will be better simply to rub them with a warm dry flannel or the dry hand beneath the bedclothes. Fresh air should be freely admitted, and the patient's diet should be as liberal as the stomach will bear. If the patient has been but a few days sick and there is very great prostration of the vital energies, beef-tea, chicken or mutton broth may be given, if the stomach does not reject it.

YELLOW FEVER.

The yellow fever is a disease of hot weather and warm climates, beginning the latter part of summer or fore part of autumn, and disappearing with the occurrence of frost. It seldom appears north of the fortieth degree of latitude, owing, as it is supposed, to the summer being too short, and it is confined, to a great extent, to the inhabitants of cities, towns, forts, and to the crews of ships; although it occasionally occurs in rural districts. It occurs more frequently in towns upon the seacoast, or upon streams emptying into the ocean, and it is confined almost exclusively to the intertropical regions, and the southern portion of the northern temperate zone of the American continent, and southwestern Europe, and western Africa, while it is almost unknown in southeastern Europe, eastern Africa, or southern Asia.

Symptoms.—Premonitory symptoms, such as loss of appetite, debility, aching in the back and limbs, may or may not precede the attack, which frequently commences in the night, sometimes with, in other instances without, chills or chilliness. Severe pains in the back and limbs are among the first and most prominent symptoms of the early stage of the disease. The skin soon becomes hot and dry, the pulse frequent, respiration hurried, the face flushed, and the eyes red and watery, a white fur appears upon the tongue, which is usually moist at the commencement; the throat is sometimes sore, and nausea and vomiting may attend the disease from the commencement, but generally these stomach symptoms are not fully developed until after from twelve to twenty-four hours, when they become very prominent. There is tenderness in the region of the stomach, on pressure, and a constant feeling of weight and oppression with burning pain; the stomach becomes very irritable, rejecting everything that is swallowed, and throwing up its own secretions, when undisturbed, accompanied by great distress, owing to the tenderness of that organ. The patient craves cold drinks, the bowels are costive, and the head and eyes ache; the mind is often disturbed, and delirium is not uncommon, sometimes violent; in some instances there is stupor. These febrile symptoms continue with little or no remission, for a period varying from a few hours to three days, or even longer in some cases; the more severe the attack the shorter the duration of the fever, as a general rule. When the fever abates the skin becomes cooler and softer, the pulse and respiration nearly natural, the headache and pain in the back and limbs disappear, the stomach becomes comparatively quiet, and the patient feels relieved.

In mild cases the patient may steadily recover when the fever abates, but we may know that the great struggle is yet to come, when during this apparent calm, there is increased tenderness, on pressure, over the stomach, and the eyes and skin begin to become yellow or of an orange color, which gradually extends over the body, and the urine has a yellowish tinge. In such cases the pulse may even be slower than natural, and in bad cases there may be heaviness or stupor.

This period of apparent abatement may last but for a few hours, or it may continue for twenty-four hours, when the stage of prostration ensues. The pulse becomes quick, and, in severe cases, irregular and feeble, the circulation returning slowly in a portion of skin where pressure has been made; the fingers and toes become of a dark purplish hue; the skin becomes yellow, and presents a bronzed aspect; the tongue becomes brown and dryish in the centre, or smooth, red, and chapped; and the teeth sometimes become covered with sordes, or crusts of dried, offensive mucus. The stomach again becomes irritable, everything swallowed is thrown up, and sooner or later a new matter is vomited, consisting at first of brown or blackish flakes, or particles, in a colorless fluid, which at length becomes black and opaque. In very malignant cases the above symptoms may occur as early as the first day. The urine is usually more natural than during the febrile stage, but it is sometimes retained or even not secreted. There is often oozing of blood from the nose, gums, tongue, and throat, and it is sometimes discharged from the stomach, or bowels, or by urine, and dark spots appear on the surface of the body, caused by its extravasation into and beneath the skin. There is often discharged from the bowels large quantities of black matter, similar to that thrown from the stomach. The patient may become indifferent to his fate; the pulse grows more feeble, the respirations slow and sighing, with occanional hiccough: the skin becomes cold and clammy; an offensive odor arises from the body; muttering delirium sets in; the eyes become sunken, the pulse extinct, and the countenance collapsed. Death may ensue quietly or in convulsions.

Instead of pursuing the dangerous and even fatal course described above, the system often reacts after the period of abatement, and a secondary fever sets in, which may be of various degrees of violence, but may always be regarded as a sign that the vital energies are not yet exhausted. This fever may terminate more or less speedily in health, it may soon end in fatal exhaustion, or it may assume a typhoid form, and continue two, or three, or even four weeks. If the patient dies, it is generally on the fourth, fifth, or sixth days, but death may ensue as early as the the third, or not until the ninth or tenth day, and in typhoid cases even much later. Such are the usual course and symptoms of this fever; but this disease is subject to great variations, often, no doubt, from being complicated with typhus and remittent fevers. Very little is known in regard to the cause of yellow fever. It is evidently an epidemic disease, and perhaps to a limited extent contagious; in this respect about on a par with typhus fever.

Treatment—Dr. Holcombe, of Louisiana, to whose writings I am largely indebted for the following directions for the treatment of this disease, in an article on yellow fever, in the North American Journal of Homœopathy, speaking of the epidemic of 1853, says: "The friends of homœopathy, the rational, specific system of medicine, the new dispensation of science, awaited with anxious hope its trial in this frightful malady. Nor was the confidence engendered by its success in cholera, inflammation of the lungs, and other dangerous diseases, misplaced in this. Before passing to the treatment of yellow fever, I cannot forbear making a few strictures on the methods by which allopathic physicians flatter themselves they can encounter this formidable disease. No outsider could be more severe on the whole school than the adherents of different practices in it have always been, and still are on each other. They harmonized in little but in blistering the epigastrium and abusing homœopathy. There were several theories in vogue during the present epidemic, but they were the old ones revamped, with little revision and no amendment. The wonderful advances in chemistry, physiology, and pathology, gave no new light to the medical management of yellow fever. The dominant molochs of allopathy, the lancet, calomel, quinine, and 'expectant medicine' each had his altar, and each received a satisfactory quota of victims."

Camphor: If the chill at the commencement of the disease is very severe and long continued, drop doses of the tincture or spirits of *Camphor*, in a little sugar and water, may be given every ten minutes until it is relieved.

Aconite: This remedy is required during the febrile stage, when the skin becomes hot and dry, the pulse full, and the eyes are red, with severe pain in the head and back. It should generally be continued until the febrile stage is relieved; and, if perseveringly used, it will often materially lessen the prostration which follows the fever. It should generally be given alternately with *Belladonna* at intervals of one half hour.

Dose of this or either of the following remedies, see page 7.

Belladonna: This remedy should be given during the febrile stage, alternately with *Aconite*, a dose every hour, and a dose of the latter remedy between, when the patient is awake. *Belladonna* may be continued when the fever abates, especially when the pain in the eyes, head, and back, lingers; in such cases it should be given alternately with *Arsenicum* during the remission. It will also be required later in the disease if much fever follows the remission, with delirium or pain in the head and back.

Ipecac: If there is nausea and vomiting during the first febrile stage, a dose of *Ipecac* may be given after every effort at vomiting, but the regular administration of *Aconite* and *Belladonna* should not be omitted when this remedy is given, until the fever abates.

Arsenicum: As soon as the remission in the fever occurs, give *Arsenicum* every hour, when the patient is awake, and continue it until the disease is cured. This is the chief remedy after the first febrile stage is over, and should not be omitted. If other remedies are indicated, give them alternately with this. For the burning in the stomach, for the black discharges, and for the great prostration of desperate cases, *Arsenicum* is our main dependence, aided by other remedies.

Lachesis: If, notwithstanding the use of *Belladonna* and *Arsenicum* during the remission, yellowness of the skin is steadily increasing, with increased tenderness of the stomach on pressure, and the pulse becomes frequent and small, and the stomach irritable, *Lachesis* may be given alternately with *Arsenicum*, at intervals of one hour.

Veratrum: If, notwithstanding the use of the above remedies, after the remission of the symptoms is over, nausea and vomiting become excessive, a dose of *Veratrum* may be given after every effort at vomiting; and if there is much pain in the bowels, it will be another indication for this remedy.

Chamomilla · If *Veratrum* fails to believe the pain in the bowels, and even vomiting, especially in the case of women and children, this remedy may be given instead of it.

Cantharides: If the urine is retained or suppressed, or if its passage is painful, an occasional dose of *Cantharides* may be given.

Bryonia may take the place of *Lachesis*, and be given alternately with *Arsenicum*, if the disease lingers, and typhus or typhoid symptoms occur; and if, after two or three days, such symptoms seem to be increasing in severity *Rhus tox.* may take the place of *Bryonia.* For further instructions in such cases, consult the sections on typhus and typhoid fevers.

If the patient has been intemperate, an occasional dose of *Nux vom* will be useful; also when there is great oppression at the stomach without vomiting. For sleeplessness, a dose of *Belladonna* or *Coffee* may be given at bedtime. It will not be best to disturb the patient while asleep, for the purpose of giving him medicine, excepting when there is an unusual tendency to sleep. If there are severe pains in the bowels, cloths wrung from hot water may be applied. If diarrhœa occurs, give *Colocynth,* and if it does not relieve, give *Phosphorus.* If the passages are slimy or bloody, with straining, give *Mercurius viv.*, and consult the section on dysentery.

Diet.—In all cases, if there is not already irritation of the stomach, there is a great tendency to it, therefore the utmost care is required in regard to diet. During the first or febrile stage, nothing should be allowed but rice water, barley water, arrow-root, thin gruel, or weak black tea, with a little milk and sugar in it. During the second stage, nothing more should be allowed, unless the patient has a great craving for food; in that case a teaspoonful of thin fresh cream may be given once in three or four hours, in addition to these drinks. Even after the fever and irritation of the stomach have abated, it is necessary to use the utmost care in returning to a more substantial diet. The above drinks may then be made thicker and more nourishing, and after a few days the patient may be allowed to chew a piece of beef-steak and swallow the juice. For further suggestions, consult the paragraph on diet, in the section on typhoid fever, for the same care is required here as in such cases of that disease as are attended with irritation of the stomach and bowels.

The room should be well ventilated, sun-light should be freely admitted, if the patient has no intolerance of light, and the utmost attention should be paid to cleanliness. The surface of the patient's body may be freely sponged with tepid water, but during the stage of prostration it must be done beneath the bed-clothes, without exposure to the air.

The statistics thus far collected, show that the mortality, when this disease is treated homœopathically, rarely if ever exceeds ten per cent., and often does not exceed five or six per cent.; whereas, under allopathic treatment, it often exceeds twenty five per cent., and is rarely less than fifteen. This disease is a formidable one, and a homœopathic physician should always be called when practicable; but it is safe to say that it is always better to trust to the judgment of a friend, or layman, and a homœopathic book and case of remedies, than to send for an allopathic physician.

INFLAMMATORY FEVER.

Symptoms.—"Rigors, sometimes severe chills followed by burning heat; pulse strong, hard, and greatly accelerated; dryness of the skin, mouth, lips, and tongue; the latter generally of a bright red, in some cases lightly coated with white, thirst, urine red and scanty, constipation, respiration hurried, in accordance with the pulse, amelioration of symptoms as the pulse assumes a more natural state. It runs its course with rapidity, rarely exceeding fourteen days, and progresses with regularity to a crisis, which shows itself in profuse perspiration," or flow of urine, a diarrhœa, or hemorrhage from the nose (Laurie's Practice) Such a fever as is described above, uncomplicated with local inflammation, is a very rare disease in this country. Typhus or typhoid fever sometimes commences with symptoms similar to the above, but the true character of the disease is manifested in a few days, when the characteristic symptoms of the fever manifest themselves.

Treatment.—*Aconite* is the chief remedy and may be given every hour. If there is pain over the eyes, with shooting pains in the head, and in different parts of the body, *Belladonna* may be given after the patient has taken six or eight doses of *Aconite.* If the headache is dull, with pains in the back and limbs, if there is constipation and hurried respiration, give *Bryonia* once in four hours, and *Aconite* every hour between.

HECTIC FEVER.

This fever is caused by some form of internal or external local chronic disease. It commences slowly, with lassitude, impaired appetite and gradual emaciation; the skin looks pale, with the exception of the hectic flush upon the cheeks; chilliness, followed by heat of skin, flushing of the cheeks, and a burning sensation in the palms of the hands and soles of the feet—not always followed by perspiration—occurs at irregular intervals. These slight paroxysms of fever may occur once or twice in twenty-four hours, usually at about the same period of the day; and one of them often occurs towards evening, reaches its height about midnight, and goes off in a free perspiration the latter part of the night. The pulse varies from ninety to one hundred and twenty. The paroxysm, when there is but one a day, sometimes occurs in the forenoon, and when there are two a day, one of them generally does. As the disease progresses the pulse becomes excited continually; after the disease is fully developed the appetite is sometimes better for a temporary period, but as it progresses the stomach often becomes irritable, and vomiting of food is not uncommon. The tongue and throat, in the latter stages of the disease, often become tender, and covered with a thrush-like exudation, and there is often in this stage a watery diarrhœa; earlier in the disease the bowels may be regular or costive. There is generally great thirst, and the urine is high colored. Swelling of the feet, ankles, and legs is common toward the termination of the disease. The mind is often clear, and the patient hopeful until near the close of the disease, when mild delirium is not uncommon.

Hectic fever may be distinguished from intermittent fever by the irregularity in the return of the paroxysms; the excessive sweats the latter part of the night, the continued frequency of the pulse, the clearer complexion and brighter eye, and the comparative absence of headache; also by the presence of chronic organic disease.

Treatment.—This will depend almost entirely upon the character of the organic disease of which this fever is but a symptom, and it would be impossible to treat it with a reasonable prospect of success, without a knowledge of the disease which has caused a given case of it. When the disease has been caused by a profuse secretion or formation of matter or pus, *Phosphorus* may be given at night, and *China* in the morning; and if these remedies do not relieve the symptoms, *Silicea* may take the place of the *Phosphorus* in a few days. A dose of *Mercurius* at bedtime will often relieve, temporarily at least, the night sweats; a dose of *Aconite* given in the morning by lessening the fever will often have the same effect on the night sweats. Corn-coffee is often useful as a drink. An abundance of sun-light and fresh air is all important. The diet should be as nourishing as the digestive organs will bear. Corn-bread should be used, or what is better, bread made from canel and shorts, or coarse wheat or ryè flour, including everything between the superfine flour and the very bran, as in such flour will be found an excess of *Phosphoric acid* and other mineral substances, as well as oil and gluten, which hectic patients need.

CHAPTER II.

DISEASES OF THE SKIN.

ERUPTIVE FEVERS—ACUTE AND CHRONIC ERUPTIONS.

SMALL-POX.

THIS is one of the most contagious diseases to which the human family is subject. It appears to have prevailed in India and China from time immemorial; but was unknown in Europe until after the commencement of the Christian era.

About twelve days usually intervene between the exposure and the commencement of the disease. Sometimes the attack may be two or three days earlier or later. There are two forms of small-pox: the confluent, where the pocks are so thick as to run together, and the distinct, where they are separate; then we have varioloid, or small-pox modified by vaccination or constitutional predisposition. Exposure to varioloid may give rise to either varioloid or small-pox, and exposure to small-pox may cause either confluent or distinct small pox, or varioloid; all depending on the susceptibility of the individual exposed. There are three stages to the disease, the febrile, the eruptive, and the declining stage.

Symptoms.—Chills followed by fever, with frequent pulse, hot skin, headache, uneasiness at the pit of the stomach, sometimes vomiting, and intense pain in the small of the back, with great muscular weakness, are among the first symptoms. The pain in the back resembles rheumatism, but differs from the latter by not being seriously aggravated by moving the body. Sometimes there is wakefulness, in other cases delirium, or even stupor, and with children sometimes convulsions. Occasionally there is great irritation of the stomach, excessive vomiting, and even inflammation; sometimes there is diarrhœa. At the end of forty-eight hours from the commencement of the chills, sometimes a little later, minute pimples, sensibly elevated above the surface of the skin, make their appearance, first on the face, then on the neck and arms, and by degrees extend over the body, and on the lower extremities last. It usually requires from one to two days from the commencement of the eruption on the face until it appears on the feet. When the eruption has made its appearance over the entire surface, if the case is a mild or distinct one, that is, if the pimples over the face and chest are not so thick as to run together when they become pustules or pocks, the fever generally abates; but if the case is to be a confluent one, the fever keeps on with very little mitigation on the appearance of the eruption. The second stage commences when the eruption has made its appearance over the entire body. The minute pimples gradnally enlarge, and at the end of twenty-four or thirty-six hours from their first appearance, a little clear fluid may be seen at the apex or top of each pimple, which has therefore been converted into a vesicle; on the third or fourth day the pocks are distinctly formed, being round and flattened on the top, in the centre of which is often a little depression. They are hard to the touch and are generally surrounded by a red circle From this period they gradually become larger, and their fluid contents become opaque, and at length purulent, when they are called pustules. When this takes place, they lose their depressed appearance and become convex. Those on the face become fully developed, and begin to turn on the eighth day of the eruption, but it is two or three days later before the same change takes place on the lower extremities. If the fever abated when the eruption made its appearance, it returns about the eighth or ninth day in all cases where the eruption is at all extensive. The declining stage generally commences about the eleventh or twelfth day, when the pustules begin to become brown and dryish, and the inflammation of the skin abates. On the fourteenth or fifteenth day, the scales begin to fall from the face, but from the extremities three or four days later. The eruption often makes its appearance on the mucous membrane of the mouth, nose, and eyes. As the eruption declines, the fever abates, the appetite returns and the patient steadily improves.

VARIOLOID OR MODIFIED SMALL-POX.—This disease usually commences with more or less fever, with pain in the small of the back, and nausea, which symptoms generally terminate on the third day, when the eruption makes its appearance. It generally commences on the face but not always; there may be a good many pimples or but a few; and the pimples sometimes disappear without becoming vesicles, but much more frequently they change to vesicles, and even imperfect pustules; and begin to decline on the fourth or fifth day of the eruption, forming hard tubercles which soon disappear. Sometimes the vesicles are scarcely at all depressed in the centre, or at least only occasionally one presents this appearance. In other cases the eruption becomes distinctly pustular and convex at the top like small-pox, but stops one or two days sooner, say on the sixth or seventh day of the eruption instead of on the eighth or ninth day. It is of no particular moment that varioloid be distinguished from small-pox, for the same care is required to prevent the exposure of the unprotected in the one case as in the other, for both will communicate genuine small-pox. There is every variety between the most malignant case of confluent small-pox and the lightest case of varioloid. It is very important that this disease is not mistaken for chicken-pox, and I shall give the distinctive symptoms in the section on that disease, to which the reader is referred.

Treatment.—First: The preventive treatment. Homœopathic remedies will not prevent this disease when given internally with any degree of certainty, nor will hydropathic measures prevent it. I make this statement in order to guard the reader against making, to his sorrow, a mistake which has cost more than one life, to my certain knowledge.

Vaccination is the only safe and reliable preventive, and this will rarely fail if the individual has been recently vaccinated with good fresh matter from a healthy person. It is generally better to take vaccine matter from the arm of a child, and it is all important that the child should be healthy, free from all eruptive and glandular diseases, and free from any hereditary tendency to scrofula, consumption, cancer, or chronic eruptions; therefore the most careful inquiry should be made in regard to the health of the parents of the child, for scrofulous parents frequently have healthy *looking* children. With such precautions there is no danger of injury from vaccination, and it is strictly a homœopathic remedy for the prevention of small-pox, as it causes a similar disease and thus destroys the susceptibility to that fearful and loathsome malady. If there is no danger of exposure to the disease it is not best to vaccinate a child until it is six months or a year old. Children which are vaccinated within the first year will require to have the operation repeated within one or two years, for a single vaccination does not always destroy the susceptibility to the disease, and they will be liable to have varioloid, at least, if exposed, if not vaccinated; and all who are vaccinated during childhood should be vaccinated after they arrive at puberty, or man or womanhood; and again by the time they are thirty or forty years of age. If an individual has been exposed to small-pox, if he is not well protected by having been recently *vaccinated*, the operation should be immediately performed, without regard to age, state of health, or condition; for no consequences which will result will be so much to be dreaded as the small-pox, and if the vaccine matter will work, the patient would be very sure to have either small-pox or varioloid. If the patient is vaccinated within seven or eight days after exposure, it will generally prevent the disease, but he may have the operation performed later and be benefited.

It is always very desirable to prevent pitting over the face and neck; for this purpose rub three parts of *Carbonate of zinc* and one part of *Oxide of zinc* in a mortar, with *Olive oil*, to the consistency of a thin paste, and apply it over the face and neck once or twice a day, so as to form a somewhat firm coherent crust, which, if it is applied as soon as the eruption makes its appearance, will prevent its development and lessen the fever and general irritation.

During an attack of small-pox or varioloid the patient should be kept comfortable, neither too hot nor cold; and his diet should be light, and his drinks cold, during the first stage at least.

Aconite: This is perhaps the most important remedy during the febrile stage, and may be repeated every hour. If there is great nervous excitability, especially with children, an occasional dose of *Coffea* may be given instead of *Aconite*.

Dose of this or other remedies, see page 7.

Belladonna: If there is severe headache, delirium, or symptoms of convulsions, this remedy should be given alternately with *Aconite* one hour apart.

Tartar Emetic: If during the febrile stage there are excessive nausea and vomiting this remedy may be given after a few doses of *Aconite*, or alternately with *Aconite*, if the fever remains high with hot skin. *Tartar emetic* is one of the best remedies which can be given during the eruptive stage, and may be continued until the pocks are fully developed.

Bryonia: If during the febrile stage there is violent pain in the back, which is not relieved by *Aconite* or *Belladonna*, *Bryonia* may be given once in two hours during the forepart of the day and *Aconite* every hour during the evening and night, until the fever and back-ache are somewhat relieved, when *Tartar emetic* may be given in their stead.

Mercurius viv.: When the pocks are fully developed, or when they begin to become opaque, this remedy may take the place of *Tartar emetic*, and be given once in two hours until the pustules begin to dry and become brown over the face and body.

Sulphur may follow *Mercurius* once in two or three hours until the scabs are all separated.

The above are all the remedies usually required, but if during any stage of the disease the symptoms assume a malignant character, which may be known to be the case if the pulse becomes small, the extremities cold, and dark spots appear on the skin, or the teeth are covered with crusts or sordes, *Rhus tox.* may be given once in one or two hours, and if it does not relieve the tendency to dissolution *Arsenicum* may be given alternately with it one hour apart. If the breathing becomes difficult and hoarse, with a hoarse cough, *Hepar sulph.* should be given alternately with *Aconite* at intervals of one hour, and if these remedies do not relieve the difficulty of breathing and cough *Lachesis* may take their place. Cloths wrung from water as warm as the patient can bear may be applied over the neck and chest until these symptoms are relieved. If diarrhœa occurs *Phosphorus* may be given, and if it does not afford relief in a few hours give *China*. When the scabs begin to separate, wash the body once or twice a day with tepid water, or with tepid water and bran.

The patient should not be allowed to go out or into the company of the unprotected who may be exposed, until all the scabs are separated and removed from every part, and he has been thoroughly and repeatedly washed. It matters not how light the case of small-pox or varioloid may have been, nothing can justify the patient in exposing others.

Varioloid requires the same remedies as small-pox.

CHICKEN-POX (VARICELLA)

This is a contagious disease, and perhaps sometimes epidemic, and confined in a great measure to children. The eruption is often the first symptom noticed, in other cases a fever of greater or less severity with some headache precedes the eruption for from a few hours to one or at most two days, and goes off when the eruption appears. The eruption usually shows itself first upon the shoulders, back, and breast, and extends over the face, head, and extremities. The pocks may be numerou or but few. Small, irregular-shaped, transparent vesicles make their appearance on a slightly red surface, and rapidly enlarge to a sixteenth or an eighth of an inch in diameter, sometimes even larger. There is more or less itching, causing the child to scratch, and as the vesicles are very delicate many of them are ruptured in this manner, and also by the garments. At the end of three or four days those which are not ruptured become opaque and present a pearly aspect when they begin to dry up, forming small brown crusts which separate, and fall off at the end of eight or nine days. Scratching and rubbing the vesicles sometimes cause ulceration of the skin, and the formation of large scabs which may leave pits when they separate.

It is very important to distinguish varioloid from this disease, although sometimes difficult, and almost impossible even for a physician to say with absolute certainty to which form of disease a given case belongs, so near do the symptoms of the two diseases sometimes approach each other. In all doubtful cases the same care should be exercised in regard to exposing others, and in vaccinating those unavoidably exposed as in small-pox. But generally there is no difficulty in deciding as to the character of the disease.

In varioloid the fever is more severe and long continued, generally lasting forty-eight hours before the eruption makes its appearance; whereas, in chicken-pox the eruption is often the first symptom which attracts attention, and the fever rarely continues more than twenty-four hours before the eruption makes its appearance. The eruption in chicken-pox is more rapidly formed and developed, appears more superficial, and the vesicle is more readily broken by scratching, less regular in form, and none of the vesicles are depressed in the centre, although some of them may present this appearance from having their tops scratched off while forming, but a slight scab will make this manifest; whereas in *Varioloid* the vesicle is much firmer, and its base is more hardened and elevated, and we can generally find occasionally a vesicle with a depressed centre, but not always. Then the fact that one or the other disease is prevailing, and that the patient may have been exposed, should always be taken into consideration.

Treatment.—This disease is attended with little or no danger to life. If there is much fever, a few doses of *Aconite* may be given; if there is head-ache, *Belladonna* or *Pulsatilla*. The above remedies may be followed by *Sulphur* night and morning, during the declining stage of the disease.

SCARLET FEVER.

This is a contagious, febrile eruptive disease, which may occur at any season of the year, and not unfrequently prevails as an epidemic. Children are far more liable to contract this complaint than adults, as very few of the latter will have the disease when exposed. It is not as contagious as small-pox or measles, and many children when exposed escape entirely. The interval between the exposure and the attack varies from two or three days to three weeks. Patients may have the disease without exposure to those who are sick with it, especially when it is prevailing in the neighborhood.

Symptoms.—A fever, attended with pain in the head, back and limbs, frequent pulse and hot skin, generally precedes the eruption, for from a few hours to twenty-four, or even for a longer period in some instances, whereas in other cases the rash commences with the fever. The throat soon becomes sore and red, the tongue coated white, with little red points projecting through the coating. The edges of the tongue are red, and when the coating peels off the whole upper surface becomes red. The rash first makes its appearance on the neck, face, and breast, and gradually extends over the body and extremities in the course of twenty-four hours. It commences in very minute red points, which coalesce in broad patches in a short time, of a continuous scarlet blush, around the edges of which can usually be seen the separate red points, like those left by the prick of a needle. The rash is sometimes very abundant, covering almost the entire surface; in other cases there are only here and there scattering patches. The redness disappears under pressure, but returns when it is removed. In some instances the skin is smooth, in other cases slightly rough, like that of "goose-flesh." There is more or less burning and itching of the skin, and sometimes fine transparent vesicles make their appearance, especially on the neck, chest, and on the bends of the elbows. The fever does not abate with the appearance of the rash, the pulse becomes frequent, the skin dry and burning. The fever is worse towards night, often attended with restlessness and delirium. Vomiting is a frequent symptom at the commencement of severe attacks, and diarrhœa occasionally occurs during the course of the disease. The throat may simply present a red appearance, with slight soreness, or it may become very much inflamed, swollen within and without, with great difficulty in swallowing, and even impeded respiration. The disease attains its height, usually from the fourth to the ninth day, when, in favorable cases, the symptoms begin to decline, the fever abates, the rash fades, the throat improves, and sometimes there is a profuse perspiration, or diarrhœa, but not always. The scarf-skin soon begins to separate in scales and often peels off in large flakes where it is thick, as on the palms of the hands and soles of the feet. Troublesome itching often attends this process.

In some instances during the febrile stage in severe cases, the brain becomes seriously affected, and great restlessness, delirium, convulsions and stupor, result; or the disease may commence with stupor, and death may ensue speedily from this oppression of the brain. In some cases the inflammation of the throat is very severe, extending to the nostrils, causing obstruction to the passage of air through them, or to the larynx and windpipe, causing croupy symptoms. Patches of false membrane frequently appear on the throat, presenting a dirty white, yellowish or ash-colored appearance. There is a profuse secretion of tenacious mucus in the throat, which the patient finds it difficult to either swallow or discharge from the mouth. The glands of the neck beneath the jaw and ear become swollen, and it is not uncommon for the swelling to linger, and abscesses to form after the fever has abated, retarding recovery.

This disease sometimes assumes a malignant form, when it becomes a very dangerous malady. In some cases of this kind the disease may commence with great anxiety, faintness, and oppression, with feeble and irregular pulse, and labored respiration, pale or livid face, and cold extremities and surface, or cold in one part and hot in another. Feeble attempts at reaction may be made, and slight and irregular febrile action ensue; or, if the above symptoms are not so severe, a low form of fever may ensue, with a tendency to delirium and stupor, and a feeble circulation, with a livid or dark-red eruption, dark spots in and beneath the skin from effused blood, and hemorrhage from the nose, bowels, or urinary organs. In the worst cases, the eruption may never make its appearance, and the patient dies within twenty-four or forty-eight hours, if not rescued by treatment. In other cases the symptoms of the attack may be less violent, and the malignant symptoms may not be so manifest at first, but are more gradually developed. In such cases, instead of high fever, hot skin, and early appearance of the rash, as in the simple form of the disease, typhoid symptoms early manifest themselves; the pulse is small, the extremities incline to be cool, and the rash is postponed, sometimes to the third or fourth day, and then it is dark and scanty. As the disease progresses, there is a tendency to delirium and stupor, offensive breath, dark offensive secretions from the throat, and early disappearance of the rash. The tongue becomes brown, crusts, or sordes appear on the teeth, gums, and palate ; blood oozes from the lips, throat or other mucous surfaces. Ulcers and gaugrenous spots often appear in the throat, and an exhausting diarrhœa not unfrequently occurs. If the tendency is to a fatal termination, the pulse becomes thready and irregular, the countenance sunken, and the surface bathed in a cold, clammy perspiration, and death ensues generally within one or two weeks from the commencement of the attack. But, instead of dying, the patient may slowly improve, but recovery is often retarded by abscesses, diarrhœa, ulcerations, etc.

Few diseases leave so many unpleasant symptoms behind them as scarlet fever. Among these may be named: abscesses in the ear, often impairing hearing; ulcerations in the nostrils, causing chronic catarrh, and pain and swelling of the joints. Dropsy not unfrequently follows scarlet fever, and is quite as likely to follow mild cases as severe ones, and is liable to occur at any period for at least three weeks after the abatement of the fever. There may be dropsical swellings of the face, body, hands and feet, or dropsy of the abdomen, chest, heart, or head. When there is difficulty of breathing on lying down, with or without cough, there is reason to fear there is dropsy of the chest, which will require prompt relief. If there is heaviness and stupor, we have to fear dropsy of the brain. Rheumatism sometimes follows this affection. This disease may be confounded with measles, but the rash is much finer in scarlet fever, and generally appears within twenty-four hours after the commencement of the fever, whereas in measles it is coarser, and appears on the fourth day of the fever.

Prevention of Scarlet Fever.—It is always desirable to prevent this disease during childhood if possible, for if an individual escapes during this period of life he is not very liable to have it at a later period. When practicable, children sick with this disease should be separated from the healthy children of the same family, and children out of the family should never be allowed to visit those sick with it, or even to enter the house, or attend the funeral of a child which has died from scarlet fever. *Belladonna* first recommended by Hahnemann as a homœopathic preventive of this disease, has now been used for many years for this purpose by both homœopathic and allopathic physicians, and many writers and physicians have borne favorable testimony as to its efficacy. During the prevalence of the disease in the family or neighborhood, a dose of *Belladonna* may be given to the healthy child at bedtime for two nights, and a dose of *Sulphur* one night, and so continued until the epidemic is over.

Treatment.—Homœopathy has gained much credit from the success which has attended the treatment of this disease in accordance with its law of cure. Not that patients can always be cured by this or any other treatment, for occasionally the disease is of so malignant a character that there is very little chance of curing the patient; whereas, in a majority of cases it is so light that patients would recover without any treatment, yet there are many cases where much will depend on the treatment. There is, perhaps, no disease which varies so much in severity and fatality in different localities, and during different seasons as this. Even in the same family at the same time, we not unfrequently witness the most malignant case by the side of the mildest.

Belladonna: In mild cases of the disease this is often the only remedy required; and in all cases it will be found useful when the following symptoms exist: soreness and inflammation of the throat, with difficulty of swallowing, especially if there is spasmodic contraction of the throat; redness of the eyes, violent headache, with sleeplessness and nervous excitement or delirium; a bright scarlet color of the eruption and of the throat, are further indications for this remedy. A dose may be given once in two hours when the patient is awake, and continued during the course of the disease, unless a change of symptoms should suggest some other remedy. Also give a dose of *Sulphur* two or three times a day, but let one hour elapse between the taking of this remedy and the *Belladonna.*

Dose of this or any of the following remedies, see page 7.

Unless there is an unusual tendency to sleep, approaching stupor, it is not well to awaken the patient to give medicine, as it will increase the nervous excitability.

Aconite: This remedy is often required at the commencement of this disease, either alone or alternately with some other remedy, generally either *Belladonna* or *Sulphur*. If the symptoms are similar to those described under the head of *Belladonna*, with a very violent fever, and bright eruption, a few doses of *Aconite* should either precede the use of that remedy, or they may be given alternately with it at intervals of one or even one half hour. But if with burning heat, there is great itching, burning and roughness of the skin, with or without minute vesicles, *Sulphur* may take the place of *Belladonna*, and be given after *Aconite*, or alternately with this remedy, until such symptoms are in a great measure relieved, when *Belladonna* may be given instead of *Aconite*, and the *Sulphur* continued.

Mercurius viv.: If the above remedies fail to relieve the inflammation of the throat, and there is a profuse flow of saliva, great difficulty of swallowing, bright redness of the mucous membrane, with or without the appearance of light-colored patches in the throat, and especially if the glands beneath the jaw begin to swell, *Mercurius* is the remedy. In such cases it should generally be given alternately with *Belladonna* one hour apart.

Coffea: If *Belladonna* or *Aconite* fails to relieve sleeplessness, and great restlessness, this remedy will often succeed. Give a dose every hour until three or four doses have been taken, omitting other remedies during the time. *Tartar emetic* may be given when there is nausea, vomiting, and diarrhœa.

Apis mel.: If there is great excitement of the brain, violent headache, startings, delirium, stupor, or convulsions, which other remedies do not relieve, give a dose of *Apis* every hour.

When this disease assumes a malignant form, other remedies will often be required from the very commencement of the attack.

Camphor: Two or three drops of the ordinary tincture or spirits of *Camphor*, dropped on sugar and dissolved in half a glass of water and given by the spoonful, will answer. This remedy should be given when the disease commences with great anxiety, faintness, irregular pulse, pale or livid face, and cold extremities and surface. A dose may be given every five or ten minutes until the above symptoms are relieved, when either *Bryonia*, *Rhus tox.*, or *Arsenicum*, will generally be required.

Bryonia: If the eruption does not make its appearance, or if having appeared, it is indistinct and dark colored, *Bryonia* will be indicated, especially if the extremities are cold, with dull pain in the head and mental torpor, with or without delirium. If *Bryonia* fails to relieve the above symptoms, *Rhus tox.* may take its place, especially if the breath becomes offensive, with crusts of dark matter collecting on the teeth, and the throat is covered with dark-colored patches of false membrane.

Arsenicum: If *Rhus tox.* does not soon relieve the malignant tendency of the disease, *Arsenicum* should be given alternately with it, especially if the disease of the throat becomes dark and offensive, the extremities cold, and the pulse small and irregular with great prostration of strength. Repeat the dose every hour. If improvement does not soon follow *Lachesis* may take the place of *Rhus*.

Carbo veg.: This is our last resort if other remedies fail to check the tendency to dissolution, and the extremities become very cold, and the pulse and respiration irregular. This remedy may be given every hour.

General Measures.—Fresh air and sunlight are very important in this as in all other diseases, yet it is important to avoid exposure to currents of cold and damp air. We should study the comfort of the patient, neither keep him too cold nor too hot. Few measures will relieve the fever, restlessness, nervous excitability, and even delirium, more promptly than frequently sponging the body with water; generally tepid or warm water should be used, but if the skin is very hot and dry, and the patient craves it, and it seems grateful to him, cold water may be used. Sponge the entire body over with a wet towel several times a day, and if the patient is very restless and sleepless at night, repeat the sponging every half hour or hour until quiet sleep results. Keep the feet warm and wipe them dry after sponging. For the thick tenacious and offensive mucus which accumulates in the mouth and throat, make a tea of dried apples and let the patient gargle his throat with it and drink of it. The diet should be light if the fever is high; nothing more than gruel, rice, toast, &c.; but if the disease is of a malignant character, the patient may require beef tea, mutton broth, and even a little meat if he desires it, and can swallow it in addition to the lighter articles named above. There is no objection to the use of cold water as a drink if the patient desires it. For at least three weeks after the fever has abated keep the patient in doors, except it may be during the middle of the day when the weather is very pleasant.

Treatment of the Diseases consequent on Scarlet Fever.—For swelling of the glands beneath the ears give *Calcarea carb.* once in four hours. For ear-ache give *Pulsatilla* every hour, and if it fails to relieve, alternate it with *Chamomilla*, and as soon as the pain is somewhat relieved give *Silicea* and *Pulsatilla* four hours apart. For running from the ears give *Pulsatilla* at night and *Sulphur* in the morning, and continue them as long as the patient improves, then give *Calcarea carb.*; follow these remedies if necessary with *Lycopodium*, and afterwards give *Silicea* every night.

For the dropsical symptoms which frequently follow scarlet fever, if the extremities and abdomen seem chiefly affected, give *Helleborus* once in two hours, and if it fails to afford any relief within twenty-four hours, give *Apis mel.* once in two hours; afterwards give *Arsenicum*, if necessary. *Bryonia* and *Helleborus* are the remedies when the brain seems to be oppressed by a dropsical effusion, if *Belladonna* and *Apis mel.* do not relieve the symptoms; give them alternately one or two hours apart. For bloody urine give *Pulsatilla* once in two hours.

While it is undoubtedly generally safer to trust to a homœopathic domestic book and case of medicines than it is to employ an allopathic physician for the treatment of this disease, yet no layman should undertake to treat a severe case if the services of a homœopathic physician can be obtained.

SCARLET RASH (ROSEOLA).

This is a non-contagious eruptive disease, often mistaken for scarlet fever or measles. It is sometimes preceded for a day or two, and accompanied, by considerable febrile excitement, whereas in other cases there is very little fever. This disease has not the catarrhal symptoms, such as watery and red eyes, sneezing, stuffing and discharges from the nose, of measles, nor has it the sore throat of scarlatina. The eruption is generally of short duration, lasting but a day or two, only occasionally running on for three or four days. The eruption is darker than that of measles, and although it occurs in patches as in the latter disease, yet none of the patches assume the semilunar shape which is frequently noticed in measles. The rash is not as fine and uniform as that of scarlet fever; it usually commences on the face, neck, and chest, with small specks or patches, which sometimes run together forming larger patches one half or one inch in diameter, in other cases they remain distinct. This eruption may be caused by dentition, improper diet, sudden changes of temperature, &c. The same individual may have this disease repeatedly.

Treatment.—A few doses of *Aconite* is generally all that is required, give a dose once in two or three hours. If there is headache, or the disease occurs with teething children, *Belladonna* may either follow *Aconite* or be given alternately with it. If the disease has been caused by errors of diet give *Pulsatilla* once in two or three hours after *Aconite*.

MEASLES (RUBEOLA).

This disease is contagious; and is characterized by catarrhal symptoms, fever, and a rash. It occurs more frequently during the winter, but may occur at any season of the year. The disease rarely attacks the same individual more than once; but few escape having it sooner or later, for it pays little or no respect to age; and adults generally suffer more than children from an attack of measles. From one to two weeks generally intervene between the exposure and the attack. This disease frequently prevails as an epidemic, although at the same time contagious.

Symptoms.—Languor, aching in the back and limbs, chills followed by fever, hot and dry skin, headache, furred tongue, and loss of appetite, are among the first manifestations of the disease; but catarrhal symptoms, such as red and watery eyes, sneezing, watery discharges from the nose, slight soreness of the throat, husky voice, and a dry hoarse cough, sometimes precede the above symptoms, almost always accompany them, or are manifested soon after their commencement. The symptoms are very similar to those of an attack of catarrh or cold in the head. With children, especially while teething, convulsions frequently occur. The eruption generally makes its appearance on the fourth day, or at the end of three full days from the commencement of the fever; sometimes it appears a day earlier, and occasionally a day or even several days later. The rash appears first on the face, then on the neck and trunk, and last on the extremities. Distinct minute red spots, slightly elevated, which momentarily disappear under pressure, first make their appearance. These spots soon enlarge, coalesce, and occasionally form semilunar-shaped patches, with healthy skin between them. The amount of the eruption varies greatly in different cases, sometimes it is very extensive, in other cases but a few patches. The color is not generally as bright as the rash in scarlet fever, and is generally brighter or darker, according to the violence of the fever. The fever and catarrhal symptoms do not abate when the rash appears, but are often aggravated. When the eruption is fully developed, which occurs on the second or third day of the eruption, there are usually more or less heat and itching of the skin. The disease generally begins to decline on the eighth day of the fever, or the fourth of the eruption, when the rash begins to fade, first on the face, then on the neck and trunk, and last on the extremities; the catarrhal symptoms and the fever abate, and the patient is soon restored to health. Sometimes the whole duration of the eruption is not more than two days, whereas in other rare instances it is prolonged to a week or more. As the disease abates, thin scales separate from the surface which has been occupied by the eruption, with more or less itching.

Complications —Sometimes the fever assumes a malignant character, and typhoid symptoms early manifest themselves. In such cases the eruption is dark colored, irregular and partial, and there is great prostration of strength, and also a tendency to faintness, congestion of the lungs, and exhausting diarrhœa. Fortunately this form of the disease is very rare in this country. Inflammation of the air passages is by far the most frequent and dangerous complication. A croupy inflammation of the larynx and windpipe or trachea, or inflammation of the bronchia, or of the lungs, not unfrequently occurs during the height of the disease, or follows as the eruption abates; and if such acute attacks are not carefully treated, they are very liable to become chronic. Diarrhœa is an occasional symptom; also inflammation and abscess of the ear, chronic inflammation of the eyelids, and chronic catarrh, not unfrequently follow an attack of measles. This disease and scarlet fever, occasionally occur at the same time, when there is a mixture of the symptoms of the two diseases.

The measles in the first stage may be very readily mistaken for catarrhal fever or influenza. When the eruption makes its appearance it is liable to be mistaken for either scarlet fever or small-pox. In scarlet fever the rash generally appears on the first or second day of the fever, in measles on the fourth; in scarlet fever it is very fine and punctuated at first, and more uniform at last, and brighter colored than in measles. Then if we bear in mind that red, watery eyes, sneezing, and a hoarse cough, are characteristic of measles, we cannot well mistake the disease. But it is not always so easy to distinguish this disease from the small-pox when the rash first begins to make its appearance; but the pimples in small-pox are harder to the feel under the finger, more prominent, and soon become vesicular and depressed in the centre, when all doubt is removed. Then in cases of small-pox, which are not so severe as to be confluent, the fever generally disappears temporarily on the appearance of the eruption, which is not the case in measles, and the severe pains in the small of the back, which are almost universally present in the former disease, are absent in the latter.

Treatment.—As almost every individnal who lives to adult age is quite sure to have this disease, sooner or later, it is hardly advisable to strive to prevent children being exposed to it, unless the prevailing epidemic is of unusual severity, as it is better to have it at home beneath the paternal roof during childhood than to risk contracting the disease during adult age, often among strangers. If a child or an adult, who has never had the disease, is exposed, it is well to give a dose of *Aconite* one night and *Pulsatilla* the next, and continue them until the commencement of the attack, as the previous administration of these remedies will generally lessen the severity of the disease. For the treatment of the attack select as follows :

Aconite: This is perhaps the most important remedy for the treatment of this disease, not only to relieve the severity of the febrile affection, but also to prevent inflammation of the air passages. A dose may be given every hour or two, when the patient is awake, and continued until after the eruption is fully developed and the fever begins to abate.

Dose of this or other remedies, see page 7.

Pulsatilla, next to *Aconite*, is more frequently required than any other remedy. The following are the chief indications which should lead to its selection: A tardy appearance of the eruption, nausea, diarrhœa, hoarseness, ear-ache, inflammation of or discharge from the ears, and discharge from the nose. *Pulsatilla* should generally be preceded by a few doses of *Aconite*, or, if a high fever continues it may be given alternately with *Aconite*, one or two hours apart. In a majority of cases the above are all the remedies required, until the declining stage of the disease, when a dose of *Sulphur* should be given every night for a few days.

When the above remedies are perseveringly used it is rare that there is any serious local inflammation developed during the course of the disease. We do not expect to cut short the fever and eruption, but simply to lessen their severity and prevent local affections; and in this the homœopathic treatment is eminently successful. But if croupy symptoms occur, notwithstanding the use of *Aconite* or *Aconite* and *Pulsatilla*, *Hepar sulph.* must be given alternately with *Aconite*, one half an hour apart, and continued until the hoarseness and difficulty of breathing are entirely relieved. Large cloths must be wrung from warm water, as hot as the patient can bear, and be applied over the neck and chest, and over them dry flannel; and the wet cloths should be changed every fifteen minutes or half hour, until the patient is relieved.

If symptoms of bronchitis occur, or of inflammation of the lungs, give *Bryonia* once in six hours, and if there is much fever give *Aconite* every hour between. If at the end of four or five days from the commencement of the eruption, when it begins to decline, the cough and oppression of breathing do not abate, and the expectoration becomes opaque and less tenacious, give *Phosphorus* before tea and at bedtime, and *Bryonia* morning and noon. If, after three or four days more, the above remedies do not entirely relieve the cough, uneasiness in and oppression of the chest, give *Sulphur*, and *Pulsatilla* in the same manner, until such symptoms and all expectoration are relieved.

If, during the course of the febrile or eruptive stage, there is violent headache, startings, or convulsions, give *Belladonna* and *Aconite* alternately, one half hour or hour apart, and wring a large towel from cold water, wrap it around and over the entire head and forehead, and place several thicknesses of dry flannel over the wet cloth, so as to entirely cover it, pin it snugly so as to exclude the cold air. Wet the towel every hour until the head symptoms are relieved. For earache, or inflammation in the ears, give *Pulsatilla*, and if it does not relieve give *Chamomilla*, or *Nux vomica*. If a discharge from the ears follows the measles, give *Pulsatilla* at night and *Sulphur* in the morning, and follow them at the end of three or four weeks, if necessary, by *Calcarea carb.* every night for a week. Then omit it for a week; afterwards give, if it is required, *Lycopodium.* If a discharge from or chronic inflammation of the mucous membrane of the nose or eyes follows the measles, give the same remedies in the same manner as directed for discharge from the ear.

If the eruption suddenly disappears after having made its appearance, or if it does not make its appearance on the fourth day, give a few doses of *Bryonia*, especially if the patient complains of a feeling of a load, weight, or pressure at the pit of the stomach, or of oppression at the chest. If diarrhœa occurs during or soon after the disease, if *Pulsatilla* does not relieve it, give *Mercurius viv.*, followed, if necessary, by *China*, at the end of twenty-four hours.

If the disease assumes a typhoid character, *Pulsatilla* and *Bryonia* are the chief remedies during the first stage, and *Pulsatilla* and *Arsenicum* during the stage of prostration; give them alternately, one hour apart.

General Directions.—Keep the temperature of the sick-room comfortable, neither too hot nor cold; and be very careful about exposure to currents of cold or damp air, for a week or ten days after the disease has abated. Allow the patient to drink cold water only in small quantities at a time, but freely of warm water, milk, and sugar. Allow no stimulating drinks, or hot herb teas. Let the diet be light during the fever, nothing more than gruel, milk-and-water, rice or toasted bread, or cracker; and only gradually more nourishing as the patient improves.

ERYSIPELAS (ST. ANTHONY'S FIRE).

This disease is characterized by a spreading inflammation of the skin, sometimes involving the deeper tissues, with fever which may precede, commence with, or soon follow the local attack. Some individuals are very liable to this disease, and it occasionally prevails as an epidemic, or depends upon an atmospheric influence; and in some instances it is of a very malignant character; in such cases the fever is of a low typhus form, and there is a great tendency to gangrene or mortification. Under such circumstances the disease is, to a limited extent, contagious, which, doubtless, depends on the typhus form of fever, rather than upon the eruption, for, ordinarily, erysipelas is not contagious. Where there is a constitutional predisposition to the disease, or when it is prevailing as an epidemic, it may be excited or caused by cold, excessive heat, improper or stimulating articles of food or drink, excessive fatigue, mental emotions, etc. It frequently originates from wounds, sometimes even from slight scratches or bruises; also from ulcers burns, blisters, the sting of insects, and stimulating applications to the skin. I have known two instances arise from piercing the ears for rings. It not unfrequently results from surgical operations, and in hospital and army practice, it is one of the chief sources of danger after operations.

Symptoms.—If the fever precedes the eruption, the patient complains of the usual premonitory symptoms of fever, such as languor, uneasiness, impaired appetite, aching in the limbs, followed by chilliness and fever, headache, sometimes nausea and vomiting, and perhaps swelling of the glands in the neighborhood of the part about to be attacked; sooner or later, sometimes not until the second or third day of the fever, a small red spot, somewhat elevated, painful and tender to the touch, makes its appearance upon some part of the surface. Sometimes the appearance of such a spot is the first symptom, and the fever is only developed as the local disease progresses. The face is the most frequent seat of the disease when it does not arise from a wound or local point of irritation; although it may attack any part of the surface of the body. On the face it generally commences upon the side of the nose, the cheek, or the rim of the ear, and spreads more or less rapidly over the face, sometimes in every direction, but more generally in one. In some instances it only extends over one side of the face, but frequently it spreads over both sides and into the hairy scalp, over the head and down on the neck. As the inflammation travels from point to point, it frequently happens that as new portions of the skin are involved, the disease abates in the parts first affected. The skin is red in the part diseased, more or less elevated, and harder than the sound skin; if the cellular tissue, and other structures beneath the skin, become involved, the swelling may be very great, so as to close the eyes and almost obscure the features. The pain is of a burning, smarting, pricking character. If the inflammation of the surface of the skin is very violent about the third or fourth day, vesicles or blisters frequently appear on the diseased parts. If the scalp is involved, there is frequently violent headache, delirium, or a tendency to coma or stupor. When the erysipelatous inflammation extends to the cellular and other structures beneath the skin, as it not unfrequently does when the face and especially when the extremities are the seat of the disease, it is not uncommon when the inflammation is not checked by treatment, for it to cause death of the cellular tissue which connects the skin to the muscles, and which surrounds the latter, and for large collections of matter to form beneath the skin, which when evacuated, either by ulceration or the lancet, escape with shreds of the cellular structures. In such cases, when recovery takes place, it is often with more or less deformity and inability to use the parts, owing to adhesions between the muscles, or between the muscles and skin. As the inflammation of the skin abates, the scarf-skin separates in scales. Erysipelas sometimes shifts from one part of the skin to another, and sometimes from the skin to internal organs. When the disease arises from wounds, it may terminate in gangrene, inflammation of the veins, or deposits of matter in different parts.

Treatment.—He alone who has treated, and seen this disease treated by both methods, can realize the wonderful superiority of the homœopathic over the empirical treatment of allopathy.

Aconite is one of the most important remedies in all cases where the fever is high, with great heat and redness of the diseased part. If given alone, a dose may be given every hour or two when the patient is awake.

Dose of this, or other remedies, see page 7.

Belladonna: Next to *Aconite*, this is the most important remedy, whether the disease involves simply the skin, or extends to the deeper structures. In all acute attacks, it should either be preceded by several doses of *Aconite*, or be given alternately with it, one hour apart. If the skin is hot, the pulse full, and the diseased part very red, with but little or with much swelling, they should be continued for at least two or three days. At the end of this period, if vesicles or blisters appear, or even if they do not, and the patient does not seem to be improving, *Rhus tox.* may take the place of *Aconite*, and be given either alone or alternately with *Belladonna*, two or three hours apart. If, at the end of twenty-four hours more the patient is not improving, omit the *Belladonna* for a time, and give a few doses of *Hepar sulphuris* instead of it. If, in any case, matter or pus forms, give *Silicea* once in four hours.

If the disease has been caused by a wound, or by an ulcer or sore, if the pulse is full and the surface hot, give *Aconite* every hour for twelve hours; after which, if the symptoms are not better alternate it with *Rhus tox.*, one or two hours apart, and continue these remedies until the fever and swelling are relieved, or if, at the end of twenty-four hours, there is no improvement, omit the *Rhus tox.*, and give *Belladonna* in its stead. If, at the end of three or four days from the commencement of the attack, the symptoms are not in a great measure relieved, give *Hepar sulph.* and *Rhus tox.*, alternately, two hours apart.

If at the commencement of the disease, or at any time during its course, it assumes a malignant character, which may be known by the fever assuming a typhoid form, and the eruption changing to a purple or livid hue, with a slow return of blood to the part after it has been pressed, or the appearance of small blisters filled with a darkish or reddish fluid, other remedies will be required. In fact, in such cases, *Aconite* will be of very little use, and *Belladonna* will not generally be required, unless it may be a dose or two to quiet active delirium early in the disease.

Give *Lachesis* and *Rhus tox.* alternately one or two hours apart, as soon as any of the above symptoms occur, even if it be at the commencement of the attack. If the extremities are cool, the pulse small, and there is great prostration of strength, with offensive breath, early in the disease, with an intense burning pain in the part diseased, you have a malignant attack which will require the above remedies from the very commencement. If at the end of two or three days the symptoms are not improved, omit the *Rhus* and give *Arsenicum* alternately with *Lachesis* one or two hours apart, and continue them until the disease is relieved, unless symptoms of mortification ensue, or sinking of the vital powers, denoted by a small and perhaps irregular pulse, and cold extremities. If such symptoms appear, omit the above remedies, and give *Carbo veg.* every hour.

In all cases, in the declining stage of the disease, after all the acute symptoms have been relieved, a dose of *Sulphur* may be given every night. Erysipelas cannot always be cured in a day, it may require several days, and the remedies must not be changed too often, for if they are, the patient may fail to get any relief.

General Directions.—As a general rule very little benefit will be derived from local applications. Internal remedies are far more efficacious than external, and the latter often interfere with the action of the former. One of the very best which can be applied, is simply dry wheat starch, finely pulverized, and there is no objection to its use. The diet should be light, nothing more than gruel, rice, toasted bread, and cracker, until the fever has abated, and there is a return of appetite, when it may be gradually made more nourishing. In a malignant attack, if the vital forces seem to be giving way, it may be necessary to resort to beef tea or mutton broth.

ERYSIPELAS, CAUSED BY POISONOUS VEGETABLES.—Poison ivy, oak, or sumach, when brought in contact with the skin, will cause an erysipelatous inflammation on many individuals. Some are so susceptible that an eruption will be caused even by the odor or exhalation from these vegetables. The skin becomes red, burns and itches, and vesicles soon form. The fluid contained in these vesicles seems to be poisonous, and by scratching and rubbing, and afterwards handling other parts, the disease is often communicated from the hands, ankles, or feet, to the face, genital organs, and other parts. The disease, without treatment, is tedious in its duration, and often causes obstinate ulcerations. It is a singular fact that while some individuals are very susceptible to the action of these poisons, others are not at all so, and can handle these vegetables with impunity.

Treatment.—*Bryonia* is perhaps the most important homœopathic remedy we have. A dose may be given once in from two to four hours, and the remedy may be continued for several days. If there is much swelling and inflammation of the skin *Belladonna* may be given alternately with *Bryonia*, two hours apart, until the acute symptoms are relieved. Give *Hepar sulph.* night and morning, as soon as the vesicles begin to dry, and continue it until the skin is healthy.

SHINGLES (HERPES ZOSTER).

This is a vesicular eruption, occurring on one side of the body, in a majority of cases the right side. The band of vesicles rarely extends more than half way around the body, although they sometimes extend up to the arm or down on the thigh. Sometimes the eruption is preceded for two or three days by febrile symptoms, and pains through the side and chest. Minute vesicles or blisters make their appearance, which enlarge to the size of half a pea, and often run together, attended with burning, smarting pain. The contents of the vesicles at first are transparent, but in the course of three or four days they become opaque, when they gradually dry up. Successive crops of vesicles may appear and prolong the disease for two or three weeks, although it generally subsides within one or two weeks.

Treatment.—*Rhus tox.* may be given once in two or three hours, and a dose of *Hepar sulph.* night and morning. If at the end of twenty-four hours the fever, pain in the chest, and soreness, are not relieved, in a great measure, omit the *Rhus.* for one day, and give *Belladonna* once in two hours, after which give *Rhus.* again. Continue the *Hepar sulph.* night and morning, until the scales fall off.

COLD SORES.—This is another herpetic eruption. For this affection give *Bryonia* once in two hours, and dissolve some in a teaspoonful of water, and wash the eruption with the solution.

NETTLE RASH (URTICARIA—HIVES).

This is a non-contagious eruptive disease, characterized by elevations of the skin resembling those caused by the nettle, or by a blow from a small stick, or the lash of a whip. These elevations are generally reddish about the borders, and white on their summits, although occasionally red. The eruption is attended by intolerable itching, tingling and burning, and appears most frequently upon the inside of the arms, thighs and legs; it also frequently appears over the body, and sometimes on the face. It is frequently caused by irregularities of diet, derangements of the stomach, and certain articles of food, such as shell-fish, mushrooms, honey, green cucumbers, etc. It occurs at all ages, but more frequently with children, especially with teething children. It is very uncertain in its duration, lasting sometimes but a few hours, or less than a single hour; in other instances two or three days, especially when attended with much fever. Its appearance is sometimes preceded, for two or three days, by febrile symptoms, headache, and deranged stomach, faintness, and chills, which usually disappear in a great measure, when the eruption makes its appearance. Sometimes this disease assumes an intermittent form, and in some cases it becomes chronic.

Treatment.—If the eruption is attended by fever, give *Aconite* once in two hours until the fever abates, then discontinue the *Aconite*, and give *Bryonia*, once in two hours during the day, and a dose of *Lycopodium* at night. If the disease has resulted from exposure to wet, damp weather, give *Dulcamara* once in two hours. If caused by errors in diet or by the use of particular article of food, give two or three doses of *Pulsatilla*, and afterward give *Bryonia*, once in two hours. If teething children suffer from this disease, give a dose of *Calcarea carb.* at night, and if they are feverish, give a dose of *Aconite*, once in two hours during the day, If not attended with fever, give *Bryonia* every morning, instead of *Aconite*. If the disease has become chronic, give a dose of *Calcarea carb.* every night for one month, then give *Lycopodium* for a month, and afterwards, if necessary, *Arsenicum*.

Dose of the remedy selected, see page 7.

ERYTHEMA (RED SPOTS ON THE SKIN).

This disease resembles erysipelas, but it differs from it in being less severe, less disposed to spread, generally more superficial, and attended with little or no fever. It may be accompanied by a sensation of heat and tingling, but rarely with much burning or pain. It may occur on the face, limbs, or body. It occasionally occurs during febrile diseases, also during teething. The surface of the skin is generally not much elevated, although sometimes slightly so.

There is a form of the disease which frequently attacks the front of the legs, between the knee and ankle, consisting of large oval patches, which become somewhat elevated, hard, and painful, but gradually soften, assume a bluish color, and go off in eight or ten days, without the formation of matter. This form of the disease is generally attended with some fever and various nervous symptoms.

Treatment.—*Pulsatilla* is the remedy for the last variety named, or when it is located on the front of the legs. Give a dose once in two hours. This remedy will often be found useful when the disease occurs in other parts, if the eruption is dark-colored, and without much heat. When it occurs in the course of febrile affections, or during recovery, *Arsenicum*, followed by *Sulphur*, will be found useful. Repeat the remedy two or three times a day. In the case of teething children, *Chamomilla* may be given morning and noon, and *Calcarea carb.* every night.

Dose of either of the above remedies, see page 7.

ITCH (SCABIES).

This is a contagious eruption, consisting of small pointed vesicles, which generally first make their appearance between the fingers, on the wrists, inside of the joints, and on other parts where the skin is thin. In its progress it may occupy any part of the surface excepting the face and scalp, which are rarely affected. It may occupy a large extent of the surface or only a small portion. The vesicles are generally separate and not clustered, and contain a little transparent fluid. They are attended with intense itching, especially at night in bed. This disease is attended by a small insect, which is found burrowed beneath the surface of the skin, a short distance from the vesicle. In some cases pustules form which fill with yellowish matter, and end in scabs and sores. The itch, without treatment, does not tend to a spontaneous cure, but may continue for years, or an indefinite length of time.

Treatment.—Sulphur is the chief remedy for this disease, and it may be used internally, and if necessary, externally. As this is perhaps more strictly a local disease than any other eruption, and as it is very difficult to destroy the insect by internal remedies alone, especially by the use of low dilutions, there is less objection to local applications than in almost any other disease, if they are applied early. Give a dose of *Sulphur* three times a day for three or four days. At the end of this period, after washing the body with warm water and soap, rub fresh lard freely over every part diseased, night and morning. If at the end of two weeks the disease is not nearly or quite cured, make an ointment by stirring a teaspoonful of the *Flowers of sulphur* into a teacupful of melted lard, continuing the stirring until the lard is cold. It is not necessary nor well to rub the whole surface of the body over with strong sulphur ointment. It will be sufficient to apply the weak ointment prepared as directed above, to the parts diseased every night for three nights, and afterward simply to touch the vesicles and sores, if there are any of the latter, every other night with a little of the same ointment, continuing at the same time the homœopathic preparation of *Sulphur* internally, as directed. If at the end of two weeks the disease is not entirely cured, give *Mercurius viv.* night and morning for ten days, then *Carbo veg.* for ten days, and afterward *Hepar sulphuris.*

Dose of either remedy, see page 7.

MILK-CRUST (CRUSTA LACTEA).

This is a disease of childhood, occurring most frequently between the ages of three and eighteen months. One or more red blotches appear on the cheeks, or some portion of the face ; these soon become studded with small yellowish pustules, attended with great itching. At the end of a few days, the pustules burst, and their contents dry on the skin, in the form of brittle, semi-transparent, yellowish or greenish crusts, which grow thicker from the constant secretion of matter beneath them. The crusts remain attached, from two to three weeks, and when they fall off the surface of the skin is red and shining. The disease may be prolonged for an indefinite period, by the appearance of fresh crop of pustules.

Treatment.—Give six globules of *Sepia* two or three times a day, and continue this remedy for three weeks, when, if the patient is not well, or nearly well, give *Rhus tox.* and *Sulphur*, alternately, forty-eight hours apart, until the disease disappears; or if they fail to cure, give *Mercurius cor.* night and morning.

SCALD-HEAD (TINEA CAPITIS—FAVUS).

This is a very offensive and obstinate disease, and is, to a certain extent, contagious. It is often compounded with eczema and lichen, and the reader will do well to consult what is said under the head of the above diseases, in any case of disease of the scalp for which he may wish to select the proper remedy.

Symptoms.—Small, elevated, dry spots or crusts, about the size of a pin's head, of a yellow color, seated on the surface of the skin, which is depressed by them, make their appearance on the scalp, or in the edge of the hair. These crusts are concave or cup-shaped, externally, and convex on the surface, which adheres to the skin. These gradually enlarge, until they are from one eighth to one fourth of an inch in diameter, still presenting upon their free surface the cup-shaped appearance, except when they unite in large masses, when the entire surface is covered with alternate elevations and depressions, around the edges of which will be found some of the concave crusts. The whole head, forehead, neck and parts of the trunk, in some cases, become covered with these crusts. The crusts of favus are of a pale yellow color, hard, dry, and break with a short fracture, presenting within a mealy appearance. When the eruption first appears, there is very little itching or irritation, but as it becomes developed, small pustules form on portions of the skin not affected, which give rise to a copious discharge, and there is a great itching, tingling, and heat, and an offensive odor, resembling that of mice. Under the microscope, the crusts of scald-head present the appearance of a vegetable growth. The disease is contagious, but may occur without exposure from neglect of cleanliness, unwholesole diet, want of pure air and sunlight. It occurs in children from two to twelve years of age.

Treatment.—Cut the hair with a pair of scissors close to the head, and apply a large linseed meal poultice every night, washing it off in the morning with soap and water, and brush the head carefully with a soft hair-brush, and continue these measures until the crusts are all removed. Give internally at the same time one of the following remedies, commencing with *Sulphur*, every night for one month, then give *Calcarea carb.* for a month.

Hepar sulph.: This is one of the best remedies for this disease. Give a dose every night and morning, and continue the remedy for three weeks; then give *Lycopodium* every night for two or three weeks; after which, if the patient seems to be improving, give *Hepar sulph.* again for the same length of time, and after that *Lycopodium.* To cure this disease a persevering treatment is required. *Sepia* and *Sulphur* may follow the above remedies if necessary, and may be given in the same manner. If other remedies fail, give *Arsenicum* three times a day, and continue it several weeks; only twice a week omit one dose, and give a dose of *Rhus tox.* instead.

The diet should be light but nourishing, principally bread made from unbolted flour, milk, and vegetables; no pork, and very little meat of any kind. Fresh air, out-door exercise, and sunlight, are all important.

ECZEMA (SCALL OR HUMID TETTER).

This is a very frequent disease characterized by the eruption of numerous minute transparent vesicles, closely set on an inflamed surface, generally attended with intense itching and burning pain. On the second or third day after their appearance, the vesicles become opaque, and either dry up or burst, and become converted into thin crusts, from beneath which a thin watery fluid exudes. When these crusts are removed, or fall off, the surface looks glassy and bright red, and there oozes from it a watery fluid. In acute attacks there may be very little inflammation of the portion of skin occupied by the vesicles, or it may be very red and highly inflamed; there may be no fever, or a high fever, at the commencement of the attack. Eczema may be seated on any part of the body. It may occupy a large extent of surface, or but a small space. When it appears on the scalp or face, in the case of children, it is often mistaken for scald-head, or tinea capitis; but it can be distinguished from the latter disease by the absence of the concave or cup-like appearance of the crusts, and by the presence of the profuse thin, watery discharge which sticks the hair together. Eczema frequently commences behind the ears, and in the edges of the hairy scalp, also on the forehead and cheeks. In chronic cases this watery discharge is rapidly dried into scales, which are pushed forward by the hair as it grows. In some cases pustules form here and there, so that we have in connection with the watery discharge more or less pus or matter. The chronic form of the disease is quite common, and is one of the eruptions frequently denominated salt-rheum. It appears frequently on the back of the hands, fingers, arms, back of the ears, and around the nipples. When the disease becomes chronic the skin becomes swollen and thickened, assumes a dark crimson hue, with numerous deep cracks or chaps, which discharge a bloody, watery fluid. From constitutional disturbance, or the action of any local cause, the parts are apt to become tense and painful to the touch, when there escapes from them a profuse watery discharge. If the disease is extensive, after a time the general health becomes impaired, the digestive organs deranged, and general debility ensues.

Eczema may occur at any period of life, from the earliest infancy to old age, and it affects females more frequently than males. It is not contagious. A predisposition to this disease sometimes seems to be hereditary. It may be caused by the direct rays of the sun, turpentine liniments, the alkali in soap, or by the handling of sugar. When caused by soda or potash it is termed the washerwoman's itch; when by sugar, the grocer's itch. It occurs not unfrequently on the legs of aged persons, especially when the veins are enlarged, and often degenerates into troublesome ulcers. The use of mercury, in large doses, may cause this eruption. When this disease appears on the fingers it is very liable to be mistaken for the itch, but can be readily distinguished, if we bear in mind that in the latter disease the vesicles are solitary, or stand alone, are large and cone-shaped, whereas in eczema they are crowded together, small, and more frequently seated on the back of the fingers than between them. Eczema is rarely dangerous to life.

Treatment.—Few diseases are more troublesome, or obstinate, than this, especially when chronic. It requires a persevering and long-continued treatment.

Aconite: This remedy will be required when an acute attack of eczema is ushered in by fever, local heat, and swelling of the affected part. A dose may be given once in two hours.

Dose of this or other remedies, see page 7.

If the disease has been caused by the rays of the sun, or by heat, it is sometimes called prickly heat. If any fever attends such cases, *Aconite* may be given three times a day for a few days, afterward give *Belladonna* night and morning. If the direct rays of the sun on an exposed surface of the skin, have caused the eruption, give *Arnica* internally, and drop five or six drops of the tincture into a tablespoonful of water, and wash the parts three or four times a day.

Dulcamara: If the eruption is attended by fever, *Dulcamara* should either follow *Aconite,* or be given alternately with it, and continued several days. *Dulcamara* will often be found useful in chronic cases, when it should be repeated night and morning, and continued as long as there is any improvement.

Mercurius cor.: This is perhaps the most important remedy we have, after the acute symptoms have been somewhat relieved by the above remedies, especially when the disease occurs during childhood, and occupies the scalp or face. A dose may be given once in six hours, and the diseased parts may be washed once or twice a day, in a spoonful taken from the same solution which is given internally. This remedy should be continued in recent cases for one or two weeks at least, and in long-standing cases, night and morning for one or two months. *Apis mel.* may follow *Mercurius cor.*, if it is needed; give a dose night and morning and oontinue as long as there is any improvement.

Sulphur should follow the above remedies in recent attacks, and may precede them in chronic cases, one dose every night. If there are scattering pustules discharging matter or pus, in connection with the watery discharge of eczema, give *Sulphur* one night and *Rhus tox.* the next for three or four weeks, and follow these remedies by *Hepar sulphuris* night and morning if necessary. If irritation of the urinary passages attends this eruption, give *Apis mel.* night and morning.

Arsenicum is a very important remedy in obstinate cases; give a dose night and morning, and continue it for several months, substituting *Dulcamara* occasionally for a week.

When the disease occurs on the legs of aged persons, give *Arsenicum* night and morning and follow it with *Carbo veg.* at the end of a month.

General Directions.—Do not use soap in washing; use simply tepid water, or water containing a small quantity of carbonate of soda, and dry the surface well after washing. In eczema of the scalp, the hair should be cut close with a pair of scissors, and if the head is covered by scurfy crusts, poultice it with linseed meal and wash with tepid water, with or without a little soda, until the crusts are removed. In chronic eczema, great benefit often results from the nightly application of a poultice of slippery-elm bark, prepared with warm water. Children, after the period of nursing, should be kept on a bread-and-milk diet, not bread made from superfine flour, but from the second and third runnings, which contain the dark and nutritive portions of the wheat, phosphoric acid, &c., which children affected with this disease need. It is not always safe to dry up suddenly the secretion which attends this disease by external applications, for fatal internal disease not unfrequently results from such treatment.

PEMPHIGUS (WATER BELBS).

This eruption is characterized by the appearnce of round or oval red spots, upon which blisters from the size of a pea to that of a hickory-nut, or even larger, make their appearance, often preceded by chills and fever, and loss of appetite. It may appear on the thighs, abdomen, arms, hands, and other parts.

Treatment.—*Hepar sulph.* alternately with *Rhus tox.*, two or three hours apart, are generally the remedies required for the acute form of the disease. Give one at night and the other in the morning when the affection has become chronic.

LICHEN.

This disease is characterized by the development of numerous minute pimples of the color of the skin, or of a reddish hue, in clusters or scattered over the surface of the skin, attended with itching or tingling and heat, and terminating either in the separation of scales or scurf, or in superficial ulcerations. The simple form of the disease is rarely attended with much fever, but minute pimples, about the size of a pin's head, make their appearance in irregular patches on the extremities, neck, face, or breast, and may spread over a large extent of surface, or be comparatively limited. The pimples become fully developed on the third day, and by the seventh or eighth day they fade, leaving on their summits minute scales. As all the patches do not appear at the same time, the disease is generally prolonged for two weeks, and in chronic cases, by successive crops of pimples for months and even years. There is a severer form of the disease, in which the pimples are clustered in large patches, are small, very red, and the skin is inflamed. It occurs most frequently on the outer surface of the limbs, forehead, and on the cheeks, and is attended by smarting, burning pain, especially at night, and is preceded by considerable fever, which abates when the eruption appears. In a few days the points of the pimples become slightly ulcerated, and pour out a watery fluid, which dries and forms thin yellowish scales or scabs. The disease may terminate in a fortnight or three weeks, or it may be prolonged for months, or even for several years, with occasional remissions during cold weather. In chronic and severe cases the skin is apt to become thickened, of a dark, livid color, uneven on the surface, and chapped or cracked, and discharges a thin, watery fluid. When it occurs on the back of the hands, and even when it appears elsewhere it is one of the eruptive diseases usually denominated salt-rheum. This disease, when there is a thin, watery discharge, often resembles eczema, but the skin is more swollen, thickened, and uneven, and the watery discharge is less than in eczema, and the itching is more intense. Bear in mind that lichen commences with pimples which may, in the course of a few days, ulcerate and discharge moderately; bnt eczema commences with vesicles which secrete a profuse watery fluid. The disease denominated ringworm is often but circular patches of lichen; in other cases it is a vesicular or herpetic eruption

Lichen is frequently caused by heat, when it is called *prickly heat*. It may be caused by stimulating drinks and food, stimulating substances applied to the skin, chronic inflammation of the stomach, derangements of the stomach and bowels, &c.

Treatment.—If the eruption is preceded or accompanied by fever, give a dose of *Aconite* once in two hours until it abates. Even if there is not much or any fever, this remedy will often be useful, especially if the disease has been caused by heat, and there is intense itching and burning.

Dose of any of the following remedies, see page 7.

Bryonia: This is generally the most important remedy in all recent or acute attacks, after *Aconite*, or when the symptoms do not require *Aconite*. Give a dose once in two hours. If the patient is not better at the end of three days, especially if new crops of pimples are making their appearance, give *Dulcamara* once in four hours.

Sulphur may follow the above remedies as soon as the symptoms are in a great measure relieved, or if they fail to relieve; also in chronic cases, give a dose every night, and continue this remedy for a week, then omit it for a week, after which give *Lycopodium* for a week, then omit, and at the end of another week give *Sulphur* again, and so continue.

A tepid bath may be employed daily for the relief of the itching and burning, and after the skin has been well dried, the seat of the eruption may be smeared over with *Olive oil*, or *Cold cream*. In chronic cases, the surface of the eruption may be moistened with water, and then rubbed over, lightly with *Glycirine* once or twice a day. Patients affected with this disease should use very little salt.

ITCHING OF THE SKIN (PRURIGO).

This disease is characterized by an intense itching of the skin, without any eruption, or with a very slight appearance of pimples, sometimes quite large pimples, but without redness of the skin, or fever. The disease is not contagious, and is generally chronic.

Treatment.—Give a dose of *Sulphur* every night for two weeks, and if the patient is then improving, continue it, but at longer intervals—once in three nights. When *Sulphuris* fails to benefit, give *Nux vomica* night and morning as long as improvement follows; then give *Hepar sulphuris* every night, and afterwards *Dulcamara*. If the disease is on the scrotum, give *Sulphur*, aud then *Dulcamara*. If on the vulva, give *Sulphur* as directed above, then *Sepia*, and afterward, if necessary, *Calcarea carb*. Wash in all cases, frequently with warm water, and use a warm bath two or three times a week.

RINGWORM.

This disease is frequently a variety of lichen, or simply an eruption of pimples in a circular form, without any vesicles; when this is the case, consult the section on lichen, and follow the general and local treatment there recommended. In other cases, the disease is a vesicular eruption (*Herpes circennatus*) characterized by the appearance of very minute vesicles, closely set, and forming circles, often with healthy skin in the centre.

Treatment.—Give a dose of *Sulphnr* night and morning for three days, and then give *Sepia* in the same manner for a week, when, if there is no improvement, you may give *Calcarea carb*. every night. *Arsenicum* may be required in obstinate cases.

CHILBLAINS.

This affection generally attacks the feet, and results from sudden changes of temperature in the part, which causes the skin to become inflammed, swollen, and painful.

Treatment.—Give *Pulsatilla* at night and *Arsenicum* in the morning. Put one teaspoonful of *Arnica tincture* into a cup of water, and wash the parts once in three or four hours.

CORNS.

Some persons are much more liable to suffer from corns than others. The disease is generally, in fact always, caused by wearing tight shoes. The external layer of the skin becomes thickened from pressure, which, by pressing on the parts beneath, causes pain, soreness, and inflammation.

Treatment.—Wear loose shoes. Carefully dissect off the corn with a sharp knife, commencing at one side and slowly cut with the point of the knife, as you raise the edge of the corn with a finger nail of the other hand or a hook, between the almost transparent corn, and the whitish surface of the true skin; and if you have patience and are careful, you can remove the corn entirely, without drawing blood or causing pain. Then wet a soft rag in *Arnica water* prepared as directed for chilblains, and wind round the toe or foot. Give *Calcarea carb.* alternately with *Sulphur*, at intervals of three or four days, to prevent a return of the complaint.

BOIL (FURUNCULUS).

This is an inflammation of the skin, and of the areola tissue beneath it, ending, if not subdued, in the death of the latter, which separates and escapes in the form of a slough or core, with pus. The swelling is of a conical shape, and if left to itself, breaks at its apex.

Treatment.—Put twelve globules or one drop of *Arnica tincture* into a glass of water, and give a teaspoonful of the solution once in six hours, and wash the boil in the same solution. If, at the end of twenty-four hours, the inflammation is not abating, omit the *Arnica* and give a dose of *Belladonna* three times a day, and if this remedy does not check the progress of the disease within twenty-four hours; give *Mercurius viv.* alternately with it, at intervals of two or three hours, and apply a poultice of bread and milk, or of linseed meal. If the pain is throbbing, and you have reason to think that matter has formed, give *Hepar sulph.* night and morning, and *Belladonna* once in four hours in the intervals, until the abscess breaks.

To remove the predisposition to boils give *Sulphur* at night and *Belladonna* in the morning for a week, then give them alternately, at intervals of three or four days, for two or three months, if the patient has suffered long from the disease. Afterward give *Lycopodium* once or twice a week.

CARBUNCLE (ANTHRAX).

This disease bears some resemblance to a boil, but the swelling is generally larger, darker, and more spongy. The cellular tissue beneath the skin early becomes gangrenous, or mortifies, and as the disease progresses, several openings form through the skin, through which a thin, offensive matter issues, with portions of dead cellular tissue. Typhoid symptoms are early manifested, and the disease, especially when it attacks the aged, or those of bad habits, or of a depraved constitution, is attended with great danger to life. The usual seat of carbuncle is on the back, neck, or head, although other parts may be affected. It may be small, not larger than a prune, or it may be as large as a tea-saucer, or even larger in some cases.

Treatment.—At the commencement of the disease give *Silicea* night and morning, and give *Belladonna* once in two hours in the intervals, until either the inflammation and swelling are relieved, or you are satisfied that they are not likely to check the progress of the disease. Then omit the *Silicea* and give *Arsenicum* alternately with *Belladonna*, at intervals of two hours. If, notwithstanding the use of the above remedies, several openings make their appearance, through which a thin matter oozes, the skin should be freely divided over the dead substance beneath, so as to allow the slough and matter to escape readily; then apply a poultice of bread and milk, or linseed meal, until the dead tissue is separated and discharged. If symptoms of great debility ensue, omit the *Belladonna*, and give *China* once in four hours. If there is burning pains, give it alternately with *Arsenicum*, once in two hours. To heal up the sore or ulcer which remains, give *China* in the morning and *Silicea* at night.

Dose, see page 7.

The diet should generally be nourishing, especially after the first few days; milk, beef, or mutton, or beef tea, toast, mashed potatoes, &c., used with moderation.

FELON—WHITLOW (PANARI).

This disease is an inflammation, resulting in the formation of an abscess on the fingers, or in the palm of the hand. It frequently attacks the balls or ends of the fingers; also the spaces between the joints. The inflammation may commence in the skin, or the fleshy part beneath the skin, or deeper among the sheaths of the tendons or chords; or, again, in the external covering of the bone, or periosteum. One form of this disease extends around the roots of the finger-nails, and is therefore called a run-around. The disease is very painful. There is often heat and swelling of the whole hand, with violent throbbing of the arteries. It usually commences with a pricking pain, as though a splinter were in the part.

Treatment.—Give *Silicea* once in six hours, and if, notwithstanding the use of this remedy, the hand becomes hot, and the patient feverish, give a dose of *Aconite* every hour between the doses of *Silicea.* Often *Silicea* alone will cure the disease if given early.

Dose, see page 7.

At the very commencement of the inflammation wet a strip of cotton or linen cloth, half an inch wide, and six inches long, in *Arnica water*, or a spoonful of water containing a few drops of *Arnica tincture*, and commence at the end of the finger and wind it around the finger as snug as the patient can bear, without causing much pain, and allow it to remain, if it affords relief at the end of one or two hours. If the disease has been continuing unchecked for several days, and the pain is throbbing, the sooner it is freely lanced the better, for if this is not done when the disease is on the end of the finger, the bone is very liable to be destroyed, and come away after a long period of suffering; or if the disease is nearer the hand, between either of the joints of the finger, the matter is apt to follow down among the tendons, into the palm of the hand, and cause much suffering and deformity. As soon as it is evident that the formation of an abscess cannot be avoided the parts should be freely laid open, and a poultice of bread and milk, slippery elm, or linseed meal, applied. Any physician can perform the operation. Continue the *Silicea* afterward.

ULCERS.

These may arise from external injuries, the action of chemical agents, &c.; or they may arise from internal or constitutional causes, scurvy, a scrofulous or cancerous diathesis, the poisonous action of mercury, and of the venereal virus. They are frequently caused by the sluggish circulation, which results from enlarged or varicose veins on the lower extremities. Ulcers caused by external agents will generally disappear readily if there is no constitutional predisposition, but if they fail to heal, proper internal remedies must be given..

Treatment.—If the patient has symptoms of scurvy, such as swollen and bleeding gums, fetid breath, livid spots on the skin, and swelling of the lower extremities give *Carbo veg.* night and morning for one week, and *Arsenicum* the next week, and so continue. Follow the general directions you will find in the section on scurvy.

Dose, see page 7.

If the patient has scrofulous symptoms, such as swelling of the glands of the neck or arm-pits, chronic inflammation of the eyes and lids, chronic discharges from the ears and nose, give *Sulphur* every night for one week, and *Calcarea carb.* for the next; afterward give *Hepar sulph.* and consult the section on scrofula.

For cancerous ulcers give *Sulphur* every night for a week, then

Arsenicum night and morning for a month, and longer if the ulcer improves; afterwards give *Silicea*. Consult a homœopathic physician.

If an abuse of mercury has been the cause of the disease, give *Sulphur* night and morning for two weeks, then *Hepar sulph* until the ulcer heals. If the disease has been caused by syphilis or the venereal disease, *Mercurius viv.* is the main remedy. Give a dose night and morning, omitting it every third week, substituting *Lachesis*.

For ulcers on the legs connected with varicose or enlarged veins, or for varicose veins without ulcers, give *Pulsatilla* night and morning, and apply every morning a bandage moistened in half a teaspoonful of *Arnica* to a cup of water, to the foot and leg, commencing at the toes and ending at the knee. Call on a physician and let him show you how to apply it properly. At the end of two weeks omit *Pulsatilla* and give *Carbo veg.* night and morning, and continue it as long as the ulcer improves. *Arsenicum* or *Lachesis* may follow *Carbo veg.* in such cases.

When there is a burning sensation in an ulcer, give *Arsenicum* night and morning, and follow it with *Carbo veg.*; if there is itching give *Sulphur*, followed by *Hepar sulphuris*.

For fistulous ulcers give *Sulphur* night and morning for a week, then *Calcarea carb.* for two weeks; and afterward, if necessary, *Silicea* until it is healed. Also, confine with a bandage, a compress of cotton or cloth, so that it shall press firmly upon the portion of the cavity, or track from which the pus comes farthest from the external opening, so as to bring the two sides of the cavity in contact and allow them to heal; leave the opening free.

If ulcers are irritable and painful apply soft rags or cotton wet in warm water. If they are indolent, or inactive, apply cloths wet in cold water, and several folds of dry flannel over them—change once in six hours. If the ulcer seems to be doing well and the matter is thick and healthy, apply a soft cloth with a little simple cerate or mutton tallow, spread upon its surface; do not remove it more frequently than once in twenty-four hours, unless the discharge is very great, and then do not wash off the matter from the surface of the sore, as it is nature's dressing

If the ulcer is on one of the lower extremities, the cure will be expedited by keeping the limb in a horizontal position.

When an ulcer is in a healthy condition, the healing process can often be hastened by drawing the edges towards each other by the means of straps of adhesive plaster, so as to lessen the extent of surface to be healed over.

ABSCESSES.

Abscesses may form on almost any part of the body, and also in internal organs. They result from local inflammation. Such inflammation may be slow or rapid in its progress; usually several days intervene between the commencement of the inflammation and the formation of pus, sometimes weeks, and even months.

Treatment.—For local inflammation which threatens to result in the formation of an abscess, give *Belladonna* when there is heat, redness, and swelling of the parts. If there is fever and thirst, give *Arnica* alternately with *Belladonna.* If the above remedies fail to check the inflammation within two or three days, give *Mercurius viv* once in three or four hours. If the pain becomes throbbing, and slight chills occur, give *Lachesis*, and if no improvement follows at the end of twenty-four hours, give *Hepar sulph.* If an abscess is slow in coming to a head, without being very painful, give *Sulphur* at night and *Silicea* in the morning for a week, then omit the *Sulphur* and give *Hepar sulph.* at night. After the abscess breaks, give *Silicea* every night and morning.

If the swelling is very painful during the formation of an abscess, apply a bread-and-milk or linseed poultice, and change when it becomes cold; or apply cloths wrung from cold water, and put over them dry flannel, so as to exclude the air and excite perspiration; change once in four hours.

RED-GUM AND TOOTH-RASH.

(STROPHULUS.)

These are but varieties of lichen. The former consists in an eruption of pimples, and is peculiar to children during the early periods of life, occurring most frequently a few days after birth The pimples are generally of a reddish or crimson hue, and scattered on the surface over the face, back of the hands and arms, and sometimes on the body, intermingled with small red patches of skin The eruption begins to fade in two or three days, and has disappeared at the end of a week or ten days. This disease is generally caused by keeping the child too warm, by the irritation of flannel, or by the action of the atmosphere on the delicate skin of a new-born child.

The tooth-rash is caused by teething; the pimples may be red, white, or the color of the skin, and are numerous, in patches, and attended with itching, and sometimes with fever. The pimples gradually disappear in the course of ten days or two weeks, but fresh patches may be developed as the old disappear, and the disease be prolonged for months.

Treatment.—For the red gum, keep the surface of the body cool—not cold, and omit flannel. Wash the surface with tepid water, or milk-and-water, and give *Aconite* once in twelve hours, and at the end of two or three days, give *Sulphur*—one dose a day. For the tooth-rash, use the same external measures, and give *Aconite* at night and *Bryonia* in the morning, for a week, then give *Sulphur* every night.

CHAPTER III.

ACUTE RHEUMATISM.

THERE are two forms of this disease; one inflammatory, attended with fever and local inflammation, one or both; the other nervous, often without the least sign of fever or even local inflammation. In inflammatory rheumatism, the fever sometimes precedes the local inflammation, but much more frequently the first symptoms are local, and in a majority of cases seated in the extremities, generally, but not always, in the lower extremities first. The first local symptom may be acute pain, or it may be simply uneasiness and stiffness in a part, soon followed by soreness and pain, especially on motion. If the pain is severe at first, it often abates somewhat when the swelling commences, but extreme soreness and pain on motion remain. The swelling is generally tense and elastic; the skin may be unchanged in color, or reddened of a light rose color. The disease may involve almost the entire exterior of the body at once, but more frequently it commences in one or more limbs, or parts of the body. It not unfrequently changes somewhat rapidly from one part to another, abating where it first commenced, in other instances it extends to other parts without abating in those previously involved. Sometimes parts are attacked several times before the disease abates. A whole limb may be involved, or only the joints; in some instances the muscles between the joints are chiefly affected. The pains are usually tearing or rending, often with shootings, and movement almost always causes great suffering. The febrile symptoms are generally, but not always, in proportion to the local symptoms, and soon follow the latter. The pulse is full and strong, but not very frequent, in a majority of cases ranging from ninety to one hundred, and the surface is not as hot as in many other febrile affections, and is sometimes bathed in a profuse perspiration, which does not relieve the sufferings. The tongue is generally white and coated with a thick fur, the stomach quiet, and the bowels constipated, the urine scanty, high-colored, and depositing a sediment on cooling. The fever is usually remittent, and worse in the evening or at night, when the pain is also worse. The disease sometimes changes from external parts to internal organs, especially to the membranes upon the external and internal surfaces of the heart, causing pain, oppression, palpitation, and faintness.

It is not uncommon to have a local inflammatory rheumatic affection either so limited, or so slow in its progress, as not to cause fever. It may involve one or more joints, but this variety of the disease often attacks the muscles, sometimes but a single muscle, causing pain, soreness on pressure, and pain on motion. The muscles of the scalp, the eye, face, neck, chest, back, sides, abdomen, and hips, are frequently thus affected. The stomach, bowels, liver, kidneys, uterus, and testicles, are not exempt from a liability to this disease. The previous or present existence of rheumatic inflammation in other organs or parts, will aid us in distinguishing this from other diseases.

Nervous Rheumatism.—This form of the disease is evinced by pain, or other disordered sensations, in organs or parts, and derangements of function or of motive power. It may affect almost any part of the body, and often resembles neuralgia. It may cause colic, spasms in the stomach, palpitation of the heart, headaches, dizziness, buzzing in the ears, earache, toothache, and a great variety of other symptoms of a nervous character, which may be known to be of a rheumatic nature, or at least complicated with rheumatism, in all cases where such symptoms alternate with rheumatic disease of the joints or muscles, appearing when such rheumatic affections are relieved, and disappearing when the joints or muscles become again affected.

In regard to the cause of rheumatism we know little; we simply know that there is a certain predisposition existing with many individuals, which renders them liable to attacks of this disease on exposure to cold when the body is hot, or to wet and damp weather, or currents of air, changes of weather, or any of the causes which develop colds or inflammatory diseases in others. Rheumatism is not a hereditary disease; it occurs frequently during childhood, and among those exposed to hardships, privations, and accustomed to excessive labor; in all these respects it differs essentially from its next door neighbor, the gout.

Treatment.—In few diseases is the superiority of the homœopathic treatment over the allopathic more manifest than in many cases of acute rheumatism; not that this disease is always easily cured by onr treatment, but allopathy has a knowledge of but few remedies which hold a specific relation to this affection, and does not possess the science requisite to guide, with any considerable degree of accuracy, in the administration of those she uses; therefore she can do little or no good in a large proportion of cases, and very many linger on for months, and in not a few instances the disease becomes chronic; whereas homœopathy has a knowledge of many remedies, and a law to guide in the selection of the right one, therefore she is able to cure promptly most cases, and it is rare that the disease becomes chronic under this treatment.

Aconite.—This is a very important remedy in most cases which are attended with fever and swelling, and should be continued once in one or two hours until the severity of the symptoms is somewhat relieved. It will be found useful when the skin is moist as well as dry, provided it is hot and the pulse full. It should generally be followed by one of the remedies named below.

Dose of this, or other remedies, see page 7

Belladonna is next in importance to *Aconite*, when the fever is of an active Inflammatory grade, and may be given once in two hours after the latter remedy, especially when the pains are shooting and burning, and the surface over the part diseased is red and shining, and there is much swelling, and the patient is worse at night. If a high fever persists after you commence giving *Belladonna*, omit the latter remedy during the evening and night, and give *Aconite*, returning to *Belladonna* in the morning. *Aconite* and *Belladonna* should be continued until the severity of the febrile and general inflammatory action is in a measure relieved, when, if the local symptoms do not steadily abate, you can select one of the following remedies, and give instead of *Belladonna*. *Belladonna* is also useful for nervous rheumatism, when the pains are sharp or shooting.

Bryonia: After the acute symptoms have been somewhat relieved by *Aconite*, or this remedy and *Belladonna*, and in cases not attended by much fever from the commencement, no remedy is so frequently required as *Bryonia*; if there is much fever lingering, it is well to give a dose once in four hours, and *Aconite* every hour between. *Bryonia* will be found especially useful when motion or moving the part diseased, causes stitching, catching tearing or shooting pains, also when there is profuse perspiration. It is one of the best remedies for nervous rheumatism, when the symptoms are aggravated by motion, and are worse at night, or in the morning. It may be given once in two hours, when the patient is awake, excepting when *Aconite* is required.

Rhus tox.: If *Bryonia* fails to relieve the symptoms in acute rheumatism, *Rhus tox.* should generally follow it. It may take the place of the former remedy at the commencement, if the disease has been caused by exposure to wet, or cold damp weather. In cases not attended with fever, or where it is very slight, *Rhus tox.* should be selected when the symptoms are relieved by exercise or motion. The pain and stiffness may be very great upon first attempting to move the part after rest, or when awaking in the morning, but if these symptoms are lessened after moving for a while, *Rhus* is particularly indicated, whereas, if they are increased, as the patient continues to exercise, *Bryonia* is the remedy. A dose may be given once in two hours.

Pulsatilla should be given when the pains shift rapidly from one joint or part to another; when there is a sensation of numbness or lameness of the affected part, or a feeling of coldness at every change of weather. Also when the pains are aggravated in a warm room, and relieved by cool air. It is more frequently required for women and children, and persons of a mild or phlegmatic temperament than for others. A dose may be given once in two hours.

Nux vomica: When there are costiveness, great sensitiveness to the open air, and numbness of the affected parts, with drawing pains in the muscles, *Nux vom.* may be given once in two hours. It is especially useful for those addicted to the use of alcoholic and fermented drinks; also for nervous rheumatism; but rarely of much service at the commencement of very inflammatory attacks.

Chamomilla, in the case of women and children, and for sensitive men, will often be found useful when there are drawing, tearing, continuous pains, which are worse at night, with great restlessness and tossing about.

Mercurius viv. should be selected when the pains seem to be in the bones, also when they are in the joints and muscles, if there is a profuse perspiration which affords no relief; and when there is a feeling of coldness in the affected parts, and the pains are burning or tearing, and worse in cold or damp weather, and also worse at night. Repeat the dose once in two or three hours.

Arsenicum may be given when the pains are burning and tearing, worse at night, aggravated by cold, and relieved by warm applications. This remedy is especially indicated when there are paroxysms of pain, which are intermittent. When the heart becomes involved, after the use of *Aconite*, *Belladonna*, and *Bryonia*, or *Rhus tox.*, *Arsenicum* becomes our main remedy. It may be given alternately with *Bryonia* or *Rhus tox.* Repeat once in two hours.

Arnica is the remedy when there is a sensation as if the parts diseased were resting upon something very hard, with violent pains as if contused. Give a dose every hour, and put a teaspoonful of the tincture into a teacupful of water, wet a cloth in it and lay it on the diseased part, and over the wet cloth place four or five thicknesses of dry flannel so as to exclude the cold air; change once in six or eight hours.

Ignatia is the remedy when there is a sensation as if the flesh were loose on the bones in consequence of blows, or a contused feeling, and when the local symptoms are temporarily relieved by a change of position. Give a dose once in two hours.

China is often a valuable remedy after the acute symptoms have been relieved, when there is great weakness and profuse perspiration, also in intermittent cases. Repeat the dose once in four hours.

CHRONIC RHEUMATISM.

This is a very obstinate disease. It generally results from an uncured acute or a sub-acute attack. It may be limited to one part, or extend to several; it may be fixed or shifting. If the muscles are involved, they often waste away and become contracted, and in old cases there are frequently stiffness, distortion, thickening, and immobility of the joints, especially of the hands and fingers.

Treatment.—Several of the remedies named for acute rheumatism, will be found serviceable, especially *Belladonna*, *Bryonia*, *Rhus tox.*, *Mercurius viv.*, *Pulsatilla*, and *Nux vom.*, and the indications for their use there given, are sufficient.

Sulphur: In all cases of acute and sub-acute rheumatism, which linger and threaten to assume the chronic form, *Sulphur* should be given; also when chronic rheumatism has been caused by an abuse of calomel or mercury. It may be given night and morning. If *Sulphur* fails to relieve such cases *Hepar sulphuris* may be given in the same manner. *Lycopodium*, *Lachesis*, *Phosphorus*, *Sepia*, and *Calcarea carb.* may be used in turn, giving a dose night and morning, and continuing the remedy for at least two weeks, and longer if the patient improves. Electricity, carefully applied, is often of service, and also vapor baths, and warm bathing; but it is better to consult a homœopathic physician, when practicable, than to attempt to treat the disease simply by the aid of a domestic book and case. Rubbing over and pressing upon the parts diseased, gently pressing or slapping them with the hand, and moving the parts, or bending and extending the joints, are exercises which are of great importance, in chronic cases, when properly applied.

GOUT.

This is not a very frequent disease in this conntry, except in instances where it is hereditary. It is caused by high living, especially by the use of high-seasoned animal food by those who do not labor or pursue an active life, and by the use of vinous and fermented drinks, or malt liquors, such as porter, lager beer, &c. Gout seldom occurs before the age of thirty, and is much more common with men than with women; and the attack is more liable to occur during the spring or autumn than during either summer or winter. The first attack generally commences suddenly during the night; the patient awaking about midnight, with an acute pain in the first joint of the great toe of one foot, which by the morning becomes much swollen, of a bright red color, and very sore to the touch. Slight chills followed by fever and restlessness attend the local disease. Toward morning there is often a remission of the pain and fever, and the patient obtains some rest, but in severe cases there is but little if any relief until the second morning, when the pain abates and the part diseased becomes more swollen, but less red and firm, and when pressed by the end of the finger a pit or depression remains for a time after it has been removed. The pain, fever, and restlessness, return the following night, but again abate in the morning; and thus the disease continues, but steadily abating in severity until the patient is restored to his usual health, at the end of from five to ten days, if the disease is not arrested sooner by treatment. Some swelling often remains for a time, and the scarf skin generally peels off, which is attended by itching. There is thirst during the fever, the urine is scanty, and deposits, on cooling, an abundant brick-dust sediment. If the patient does not entirely change his manner of living, the first attack is but a foretaste of the future, and at the end of from one to two or three years he has a return of the disease; and afterward the attacks gradually become more frequent, and also both great toes and other joints of the foot, the ankles, knees, elbows, wrists, and many other parts may suffer in their turn; or several may be affected at the same time. After the patient has had several attacks, the disease may commence in other parts; and even the first attack does not always commence in the first joint of the great toe, but sometimes in the ball of the foot, or the ankle, and occasionally in one of the finger joints, or in the wrist. Gouty subjects are extremely subject to heart-burn and sour stomach at all times In chronic cases earthy or chalky matter is frequently deposited within and around the joints, muscles, and ligaments, impairing their functions and causing deformity.

Gout bears quite a resemblance to rheumatism, and sometimes both diseases exist at the same time. Gout attacks high livers, the indolent, but children are generally exempt; whereas rheumatism is common among those who work hard, are much exposed, and children frequently suffer from this disease In gout, the fever is more variable, and there is little disposition to sweat; whereas in rheumatism the fever is more constant, and there is often profuse perspiration. The hands and feet are much more liable to be affected, and leave the rest of the body free, in gout than in rheumatism.

Treatment —We are first to strive to relieve the attack if the patient is suffering from one, and then to prevent a return of the disease, for it is almost sure to return if the utmost care is not used to prevent it.

Aconite may be given every hour in all cases where there are much fever and heat of the skin, and continued until these symptoms are removed.

Dose, see page 7.

Bryonia: After a few doses of *Aconite*, *Bryonia* should generally be given once in two hours during the day, and *Aconite* during the night, until the acute symptoms are relieved. If these remedies do not relieve the symptoms within two days, *Rhus tox.* may take the place of *Bryonia.*

Nux vomica: As soon as the acute symptoms have been somewhat relieved by the above remedies *Nux vom.* may be given, especially when the stomach is sour, or otherwise disordered, the bowels costive, and if the patient is addicted to the use of stimulating drinks, give a dose once in two hours.

Pulsatilla: If *Nux vom.* fails to relieve the symptoms named, *Pulsatilla* should be given; and this remedy may be administered instead of *Nux vom.* when the bowels are loose, or if the patient is of a mild temperament or a female.

To prevent a return of the paroxysms, or to cure chronic gout, *Nux vomica* and *Pulsatilla* will be found very efficacious, and should be administered when there is the slightest derangement of the digestive organs. If the stomach is sour or the bowels are loose,

Pulsatilla may be given every night; but if the bowels are constipated, and the patient is subject to the piles, *Nux vomica* every night will do better. In addition to the above remedies *Calcarea carb.* may be given every morning when there are earthy concretions about the joints, and when there is irritation of the urinary passage, with an earthy sediment in the urine, especially if it is light colored; whereas if the sediment in the urine is reddish, like brick dust, or even yellowish, give *Lycopodium* in the morning instead of *Calcarea carb.*

But if a patient expects to get a permanent cure of this disease, or even anything like satisfactory palliative relief, he must change entirely his manner of living in the intervals between the attacks, for the same course of life as that which induced the disease in the first instance, if continued, will most certainly bring on a return of the symptoms, in spite of remedies. There is but one course which can save the patient from untold sufferings, and the longer it is delayed, the less efficacious will it prove No sudden changes should be made, for they will not always be tolerated, but gradually, as his digestive organs will bear it, the patient must cease entirely to use alcoholic, vinous, and fermented drinks, and all stimulating condiments, and use very little animal food, and never eat meat more than once a day at most, and very temperately then. Regular systematic exercise is all-important, so as to keep the digestive organs in a healthy state.

NEURALGIA.

This is a disease of the nervous system, and consists of severe paroxysms of pain, of a purely nervous character, unattended by inflammation, lasting from a few minutes, or even seconds, to several hours, days, or weeks, in different cases. There are always more or less perfect remissions when the paroxysms continue any considerable length of time, generally occurring at irregular intervals. Sometimes, especially in sections of the country where intermittent fevers prevail, the disease assumes an intermittent form, and the paroxysms occur at regular intervals, once in one, two, three, seven, or fourteen days, as do those of regular intermittent fevers, and subject to the same variations. Such cases are called masked ague, as they undoubtedly arise from the poison that causes ague, and require similar remedies. Persons who have once had an attack of neuralgia, are very liable to have a return of the disease sooner or later, unless there is a resort to a persevering medical and general treatment, for the purpose of eradicating the tendency to it. The pain is generally very severe, and more or less darting or lancinating, and sometimes burning, tearing, aching, beating, benumbing, or tingling. In some instances it seems like electric shocks, and causes the patient to start suddenly, and spasmodic twitchings of the muscles, are not uncommon. Sometimes there is tenderness of the part on pressure, especially on slight pressure; strong pressure often affords partial relief, and friction with the hand frequently relieves even when hard pressure seems to increase the pain. The paroxysms may come and go off suddenly, or gradually, and may return several times a day, or only at long intervals, and may cease entirely, or continue to recur during life. This disease may attack almost any part of the body, external or internal, but all parts are not equally susceptible. It frequently attacks the head and face, and may be confined to a single small spot or extend over half of either. When its seat is in the nerves of the jaws and teeth, it causes one of the forms of toothache; when in those of the ear, it causes earache. The eyes, temples, heart, stomach, and bowels, are not unfrequently affected, also the upper and lower extremities, the back, and walls of the chest. It frequently shifts from one part to another.

Very little is known in regard to the causes of neuralgia, but it is quite certain that a predisposition to this disease, and to its recurrence is caused by whatever tends to impair the general vitality of the system, such as exposure, excessive labor, intemperance, excesses of every kind, especially sexual excesses and abuses, indolence, and the want of pure air and sunlight. It sometimes depends upon a local irritation of, or pressure on a nerve, but the pain is often at some distance from the diseased point which causes it. Neuralgia is frequently complicated with rheumatism or gout, or at least, patients subject to the latter diseases, are very liable to the former.

Treatment.—We should not only strive to relieve the paroxysm when the patient is suffering, but also endeavor to eradicate the tendency to the disease, by remedies and general measures. For present relief during the paroxysm, one of the following remedies may be selected.

Aconite tincture, or globules saturated with tincture: This is one of the best remedies when the pains are very acute, almost insupportable, especially at night, or even during the day, if the pains are shooting, and the disease is located about the face or head. Three drops of the tincture, or twenty globules, saturated with *Aconite*, may be put into a half-pint glassful of water, and a tablespoonful may be given to an adult, but only from a half to a whole teaspoonful to a child, every ten minutes, and the parts diseased may be washed with a spoonful of the same solution until the pain is relieved; then a dose may be given three or four times a day, to prevent a return of the symptoms. The dilutions of *Aconite* will rarely relieve the symptoms, it requires generally either the prime tincture, or globules saturated with the tincture.

Belladonna: If *Aconite* fails to relieve the symptoms, *Belladonna* may be selected, or take the place of it at the commencement, when the pains are piercing and burning, with or without muscular twitching, and aggravated by a bright light, noise, a current of air, or by the warmth of bed; and if the paroxysms of pain occur in the afternoon or forepart of the night, this will be another indication for this remedy; although it may be found useful when they occur at any period of the twenty-four hours. A dose may be repeated every hour unless it aggravates the symptoms; in that case it should not be repeated, at least for several hours, or until the aggravation has passed off. After the symptoms are relieved, it may be given three or four times a day to prevent a return of the disease.

Dose of this or other remedies, see page 7.

Nux vom. will be found especially useful in case the patient is subject to the gout, or if he is addicted to the use of alcoholic and fermented drinks, or if he is a high liver, of sedentary habits; and with others when the following indications exist: Drawing or jerking pains, sensation of numbness, shocks like electric shocks, symptoms worse after a meal, also at night, and in the morning, aggravated by cold air, and reading or thinking. Give a dose every hour until the pain is relieved, and then repeat two or three times a day to prevent its return.

Chamomilla: Excessive nervous sensibility, which renders the least pain insupportable, beating and tearing pains—more frequently required for women and children than for men. Repeat the dose every half hour or hour.

Pulsatilla: Pulsative and piercing pains, aggravated on lying down in the evening, during repose, and while sitting, relieved by cold air; especially useful in the case of women, and persons of a mild disposition, but may be of service in the case of men. Give a dose every hour.

Coffea may be given when there is great nervous sensibility, tearfulness and discouragement; it may be repeated every half hour, and if it does not relieve, it may be followed by *Ignatia,* especially if the pain is partially relieved by movement, or change of position.

Bryonia: This remedy should be selected in case the patient has suffered from rheumatism, especially if the pains are pressive or drawing, tearing and piercing; and are aggravated by movement of the body. If similar symptoms occur, but are relieved by exercise or movement, *Rhus tox.* may be given instead of *Bryonia.* Repeat either every hour.

China: This is an important remedy in intermittent cases, especially when the patient has frequently had intermittent fevers. It will also relieve in other cases when there is excessive sensibility of the skin to the slightest touch, and there is a sensation of torpor and weakness in the affected part. Give a dose once in four hours.

Arsenicum is more frequently required than any other remedy when the disease assumes a regular intermittent form. In such cases it may be given alternately with *Nux vomica.* Burning or tearing pains, or a sensation of coldness in the affected parts, are also indications for *Arsenicum.* Give a dose every hour, and gradually lengthen the intervals as the patient improves.

For further suggestions in regard to the medical treatment of this disease, consult the sections on the treatment of headache, toothache, gastralgia, colic, &c.

It is all-important that the patient change his manner of living, so as to conform strictly to the laws of health; otherwise remedies will do little more than palliate his sufferings. The great essentials for health and life, are sunlight, pure air, regular active exercise, and plain wholesome food and drink, free from stimulants and stimulating condiments. Patients who persist in shunning the light of the sun, and active exercise, and live in the confined air of over-heated rooms, and eat superfine flour bread, need no expect to be cured of neuralgia. Consult the "Avoidable Cause of Disease."

SCURVY.

This disease is generally caused by the absence of fresh vegetable food. Impure air, or whatever else tends to debilitate the system or deprave the blood, will favor the development of the scurvy. Sailors, when long confined to salt meats, bread, beans, &c., are very liable to this disease. When it occurs on land, it is generally in fortifications, or toward the close of winter and during the forepart of spring, when fresh vegetables are scarce. The worst case I have ever seen on land, was caused by living entirely on bread made from superfine flour.

Symptoms.—Aching and weariness in the limbs, paleness of the complexion, swelling, tenderness, redness and bleeding from the gums, are among the first symptoms. As the disease progresses, the paleness increases, sometimes with a livid hue; hard and painful swellings appear on the lower extremities, lower jaw and hands, causing contraction, stiffness, and pain on movement. The gums become excessively swollen, sometimes so as to conceal the teeth; bleed freely, may present a blackish appearance, the teeth become loose, and in some instances fall out; chewing is very difficult, and the breath excessively offensive. Purple spots appear on the surface of the body, hemorrhage occurs frequently from the mouth, nose, stomach, bowels, and urinary organs. In desperate cases, old scars ulcerate, united fractures may separate, and the debility is extreme. The bowels are generally costive, and the appetite good. Scurvy is frequently complicated with dysentery and typhoid fever, and sometimes with congestion or inflammation of the lungs and other organs, which adds much to the danger.

"Dr. Garrod, from an examination of the composition of food, under the use of which scurvy was capable of occurring, as well as of such substances as had been proved beyond doubt to be anti-scorbutic, was led to the conclusion that the absence of potash was the cause of the scurvy. In this way he shows: 1st. That potash is deficient in scorbutic diet; 2d. That all bodies proved to be anti-scorbutic, including fresh meat and vegetables, milk, lemon juice, etc., contain a large amount of potash; 3d. That in scurvy the blood is deficient in potash, and the amount of that substance thrown out by the kidneys, is less than what takes place in health; 4th. That scorbutic patients, when kept under a diet which gave rise to the disease, recover when a few grains of potash are added to their food. The salts of potash, such as the nitrate, oxalate, and bitartrate, are well-known anti-scorbutics, but their efficacy has always been ascribed to the acid, rather than to the alkali; 5th. That deficiency of potash in the system, seems capable of explaining some of its symptoms, especially muscular weakness, as potash is a necessary constituent of the muscular system." (Bennett.)

The above conclusions of Dr. Garrod require further confirmation before we can rely upon them, but they are worthy of being borne in mind.

Treatment.—A proper diet is far more important than medicine, in fact the latter can be of little use when the former is neglected. All vegetables are not equally efficacious as anti-scorbutics. Among the most important are acid fruits of all kinds, especially lemons, limes, and sour oranges; potatoes cooked or raw are perhaps next in importance; then raw cabbage, turnips, and carrots. If in the early spring, the above vegetables are scarce, or if among emigrants in new countries or soldiers, miners, &c., they are not to be had, and symptoms of scurvy appear, it will not do to be too particular in the selection of vegetables, but any of the following which can be obtained, may be freely used: Radishes, mustard, lettuce, spinage, celery, garlic, parsley, sorrel, dandelions, and even horse-radish. In fact almost any early vegetable which is used as a salad, or as greens, may be used in cases of necessity. It is well for emigrants into new countries who cannot carry with them a supply of potatoes, cabbages, and turnips, to provide themselves with the seed of lettuce, mustard, and other early vegetables, so as to supply themselves with vegetable food as soon as possible in the spring. It is not necessary that severe symptoms of scurvy appear before there is great danger; for when the vitality of the blood has been in a measure destroyed, the patient becomes very liable to attacks of dysentery, typhus and typhoid fevers, and inflammation of the lungs, and in fact many other diseases; and in such cases they are very dangerous. Fresh meat, especially wild meat, is very useful, and should be given when it can be obtained. Lemon juice is one of the best remedies, and may be freely used when it can be obtained, in the form of lemonade. Vinegar is of little or no value and should not be used except it may be moderately on salads, cabbage or greens. Also give one of the following remedies:

Mercurius viv.: If the patient has never, or not recently, taken this remedy in large doses, give it once in four hours when the patient is awake, especially when the gums are ulcerated, the teeth loose, and there are swellings on the limbs.

Carlo veg. may follow *Mercurius*, or precede that remedy, when the breath is very offensive, and there is a burning sensation in the mouth, and great weakness. *Nux vomica* may be given alternately with *Carbo veg.* at intervals of two or three hours, in case the latter remedy fails to relieve the symptoms when given alone.

Arsenicum: This may follow the above in case they fail to benefit, or relieve all the symptoms, especially when there are burning sensations, ulcers on the edges of the tongue, swelling of the limbs, and great weakness.

Dose, see page 7.

SCROFULA.

Tuberculous consumption, enlargement of the mesenteric glands, a certain form of inflammation of the eyes, hip disease, and various other forms of local diseases, are regarded as scrofulous affections, and will be duly considered under their various heads; but the disease now under consideration consists of swelling, induration, and frequently of inflammation and ulceration of the absorbent glands of the neck, arm-pit, groin, or breasts. A single gland may be enlarged, when the swelling is generally oval; or there may be several, forming an irregular mass. The tumors may remain for months and years, and then gradually abate, or they may become inflamed, and an abscess form, which, after a time, bursts and discharges pus alone, or mixed with a curdy matter, leaving an ulcer, which discharges a thin, imperfect matter, and may be a long time healing; and when healed leaves a large, irregular scar. If these glandular swellings suddenly abate, under the use of external remedies, disease of the lungs not unfrequently follows. This affection is most frequent in children and young persons, and females are more liable to it than males, and a predisposition to it is often inherited. It is undoubtedly caused either by some defective action in the organs of nutrition, or those of secretion, one or both.

Treatment.—General measures are far more important than medicines, not that the latter may not be useful. Sunlight, pure air, and active exercise, including proper amusements, are the great instrumentalities for renovating the organism by strengthening the whole system, quickening the digestive organs, and stimulating the organs of secretion to remove all useless substances from the system. Let every individual who is tainted with scrofula in any form, or who has a child thus affected, obtain the author's work on the "Avoidable Causes of Disease," and carefully read it through, and he will find information which is far more important, not only for the prevention of the disease, but also for its radical cure, when it has already commenced, than any remedies possibly can be. Still proper remedies are useful, and very important.

Calcarea carb.: Give six globules of this remedy, or, if in powder, as much as will lie on the end of a penknife-blade, every night for one month. Then give *Sulphur* every night for two weeks; repeat these remedies if necessary. If the enlarged glands become sore and painful at any time, give a dose of *Belladonna* once in four hours, between the doses of the above remedies. If an abscess threatens, or forms, notwithstanding the use of the above remedies, give *Hepar sulph.* night and morning, until it bursts; then give *Silicea* night and morning, until the ulcer heals.

The diet should be nutritious, consisting of bread made from coarse flour, butter, milk, meat, and vegetables. Pastry and bread made from superfine flour should not be used, as the former deranges the digestive organs, and the latter contains too much starch, and not enough nutriment.

HIP DISEASE AND WHITE SWELLING.

These are scrofulous affections of the joints. In the hip disease there is an inflammation of a scrofulous character in the bones and joints, which comes on very insidiously, and, if not checked, it progrésses until the joint is destroyed, an abscess forms, and if the patient survives, it is only with a shortening of the limb and deformity. Among the first symptoms noticed are generally the following: A disposition to stumble, lameness, pain in the knee or ankle, sometimes in the thigh or hip. As the disease progresses the limb sometimes becomes elongated, and generally emaciated; the pain increases, and is often very troublesome at night; then swelling and an abscess, and finally shortening of the limb and flattening of the nates. Pressing the thigh-bone into the socket by a sudden push or blow on the foot or the upper end of the thigh-bone causes pain.

White Swelling, is a somewhat similar affection of other joints, which often results in disorganization of the joint, and anchylosis or stiff joint, if not in the loss of the limb.

Treatment.—*Mercurius viv.* is the most important remedy at the commencement of the disease. Give a dose night and morning, and if there is much pain, give *Belladonna* occasionally between the doses of *Mercurius*. *Colocynth* will also sometimes relieve the pain. Continue *Mercurius* as long as there is any improvement; but when it ceases, or the patient is apparently well, do not stop the treatment, but give *Sulphur* every night for one week, and *Calcarea carb.* every night for the next week, and so continue. If, notwithstanding the treatment, an abscess begins to form, give *Hepar Sulph.* night and morning, and after it breaks, give *Silicea* every night for one week, and *Calcarea carb.* every night for the next week, and so continue until the discharge ceases. A current of electricity passed through the hip for a short time daily, will often hasten the healing process. Treat white swellings in the same manner. A homœopathic physician should always be consulted in all cases of disease of the joints or bones when practicable, and he should be consulted early if possible.

DISEASES OF THE BONES AND PERIOSTEUM.—Bathing in cold water when the body is hot, and other causes, not unfrequently excite inflammation of the periosteum, or external covering of the bones, or of the bones themselves. If this inflammation is not soon checked by treatment, it goes on to the formation of matter, or pus, and finally to the death of the bone itself. Only the external surface of the bone may be involved, or the entire shaft may be destroyed. In the first case scales and pieces of dead bone, after much suffering, and at the end of months, are separated and work their way to the surface with the discharge; but if the entire shaft is involved before it is detached from living portions, a new bone often forms around it, from which it can only be removed by a surgical operation.

At the commencement of the disease there is deep-seated pain; soreness and swelling soon make their appearance, attended by fever, a hot skin, frequent and full pulse, and loss of appetite. This disease is often, at its commencement, mistaken for rheumatism. Syphilitic and mercurial poisoning often cause nodes or swelling and soreness of the periosteum, but the symptoms are generally much less acute than when the disease results from the other causes named.

Treatment.—At the commencement of the attack, give *Mercu-*

6

rius viv. once in two hours, and if relief is not soon afforded, alternate it with *Belladonna,* one hour apart; and continue these remedies for two days, and longer, if the patient is doing well or improving; but if there is no improvement, give *Phosphorus* once in two hours. This is a good remedy in cases where the bone is involved; and it is especially useful when the disease commences in the periosteum; and in such cases, it may even precede the other remedies above named, but if, at the end of two days, it does not relieve the symptoms, *Mercurius* and *Belladonna* should take its place. A remedy in this disease should be continued at least two or three days before it is changed, and never change as long as there is any improvement. If, at the end of four or five days, the above remedies do not relieve the symptoms, give *Silicea* once in two hours, but omit one dose in the course of the twenty-four hours, and give a dose of *Sulphur.* If, notwithstanding the treatment, an abscess forms, *Silicea, Calcarea carb., Sulphur*, and *Phosphorus*, are your chief remedies—one dose of one of these remedies a day. If the disease has been caused by syphilis, give *Mercurius viv.* once in two hours, but if it does not relieve, give *Nitric acid;* also give this remedy once in four hours when mercury is the cause.

DROPSY.

This affection may be caused by exposure; it may follow eruptive febrile attacks, especially scarlet fever, but it is very frequently caused by disease of the kidneys, heart, lungs, liver, or spleen. Dropsy of the different cavities may result from inflammation of the membrane which lines them. There are various forms of the disease named by authors, such as cellular dropsy, called anasarca; this affects the extremities, face, and body, externally to the various cavities. Next, abdominal dropsy, named ascites; dropsy of the chest, named hydrothorax. Then we have dropsy of the brain, named hydrocephalus; and dropsy of the scrotum, named hydrocele. If the disease results from inflammation of the various cavities, it is usually preceded by fever and pain in the part, but not always. For dropsy on the brain, consult the sections on hydrocephalus and inflammation of the brain. So if the dropsy is confined to the chest, consult the sections on pleurisy and pericarditis; if to the abdomen, consult the section on peritonitis. If the disease follows scarlet fever, consult the section on that disease. If there is no evidence of disease of the heart, lungs, liver, or spleen, and the lower extremities commence to bloat unexpectedly, without any cause which can be traced to organic disease, pregnancy, or scarlet fever, consult the section on Bright's disease of the kidneys. If the dropsy is caused by disease of the heart, consult the section on diseases of the heart.

Treatment.—If this affection is caused by exposure to wet or damp weather, give *Dulcamara* once in two hours. If *Dulcamara* fails to relieve give *Apis mel.* in the same manner.

In dropsy of the chest there are shortness and difficulty of breathing, which are aggravated by lying down, and during exercise, and dullness on percussion.

For dropsy of the chest, *Bryonia*, *Sulphur*, *Arsenicum*, *Mercurius*, and *Helleborus*, are the chief remedies. If they fail to relieve, give *Apis mel.*: One of these remedies may be given once in four hours.

For dropsy of the abdomen, *Apis m l.*, *Arsenicum*, *Mercurius*, *Helleborus*, *Sulphur*, and *China*, are important remedies, and one of them may be given once in four hours.

For cellular dropsy, *Apis mel.*, *Arsenicum*, *Dulcamara*, *Helleborus*, *Mercurius*, and *Sulphur*, are the principal remedies. If the disease follows scarlet fever, *Arsenicum* and *Helleborus* are useful remedies, and may be given alternately two hours apart. If they do not relieve the symptoms, give *Apis mel.* once in two hours. If this disease follows the abuse of *Quinine*, give *Arsenicum*. If it follows the abuse of *Arsenic* give *China*. If it has been caused by the abuse of mercury, give *China* alternately with *Sulphur* two or three hours apart. If it follows the loss of blood or other animal fluids, give *China*.

In all cases consult the sections on the diseases named above; ascertain if possible the cause of the dropsical effusion, for it is impossible to make a satisfactory prescription without some knowledge of the cause. Dropsy is generally but a symptom of some other disease.

CHAPTER IV.

DISEASES OF THE CHEST AND RESPIRATORY ORGANS.

INFLAMMATION OF THE RESPIRATORY PASSAGES.

THE inflammation may be confined to the nostrils, or to the larynx, trachea or windpipe, or to the bronchia or small air passages throughout the lungs; or it may commence in one part and travel to other parts, and perhaps abate where it first commenced; or it may involve all of the air passages at the same time. It may be either acute or chronic.

COLD IN THE HEAD (CORYZA).

This is a very common and annoying disease. A cold in the head may involve simply the nostrils, or it may extend to one or more of the neighboring sinuses or bony cavities existing over the eyes and in the bones of the upper jaw. Sometimes it is confined to one nostril. It is caused by the partial application of cold as to the back of the head, neck, or feet, and by sudden changes of weather. Some persons are much more liable to this affection than others, and the disease is often epidemic, being a very general attendant on influenza and the first stage of measles.

Symptoms.—The first symptoms are dryness, fullness and tickling in the nostrils, with sneezing, which are soon followed by a profuse thin watery transparent discharge, which often causes irritation of the external surface of the nostrils and the upper lip. The nostrils are sometimes closed by the swelling of the mucous membrane, and there may be heat and burning in these passages, also either a dull aching, or a stinging pain. The eyes often become red and watery from the extension of the inflammation. If the disease extends to the sinuses, or cavities over the eyes and in the upper jaw, there is a dull pain in the forehead and cheek-bones, on one or both sides, with burning and heat. The sense of smell is often impaired for the time being, and there is frequently more or less deafness. If the local inflammation is not severe, or extensive, there may be little or no fever, but in severe cases there is chilliness, pains in the head, back, and limbs, with a high fever, furred tongue, and loss of appetite. This disease usually attains its height in three or four days when left to itself, after which the symptoms abate, the secretion becomes thicker, opaque, less acrid and less copious; sometimes it becomes bloody, greenish, or even deep yellow. Sometimes for a week or two the patient constantly feels that he is getting more cold; in such cases the disease retains its acute character, and the discharge remains watery until this symptom abates. In some cases the nostrils remain dry and swollen, without any watery discharge, until thick opaque matter makes its appearance.

In the case of very young children, the stoppage of the nostrils causes difficulty of nursing, as the child cannot breathe except when he lets go of the nipple; without attention on the part of the mother, he may become black in the face, and have convulsions from obstructed respiration. The child may become discouraged in his attempts to nurse, and suffer for the want of nourishment, if he is not fed.

Treatment.—At the very commencement of the disease when there is dryness, swelling of the mucous membrane, and sneezing, give a dose of *Nux vom.* once in two hours.

Aconite: If *Nux vom.* fails to relieve, and there commences a profuse watery discharge with heat and burning, aching in the bones of the face, chills and fever, dissolve six pellets, or one drop of the tincture of *Aconite* in a tumblerful of water, stir it well, and let the patient, if an adult, drink the whole of it, and if at night, let him go to bed, cover himself up warm, and get into a free perspiration. If the first dose is given during the day, it can be repeated at night. This remedy when thus given, will rarely fail to lessen the severity of the disease. A child may take one fourth of the quantity directed above; if a very young child, give but a teaspoonful.

Arsenicum: Give a dose of this remedy once in two hours, when there is a thin watery discharge which *Aconite* fails to relieve, if there are burning heat, but little thirst, and an aggravation of the symptoms in the morning, and especially if they are palliated or relieved by warmth. Continue the remedy for at least twenty-four hours.

Mercurius viv. may be given instead of *Arsenicum*, if the symptoms are aggravated by warmth instead of being relieved by it; and also if there are great thirst, pains in the limbs, sore throat, copious watery discharge from the nostrils, and pains in and soreness of the nose and face.

Hepar sulph. is often required after the remedies already named, when they fail to entirely relieve the disease; also, if notwithstanding the above remedies, the patient feels that he is constantly getting additions to his cold. If the disease is confined to one nostril, or if a susceptibility to it has been caused by an abuse of mercury, this is an indication for this remedy. Give a dose once in three hours.

Bryonia: Give this remedy once in two hours when there is dry obstruction of the nose which has continued for over twelve hours.

Belladonna may be given either alone or alternately with either of the above remedies, if there are sharp pains through the forehead and face, with swelling and soreness of the nose and loss of smell, which are not relieved by other remedies.

If the discharge becomes thick, whitish, yellow, or green, and does not soon abate, give a dose of *Pulsatilla* at night, and of *Sulphur* in the morning, until it is relieved.

For this disease, or snuffles, in infants, oil the nostrils and upper lip, and even the nose itself with *Glycirine*, first moistening the surface with water. If you cannot obtain *Glycirine*, use *Sweet cream* or *Sweet oil.* Give a dose of *Chamomilla* once in four hours if the nostrils and lips are chapped, and the child is either very restless, or there is dullness and drowsiness. *Nux vom.* is often useful at the commencement of the disease. Also consult what is said above in regard to *Arsenicum*, *Mercurius*, and *Bryonia.*

Chronic Inflammation of the Nostrils, or Catarrh—(Ozæna).—This affection frequently follows acute inflammation, and is often a very obstinate disease. It sometimes results from measles, or scarlet fever, and in other instances it has a scrofulous origin, and it may be caused by the venereal disease. With chronic inflammation there may be dryness of the mucous membrane, heat and swelling, so as to obstruct the passage of air; if the disease affects the back part of the nostrils, there is a frequent disposition to clear them out by a sudden and forcible inspiration of air. In other cases there is a copious secretion of a whitish opaque mucus, or of a yellowish or greenish matter, which may have an odor more or less offensive, and it is often very disagreeable. Sometimes ulcers form on the mucous membrane, and occasionally, especially in syphilitic cases, the bones of the nose become diseased and die, and pieces escape with the discharge. In some cases large solid flakes of exceedingly offensive matter are occasionally discharged either from the surface of ulcers or of the inflamed membrane. The sense of smell is often impaired, and sometimes lost.

Treatment.—In all cases, especially in children, when the disease is in a great measure *confined to one nostril*, examine carefully and see if there is not a foreign substance or body in the nostril which has caused the affection; for children frequently crowd into the nostrils pebbles, beans, kernels of corn, pieces of cloth, worsted, cotton, &c.; and such substances cause inflammation, which will continue until the foreign body is removed. To remove such foreign bodies bend the flat end of a probe, or of a tape-needle, or the crooked end of a wire hair-pin, sidewise, so as to form a slight hook, and pass it into the nostril, and carry the end up over the foreign body, then press down upon it and draw it forward on the floor of the nostril. In this way you can remove, in half a minute, almost any substance a child can crowd into the nostril; whereas, if you attempt to remove it with forceps, you will generally fail.

In slight cases, especially in such as follow the acute disease, or the measles, or scarlet fever, give a dose of *Pulsatilla* every night and a dose of *Sulphur* every morning for one week; then give *Pulsatilla* one night and *Sulphur* the next, for two weeks; after which give them two or three nights apart as long as there is an improvement. If the above remedies do not entirely cure the disease, give *Calcarea carb.* night and morning for a week, then every night for a week or two, and afterwards once or twice a week.

If there is swelling of the mucous membrane of the nostrils, with heat, dryness, and obstruction, without discharge, give a dose of *B yonia* every morning, and a dose of *Lycopodium* every night, for two weeks; then give these remedies twenty-four hours apart for an equal length of time, and afterward two or three days apart.

If the disease occurs in a scrofulous habit, the above remedies will be found useful, especially *Sulphur*, *Calcarea carb.*, and *Lycopodium.* If in such cases there are ulcerations with the discharge of large offensive scales, or if the bones are diseased, *Sulphur*, followed by *Calcarea carb.*, will still be useful, but *Silicea* will often be required to complete the cure; give this remedy every night and gradually lengthen the intervals.

If the disease has had a syphilitic or venereal origin, give *Mercurius cor.* night and morning, and if the patient ceases to improve under the use of this remedy, at the end of three or four weeks, give *Nitric acid* night and morning. If the above remedies fail to relieve cases which have had a venereal or syphilitic origin, obtain at a druggist's ten grains of *Iodide of potassium*, dissolve the whole in forty spoonfuls of water, and take a spoonful three times a day. Cork the solution up in a bottle.

Chronic inflammation of the nostrils is a very obstinate disease, and requires a persevering treatment for a permanent cure. If convenient, you will do well to consult a homœopathic physician, and follow his directions.

LARYNGITIS,

OR INFLAMMATION OF THE UPPER PORTION OF THE WINDPIPE.

A superficial inflammation of the mucous membrane of this part is very common, and is the cause of the hoarseness which often occurs during a cold, especially at its commencement; but the disease now under consideration, involves the structures beneath the mucous membrane, causing swelling, and a narrowing of the passage, and, consequently, an obstruction to the entrance of air, and it is one of the most formidable and dangerous of all the diseases to which man is subject; fortunately it is not very common. It may be either acute or chronic. The acute form may occur in a person in full health, with a high fever at the commencement, or the patient may be weak and debilitated from other diseases, and have little or no fever. The causes are sudden changes of temperature, exposure of the neck and shoulders when the body is hot, the inhalation of hot or irritating vapors, an attempt to swallow hot or corrosive liquids, and the inhalation of flame in cases of burning about the head and neck. Inflammation of the throat occasionally extends to the larynx, or upper portions of the windpipe; and this affection is a frequent cause of death, in diphtheria, scarlet fever, and small-pox.

Symptoms.—Hoarseness, a hoarse cough, constriction, tenderness, and pain in the upper part of the windpipe, with difficult, prolonged and sonorous inspiration. Swallowing usually causes convulsive fits of coughing, and increased difficulty of breathing. At first there are generally chills followed by fever, flushed face, hot skin, and full pulse; but in delicate and debilitated patients there may be no fever. If the disease is not relieved by treatment, the cough becomes more painful, harsh and squeaking; the act of drawing in the breath is prolonged, wheezing, whistling, and requires a great effort on the part of the patient; expiration, or the passing out of the breath is performed easily. The patient is restless, and feels that he is on the point of suffocation; he sleeps but a few moments at a time, and awakes gasping for breath. The countenance becomes anxious and pale; the eyes staring; the nostrils raised; the lips livid; the voice reduced to a whisper; the pulse becomes very frequent, feeble, and irregular, and the extremities bathed in a cold, clammy sweat; Delirium, drowsiness, and stupor, often precede the termination of the disease in fatal cases; and death usually occurs on the fourth or fifth day, although sometimes as early as the first day, and in other instances not until the end of two or three weeks. Sometimes in hysterical females, and young children there is a spasmodic affection of the larynx, which bears some resemblance to the affection now under consideration, but in such cases there is no fever, and the attack is more sudden, and apparently alarming at its very commencement than in the genuine disease.

Treatment.—This disease requires a prompt and persevering treatment, and if the symptoms are not soon relieved by the remedies named, a homœopathic physician should be called without delay. Generally this disease will be readily cured by the early use of homœopathic remedies, but not always. If a homœopathic physician cannot be had, and notwithstanding your treatment the symptoms become alarming, the face pale or livid, the pulse small and frequent, and the extremities cool and moist, you should send for an allopathic physician, as the life of the patient can sometimes be saved, in such cases, by making an opening into the trachea or windpipe, and allowing the patient to breathe through the opening, until the inflammation is cured.

Aconite: In all cases attended with chills and fever, or fever alone, give a dose of this remedy every half hour, and if at the end of two or three hours the symptoms are not relieved, give *Spongia* alternately with it, at intervals of one half an hour. If these remedies do not relieve the symptoms within twenty-four hours from the commencement of the disease, or even twelve hours, in severe cases, omit the *Spongia* and give *Hepar sulph.* alternately with *Aconite*, at intervals of one half an hour. Do not discontinue the *Aconite* unless the pulse becomes small, and the extremities moist and cool; but if such symptoms appear, with lividity of the face, omit the *Aconite* and give *Lachesis* alternately with *Hepar sulph.* at intervals of one hour.

When this disease occurs in consumptive patients, and those debilitated by chronic diseases, or chronic laryngitis, where there is no fever, *Aconite* will not be required, but *Spongia* and *Hepar sulph.* may be given, and if they do not relieve the symptoms, give *Arsenicum* every hour.

In addition to the internal remedies, at the commencement of the disease wring a small napkin from cold water, fold it and place it over the front part of the neck, and over that five or six thicknesses of dry flannel, so as to cover the wet cloth entirely; confine the whole snugly to its place by a bandage or handkerchief around the neck; wet the napkin once in four hours. If at the end of twenty-four hours the patient is not improving, omit the cold cloths and wring a large towel from warm water, as hot as the patient can bear it without scalding, and place it on the front part and sides of the neck and chest; cover it with dry flannel. Wet the towel often, every ten or fifteen minutes, during the paroxysms of difficult breathing. If convenient give a warm bath once a day. The diet should be light, and contain no animal food or stimulating condiments.

CHRONIC LARYNGITIS,

OR CHRONIC INFLAMMATION OF UPPER PORTION OF THE WINDPIPE.

This form of disease is much more common than the acute variety just described, and is of various degrees of severity. If it is slight, and confined to the mucous membrane, it may exist for months without much inconvenience, excepting hoarseness, habitual husky cough, and perhaps slight soreness on pressure. It frequently results from a neglected cold, and may follow an acute attack. The causes are similar to those which produce the acute form of the disease. Clergymen who neglect active exercise, so that their general systems become debilitated, and especially if they do not use their vocal organs in reading, speaking, and singing, during the week, are very liable to this disease.

In aggravated forms of the disease, the mucous membrane, and cellular structure beneath it, and the vocal chords, become thickened, and even ulcerated; the hoarseness increases, the voice may be squeaking, and even lost. The cough is generally dry early in the disease, but as it advances it becomes loose, and the expectoration often contains matter or pus. Sometimes there is considerable pain, but in other cases there is little or none. A sensation of dryness, tickling, itching, smarting, or burning, is common, and if ulcers form there is often a pricking sensation, as if a sharp body were in the throat. A sudden loss of voice may occur with a slight disease affecting the vocal ligaments, or it may be simply a nervous affection; in either case it is generally soon relieved; but when the voice becomes gradually impaired until it is lost, the disease is almost always more serious. The dry, squeaking kind of hoarseness implies a more permanent and worse form of disease than the deep, loose, or rattling hoarseness, which may be the result of relaxation. Sometimes earthy concretions form in the larynx, and are expectorated. In rare instances the inflammation extends to the cartilages, or gristly structures of the larynx, and they become bony, and perhaps die, and abscesses form around them, which discharge either externally or internally, and portions of the cartilages are sometimes separated and expectorated. Respiration becomes affected sooner or later in this disease, and is generally worse during the night, and on exertion. Sometimes there are severe paroxysms of difficult breathing, and the patient is frequently unable to lie down. If the disease continues on unchecked, the patient is worn out by hectic fever, night sweats, or diarrhœa, and dies. Or he may be cut off at an earlier stage by an attack of acute inflammation; and, as was stated in the section on acute laryngitis, the disease in such cases is often unattended with fever; it is generally, in fact, in such cases, but a dropsical swelling of the parts, which threatens or causes suffocation by mechanically closing the passage. Chronic laryngitis frequently occurs during the latter stages of consumption of the lungs, and in those who die from the former disease, tubercles are often found in the lungs. This disease may result from an abuse of the vocal organs in speaking and singing, the inhalation of air loaded with dust, neglected colds, suppressed eruptions, the abuse of mercury, and the extension of syphilitic or venereal disease of the throat. Scrofulous and intemperate individuals are more liable to it than others.

Treatment.—To prevent this affection gentlemen should avoid shaving, not even deprive the upper lip of nature's covering. A man can talk all day as easily as he can walk all day, if he only does it *every day.* Very few can perform any kind of active labor but one day in the week only, without causing, sooner or later, actual disease. If the reader would avoid this disease, or get rid of it, if already affected, let him obtain and read without fail, the author's work on the "Avoidable Causes of Disease," and he will there find information more important than medicine, not but that the latter is needed, for without shunning the causes which have induced the disease, medicines can but palliate it at best.

Hepar sulph.: Give this remedy night and morning, when there is a short, hacking cough after eating, dry cough in the evening, or cough with scraping and rawness in the larynx, chronic hoarseness, or a deep, dry, hoarse cough. *Hepar* is also useful when the cough is loose, with rattling of mucus; and also when there is seated pain and soreness in one spot, which is aggravated by pressure, speech, cough, and breathing If a predisposition to this disease has been developed by an abuse of mercury, this remedy is especially indicated.

Dose, see page 7.

If it fails to relieve give *Mercurius protiod.* three or four times a day, especially if the soreness extends to the throat, and there is soreness on swallowing, and frequent inclination to clear the throat, with or without hoarseness. Afterward give *Hepar sulph.* if it is needed.

Spongia will often benefit the patient in the earlier stages of the disease, and when the symptoms have been aggravated by taking cold, especially when the cough is dry, deep, and hoarse, and the respiration squeaking or sonorous. Give a dose once in six hours.

Give *Lachesis* once in six hours when the symptoms are worse after sleeping; when the slightest pressure causes pain and cough; also when there is a dry cough, caused by tickling, and hoarseness, with feeble voice, noisy, squeaking respiration, with suffocative paroxysms.

Phosphorus is indicated by burning, roughness, painful sensitiveness of the larynx, and hacking cough caused by tickling, also by morning hoarseness and loss of voice. It will often be useful after other remedies, in the advanced stages of the disease, when there is profuse expectoration, and if diarrhœa ensues, or the disease is complicated with consumption of the lungs. Give a dose night and morning.

Calcarea carb.: Give this remedy night and morning when there is chronic hoarseness, worse in the morning, dry, hacking cough on retiring to bed, or a loose cough with profuse whitish or yellowish expectoration. It is especially useful for young subjects, and also when the cartilages are diseased.

Mercurius viv. may be given once in six hours, when the inflammation extends to the throat, and there is pain and soreness on empty swallowing, with hoarseness and cough. This remedy is especially useful if the disease has been caused by syphilis or the venereal disease. In such cases *Nitric acid* should follow *Mercurius.*

Arsenicum: Give this remedy once in six hours when there is a feeling of dryness and burning in the larynx; cough as if from the fumes of sulphur, with a sense of suffocation, and especially if the cough is aggravated by cold air.

Carbo veg. is indicated when there is hoarseness in the evening, aggravated by talking, and by cold and damp weather; also when there are tingling and itching in the larynx, with wheezing respitation; cough in the morning when rising, or on going into the open air.

Silicea will be found useful in cases where there is reason to fear the existence of ulcerations, when there is a profuse, yellowish, perhaps offensive expectoration, and when the cartilages are diseased. Give a dose night and morning.

Sulphur: If the patient has been subject to eruptive diseases, or if the disease is of long standing, give a dose of *Sulphur* every night for a week, at the commencement of the treatment: also if the disease does not seem to yield, or is only partially relieved by other remedies, give *Sulphur* a week, and as much longer as there are signs of improvement.

As this is an important, and a somewhat common and obstinate disease, I have given the chief indications for a large number of remedies. Select carefully your remedy, and do not change it in less time than one week, nor then if there is any improvement. If a patient improves under the use of a remedy, lengthen the intervals between the doses, and continue it as long as there is the slightest improvement.

HOARSENESS.—This symptom is generally caused by inflammation of the mucous membrane of the larynx or upper portion of the windpipe, and as a symptom of acute and chronic laryngitis it has already been considered. It is also present in croup or inflammation of the windpipe or trachea. But it sometimes happens that from exposure to cold and other causes, there is hoarseness without fever, soreness, or any other symptom. When this is the case give a dose of *Drosera* once in four hours, and if it does not relieve this symptom within twenty-four hours give *Belladonna* once in two hours. If there is soreness of the throat in connection with the hoarseness, give *Mercurius viv.* alternately with the latter remedy. *Pulsatilla* often does better than either of the other remedies named, in the case of females. If the above remedies do not soon relieve the symptoms, consult the sections on acute and chronic laryngitis and croup.

CROUP (TRACHIETIS)

This is one of the most alarming and even fatal of the diseases of childhood. The croup consists of an inflammation of the windpipe or trachea; the disease generally extends to the larynx or upper portion of the windpipe, and sometimes to the bronchia or air passages throughout the lungs. In some cases the inflammation is accompanied by the formation of a false membrane, which mechanically obstructs the passage of air to a greater or less degree. The croup occurs most frequently between the ages of one and twelve years; although children younger than one year, and persons older than twelve, are not exempt. It is more frequent among males than females, and is more common during cold than during warm weather. This disease is caused by exposure to cold and damp weather, when the neck, shoulders, and arms, are not properly protected by clothing. Dr. Eberlie says that during a practice of six years in a German settlement, he saw but one case, and that occurred in a family where the American style of dress had been adopted. Hot rooms, and the confinement of children indoors, are also fruitful causes of this affection. When a child is thus confined, the least breath of cold or damp air from an open window or door may cause this disease. Thin shoes and stockings, especially with children who live in warm rooms, high-seasoned food, and all stimulating condiments, favor the development of croup and bronchitis. This disease frequently occurs during the progress of scarlet fever, small-pox, and measles.

Symptoms.—Before the attack the child is often peevish, fretful and perhaps feverish; there may also be symptoms of cold in the head, and slight hoarseness. Toward evening, or sometime before midnight, the hoarseness and fever increase. In other instances, without any premonitory symptoms, the child awakens suddenly during the night, with a sensation of suffocation, with a hoarse ringing cough, hurried and hissing respiration, and a rough hoarse voice, sometimes almost as if the patient were speaking through a brazen instrument. There are great agitation, alarm, and distress; and there is usually more or less heat of skin, and frequency of pulse. The difficulty of breathing at the commencement of the disease generally depends, in a great measure, on a spasmodic contraction of the larynx, for it occurs in paroxysms. The symptoms are usually worse during the night, especially about midnight, and the patient is often quite comfortable during the day. If the disease continues on uninfluenced by treatment, generally, at some period between the second and the sixth days, symptoms of great prostration ensue, the difficulty of breathing increases, the cough becomes squeaking, the pulse small and irregular, the extremities bathed in a cold clammy sweat, and the countenance, during the severe paroxysms of difficult breathing, becomes of a livid or dusky hue. The duration of the disease, in fatal cases, is usually from three to six days, although patients sometimes die within twenty-four hours, whereas, in other cases, not until the end of nine or ten days. Cases in which the symptoms are the most violent at the commencement, are not always the most dangerous, for such patients necessarily receive prompt treatment, and the disease is often, in such cases, in a great measure spasmodic, with very little inflammatory action; and if there is considerable fever and inflammation, there is frequently very little tendency to the effusion of false membrane; whereas, in those cases which commence gradually, with a slight fever, hoarseness, and cough, the disease often progresses to the membranous stage.

before attention is seriously called to it; and in such cases the tendency to a membranous formation is often very strong. "The prognosis, in all cases of croup," says Dr. Condie, "is very serious; the probabilities are against recovery." This may be true, under the "heroic treatment" of allopathy, but it certainly is not true where patients are treated homœopathically, and bloodletting, leeching, emetics, cathartics, swabbing the throat with caustic, etc., etc., are omitted, for comparatively few patients die from this disease, under our treatment, yet they cannot always be cured.

Treatment.—The symptoms, as has been stated, are almost always worse during the night, and even when the disease is steadily progressing toward a fatal termination, the patient is often comfortable during the day, therefore give the proper remedies regularly during the day, and do not omit them, nor lessen the frequency of the doses until the last symptom has been removed. Always awaken the patient regularly to give the medicines until after midnight, then, if he is comfortable, give them only when he awakes, until morning, then give them regularly again during the day and until after midnight.

Aconite: Give this remedy every half hour until the patient has taken four doses, when, if he is improving, continue it at intervals of one hour; but if there is no improvement, give *Hepar sulph.* alternately with it at intervals of half an hour. Give these remedies during the afternoon and night, but every day during the forenoon, give *Spongia* every hour, and omit the other remedies until afternoon; then omit the *Spongia* and give *Hepar sulph.* and *Aconite* again. If you persevere in the use of the above remedies, you will rarely fail to prevent the formation of a false membrane, and the nightly paroxysms will grow less, and at the end of from one to three or four days, the patient will generally be restored to health. Do not change the above for other remedies, so long as the symptoms improve, or the nightly paroxysms grow less, even though it be but slowly.

Dose for any of these remedies, see page 7.

Lachesis: If, after using the above remedies from two to three or four days, instead of improving, the symptoms seem to be getting worse, the difficulty of breathing more constant, the cough and voice squeaking, the pulse small or irregular, and the extremities cool, give *Lachesis* alternately with *Hepar sulph.* at intervals of half an hour or one hour; and if at the end of twelve or twenty-four hours there is no improvement, omit the *Hepar sulph.* and give *Phosphorus* once an hour during the forenoon, and *Tartar emetic* during the afternoon and night. A homœopathic physician should always be consulted, if practicable, if the symptoms are not promptly relieved by the treatment.

Sometimes, as the croupy symptoms abate, symptoms of bronchitis become manifest, the breathing is hurried, the cough is loose, but not croupy, and if you apply your ear to the walls of the chest, you hear a rattling of mucus, or bubbling in the air passages; when such symptoms occur, omit other remedies and give *Bryonia* during the forenoon once in two hours, and *Tartar emetic* every hour during the afternoon, evening, and night, when the patient is awake.

Consult the section on bronchitis, if the above remedies fail to relieve.

External applications, Diet, &c.—At the commencement of the disease, wring a small napkin, or a few thicknesses of cotton or linen cloth from cold water, and apply over the front part of the neck; put over it four or five thicknesses of dry flannel, and confine all by a bandage or handkerchief, so as to exclude the cold air. Wet the cloth once in six or eight hours. If, notwithstanding the above application and the use of the remedies, the paroxysms of difficult breathing become very severe, wring large towels or cloths from warm water, as hot as the patient can bear without scalding, and apply them over the entire front and sides of the *neck and chest*, and cover the wet cloths with dry flannel. Wet the cloths every ten or fifteen minutes. A warm bath once or twice a day, is also useful. The diet should be light and without animal food.

If you would prevent this disease, or eradicate a predisposition to it in your children, read carefully the chapters on the "Conditions requisite for Physical Development and Preservation," "Use and Abuse of the Digestive Organs," and on the "Management and Education of Children," in the author's work on the "Avoidable Causes of Disease." Also give *Hepar sulph.* and *Spongia*, alternately, one week apart.

SPASM OF THE GLOTTIS, OR CROWING DISEASE.

This affection is sometimes called spasmodic croup, as there is no inflammation or fever attending it. It generally occurs in children under three years of age and those of a delicate and nervous temperament, are more liable to it than others.

Symptoms.—The attack frequently occurs during sleep, the child awaking much agitated, alarmed, and struggling for breath; there is sometimes cramping of the hands and feet, and occasionally the whole body is convulsed. These symptoms are caused by a spasmodic contraction of the opening to the windpipe or glottis, which mechanically prevents the entrance of air to the lungs. This spasm may abate suddenly and the air enter freely without any unusual sound, but more frequently it abates gradually, and the air, as it enters, causes a crowing sound. In other cases, or perhaps in the same patient the attack occurs when the child is awake, perhaps when the nurse is tossing him up and down, or when he is frightened. A patient, after having once had the disease, is very liable to a return of the symptoms, and attack may follow attack, if the disease is not cured, until at length the little patient is not free from it for a single hour, and may finally die from suffocation or convulsions. There is usually no cough, and the child breathes freely in the intervals between the paroxysms.

Treatment.— Give *Belladonna* and *Cuprum* alternately at intervals of four hours, when the child is awake, and as soon as the paroxysms cease, give the former at night and the latter in the morning. If the above remedies fail to cure the disease, give a dose of *Calcarea carb.* every morning and *Hyosciamus* once in four hours during the afternoon and forepart of the night. Keep the child quiet and avoid exciting it, or tossing it up and down.

INFLUENZA (GRIPPE).

This is an epidemic disease, which generally proceeds from east to west, or from the south northward, but sometimes the reverse.

Such epidemics usually appear at intervals, varying from two to three years.

Symptoms.—Influenza generally commences with symptoms of cold in the head, sore throat, pains in the limbs, back and head, weariness, chilliness, followed by fever, and soon afterward by cough and uneasiness in the chest. The most characteristic symptom is the great debility which attends this affection. The pulse is feeble, there is often giddiness and faintness on sitting up; the spirits are depressed, and the sight and hearing are sometimes affected. Nausea and vomiting are more common than during ordinary colds. There is usually a remission of the symptoms in the morning, and an aggravation toward night. In some instances, instead of catarrhal symptoms, there are simply violent headache, flushed face, delirium, and fever. In other instances, nausea and vomiting; and in still other cases, diarrhœa or dysentery; and all these various affections apparently caused by the same epidemic poison acting on different individuals. The duration of an attack of influenza, when uninfluenced by treatment, varies from two or three days to two weeks. A cough sometimes remains after the other symptoms are removed.

Treatment.—At the very commencement of the disease if there is great prostration, chilliness, with or without nausea and vomiting, a drop of *Camphor*, repeated at the end of an hour, will sometimes relieve the symptoms, especially if the patient covers up warm in bed, and gets into a gentle perspiration. In case there is much fever early in the disease, six globules of *Aconite* or a drop of the tincture, dissolved in a glass of water, and taken at one dose, the patient covering himself up well in bed, will either relieve or lessen the severity of the symptoms.

Mercurius, viv.: Give this remedy once in two hours, if the above remedies fail to cure the disease, and there are great prostration of strength, pains in the bones of the face, sore throat, and especially if there are symptoms of dysentery or bilious diarrhœa, or the symptoms are aggravated by warmth.

Arsenicum may be given once in two hours instead of *Mercurius viv.*, if there is little or no soreness of the throat, but a profuse watery discharge from the nose, with burning and excoriation of the nostrils, thirst, oppression of, and burning in the chest, great prostration of strength, aggravation at night and relief from warmth.

If there is much cough attending or following the disease, consult the section on cough and bronchitis, and select a remedy, and give either alone or alternately with either *Mercurius* or *Arsenicum.*

COUGH, AND COLD ON THE CHEST.

Cough may be caused by irritation or inflammation of any portion of the windpipe, bronchia or air-passages through the lungs, the air-cells, and substance of the lungs themselves, also of their external covering or the pleura. It may be caused by tubercles in the lungs, also by an elongation of the uvula or the little body which hangs down from the back part of the palate. The cough may be either acute or chronic, there may be fever attending it, or the patient may be free from fever. In this section I simply propose to treat of recent coughs, and those unattended by fever. If the disease is chronic, or of some weeks' duration, and the cough is hoarse or squeaking, and the voice is impaired, consult the section on chronic laryngitis, or chronic inflammation of the upper portion of the windpipe. If the disease is of weeks' or months' standing, and the cough at its commencement was short and hacking, and is attended with shortness of breath, consult the sections on consumption and chronic pleurisy. If the chronic cough seems to originate in the chest, and there is more or less soreness of the chest, with difficulty of breathing, and expectoration, consult the section on chronic bronchitis. If a recent attack of cough is attended by chills and fever, hot skin and frequent pulse, if the cough is hoarse, shrill, or squeaking, and the patient is an adult, consult the section on laryngitis; if a child, consult the section on croup. If the cough is not hoarse and is attended with high fever and oppression and difficulty of breathing, consult the sections on inflammation of the bronchia, lungs, and pleuræ. But when the cough has been of but few days' or weeks' standing, without fever, consult the remedies in this section.

A cold on the chest is a slight inflammation of the bronchiæ or air tubes, sufficient to cause a cough, which is at first dry, but afterward becomes loose, but without much if any fever, pain, soreness, or difficulty of breathing. It is a mild bronchitis, involving simply the mucous membrane of the air tubes, which, although sufficient to cause cough, is either not severe enough, or not sufficiently extensive to cause much fever, oppression or other alarming symptoms; still it differs from the most formidable cases of bronchitis only in the severity and extent of the diseased action, and of the symptoms, and not in the character of the disease. In all cases attended by fever and oppression of breathing consult the section on acute bronchitis.

Treatment of Coughs.—Give *Belladonna* once in two hours when the cough is spasmodic, not allowing time to breathe, or a short dry hollow cough, especially if it is caused by a tickling or itching in the throat or larnyx, and if there is a sensation of dryness in the chest. This remedy is generally most important for dry coughs It is sometimes useful when there is tenacious mucus expectorated, especially at night.

Dose, see page 7.

Chamomilla may be given once in two hours when there is a dry suffocative cough, caused by dryness, burning, and tickling in the throat and upper portion of the windpipe, and also when there is a tickling in the throat pit, and cough at night or during sleep. This remedy is often required for children.

Nux vom.: This remedy, like the two named above, is frequently required at the commencement of colds in the chest, when the cough is dry, and caused by tickling, roughness, and scraping, in the windpipe, with a spasmodic sensation, and when the cough is worse towards morning, and during the fore part of the day.

The following remedies, also, will often be found useful for dry coughs.

Rhus tox., when there is a rough scraping feeling, or tickling sensation, in the windpipe, and the cough is aggravated by cold air and relieved by exercise and warm air.

Lachesis, when the cough is worse after sleeping, also on arising from a recumbent position and in the cold air, and when it is aggravated by the least pressure on the upper portion of the wind-pipe.

Arsenicum when there is burning in the chest, with a wheezy sensation in the lungs.

Hyosciamus when the cough is aggravated by lying down, and relieved by sitting up, and if there is dryness and heat in the air passages.

Ignatia when there is a constrictive sensation as if from the vapors of sulphur, or dust, in the air passages. If this remedy does not relieve, give *Calcarea carb.*

Cina when children are troubled with worms, and are subject to a dry cough.

Dulcamara: When there is a short, hacking cough, without or with the expectoration of tenacious mucus, caused by exposure to wet, and cool, damp air.

Ipecac: When the cough is short and dry, and excited by a tickling in the throat and upper part of the windpipe, with asthmatic or wheezing breathing.

For loose coughs, some of the remedies already named, especially *Belladonna*, *Dulcamara*, and *Ipecac*, will often be useful, particularly when the expectoration is tenacious and transparent, but when it is whitish or yellowish, they will less frequently be efficacious than one of the following remedies:

Bryonia: This remedy will sometimes be found of service at the commencement of a cough, when it is dry, but generally some one of the remedies already named will do better, but when there is a profuse, or more or less free, transparent, whitish or yellowish expectoration, especially in the morning, or after eating and drinking, and the cough is somewhat spasmodic, with pain in the sides or chest, give *Bryonia* once in four hours.

Pulsatilla may follow *Bryonia*, or be given instead of the latter remedy, when there is a free expectoration of yellow or white tasteless or bitter, salt or sweet tasting mucus. If there is nausea and vomiting, with a suffocative sensation, pain and soreness in the abdomen, or involuntary passage of urine while coughing, these are indications for this remedy.

In addition to the above, if the loose cough is not relieved, one of the following remedies will often cure it:

Phosphorus: Give this remedy when the expectoration is transparent, green, or white, and of a sweetish or saltish taste, and if the cough is excited by talking, laughing, or walking in the open air. When the latter symptoms are present it will often be useful even though the cough is dry.

Give *Stannum* night and morning, if there is a very profuse expectoration of transparent or whitish, sweet tasting mucus.

Give *Sulphur* for either a dry or loose cough, if it does not yield to other remedies, especially when there is a congested or full feeling of the chest, which seems to cause the cough.

Be careful and not change the remedies too often. Select your remedy with care and give it at least for twenty-four hours, and longer if the patient improves.

If you fail to relieve the symptoms, and the disease is without fever, consult the sections on chronic bronchitis, laryngitis, and consumption.

ACUTE BRONCHITIS.

(INFLAMMATION OF THE AIR-PASSAGES IN THE LUNGS.)

An ordinary cold on the chest is the lightest form of this disease, but that affection has already been noticed in the preceding section. It now remains to consider acute bronchitis in its severer forms. The causes of this disease are the usual causes of colds; such as sudden changes of temperature, exposure when the body is hot, etc. This affection may commence with a cold in the head, sore throat and hoarseness; in other cases without any such symptoms, a sensation of coldness, roughness, or dryness, is felt in the chest, near the top of the sternum or breast-bone; then follows a sensation of heat, tightness, soreness, or pain, in some part of the chest, usually beneath the breast-bone, with a cough, which is at first short and dry, but soon becomes deeper and more urgent, and accompanied by the expectoration of a transparent, glary, saltish-tasting mucus, which does not relieve the cough, but seems to aggravate it by its irritating qualities. Chills, followed by fever, either precede, accompany, or soon follow, the above symptoms. The fever is generally worse toward evening, when the pulse is quick, the breathing short, the skin hot, the urine scanty and high-colored. If you apply your ear to the chest, at the commencement of the disease, you will hear a hissing or whistling sound, caused by the narrowing of the air-tubes from the swelling, the result of the inflammation ; gradually this whistling ceases, and you hear a bubbling sound, caused by air passing through the bronchiæ which are partially filled with mucus. If you apply your ear over a healthy chest you hear, as the air passes through the bronchiæ, a sound similar to that caused by the passage of a gentle wind through the leaves of a tree. By applying the ear to the chest, both in front and on the back, and on both sides, from the top to near the lower ribs, you will be able to judge, with considerable certainty, as to the extent of the disease, and the danger, by the extent of the mucus rattling. If it is confined to one lung, there will not be much danger, and even if a part only of one lung is free, so that you can hear the natural breathing, the danger will not be very great; but if the mucus rattling is universal over both lungs, completely masking the natural respiration, the danger will be very great. If the disease is severe, and is not arrested by treatment, the difficulty of breathing increases, there is great oppression, the pulse is quick and weak, often irregular; there is great weakness, the countenance is anxious, pale, or partially livid, the mental faculties are confused or disturbed, the tongue becomes loaded with a brown fur, the thirst intense, and the urine scanty. In this severe form of the disease the patient may die between the fourth and eighth days, during a severe paroxysm of difficult breathing, or from a steady increase of the symptoms, or else he will gradually recover. When recovery is about to take place, the difficulty of breathing diminishes, and is chiefly confined to the evening the expectoration becomes less adhesive and frothy, and at length opaque; the fever abates, the countenance improves, and either the patient steadily recovers, or the inflammation passes into a chronic form. As the disease declines and the expectoration becomes whitish, if you apply your ear to the chest, you will hear occasionally a clicking sound instead of a rattling of mucus.

In debilitated habits, where the countenance is pale, and the blood thin and watery, in adults and young children, and also in those who are debilitated from age, or chronic diseases, we sometimes have a very formidable variety of this disease without much febrile excitement. In such cases there is a profuse secretion of mucus into the bronchia, which causes great oppression of breathing, extreme debility, small, frequent, and often irregular pulse, and severe suffocative paroxysms. The expectoration in this form of bronchitis may be scanty at first, but soon becomes copious and frothy. Young children, when affected with bronchitis, swallow the mucus when it is raised into the throat by coughing and breathing, and do not eject it; it passes into the stomach and does no particular harm. Sometimes children have convulsions, twitchings, or symptoms of stupor, at the commencement of an attack of bronchitis, and if you neglect to apply your ear to the chest, you may suppose that the child has disease of the brain, until symptoms of threatening suffocation, purple countenance, small and irregular pulse, reveal the seat of the disease. In some of these cases there may be but little heat or fever.

Treatment of Bronchitis.—There are perhaps few diseases where the superiority of the homœopathic treatment over the cruel time-honored treatment of allopathy, is more marked than in the one under consideration. Very few, except the very aged or those debilitated by other diseases, or of bad habits, die from this affection; even young children, except those of very feeble constitutions, generally recover under a prompt and persevering homœopathic treatment.

Aconite: This is the first and most important remedy in all cases attended by any febrile excitement, or heat of skin. Give a dose every hour, and continue it for twelve hours. If at the end of this period, there is a violent dry cough, or spasmodic cough, or a sensation of dryness in the chest, or tickling in the throat, which excites cough, give *Belladonna*, and if fever continues, give it alternately with *Aconite*, one hour apart. *Belladonna* will still be indicated, when a tenacious and glary mucus begins to be expectorated This remedy is especially efficacious in the case of children, and it is indispensable when there are symptoms of congestion of the brain or convulsions.

Dose of this or of other remedies, see page 7.

Bryonia: If *Aconite*, or *Aconite* and *Belladonna*, fail to cut short the disease at the end of two or three days, *Bryonia* will generally be required, especially when there is a profuse transparent or opaque, whitish or yellowish expectoration, dryness of the throat, stitches in the chest, or a free perspiration. Give a dose of *Bryonia* once in four hours, and a dose of *Aconite* every hour between the doses of *Bryonia*, whenever there is any fever or heat of skin. As soon as the patient is free from fever during the forepart of the day and latter part of the night, omit *Aconite*, and only give it when there is fever. If, after the fever has been in a great measure relieved, the cough remains troublesome, with oppression of the chest, give *Phosphorus* during the afternoon and evening once in two hours, and *Bryonia* during the forepart of the day.

Tartar emetic: If the above remedies fail to check the progress of the disease, and the rattling of mucus is heard throughout both lungs, and there are great oppression and severe paroxysms of difficult breathing, give this remedy every hour. Also give it at the commencement of the disease, when in aged persons, or delicate young children, and persons debilitated by other diseases, there are great oppression without much fever, cool extremities and small pulse, and it fails to relieve the symptoms; give it alternately with *Bryonia*, one hour apart.

Sulphur and *Arsenicum* are our main reliance in desperate cases of this disease; they are rarely useful at the commencement; but when, notwithstanding the use of other remedies, there are threatening symptoms of suffocation, from an accumulation of mucus in the air passages, with rattling, give a dose of *Sulphur* every hour, until the patient has taken five or six doses, and if the symptoms improve, continue it; but if there is no improvement, give a dose of *Arsenicum* every hour.

For the declining state of the disease, after the fever has been relieved, and the expectoration has become opaque, whitish or yellowish, to prevent the disease from becoming chronic, give a dose of *Sulphur* morning and noon, and a dose of *Pulsatilla* before tea and at bedtime.

Diet, &c.—The patient should be kept in an even temperature; the diet should be light, gruel, arrow-root, rice-water, soft boiled rice, and the like. For severe paroxysms of difficult breathing, wring large cloths, from warm water, as hot as the patient can bear, and apply them around the chest, and place over them dry flannel, and change them often.

CHRONIC BRONCHITIS.

This generally follows an acute attack, although the latter may have been slight in some cases, nothing more than the mild form of the disease, or a cold on the chest. The inhalation of air loaded with dust, frequently causes this disease, therefore, needle-grinders, stone-cutters, workers in hair and feathers, are very liable to this affection. In such cases, it generally begins with difficulty of breathing; and, after a time, cough and copious expectoration make their appearance; sometimes the latter is mixed with blood and matter, or pus.

The slighter forms of chronic bronchitis are indicated only by habitual cough and expectoration, which are increased by sudden changes of weather, and are most troublesome during the winter and spring. Aged persons are very subject to this disease during such seasons of the year. In severer forms of the disease there are paroxysmal cough, difficulty of breathing, soreness, tightness, and wandering pains in the chest. The expectoration is whitish, yellowish or greenish, and sometimes contains pus or matter. If the patient happens to get a severe cold, so as to cause an attack of acute inflammation of any part of the bronchia, tenacious transparent mucus will be mixed with the opaque matter. When the expectoration is very copious there are usually prostration of strength, wasting of flesh, hectic fever, and night sweats, and sometimes diarrhœa. This affection not unfrequently follows measles, scarlet fever, and small-pox, when the irritation of the air passages which frequently attends these eruptive diseases is neglected. If you apply your ear to the chest of a patient suffering from chronic bronchitis you will hear over different parts mucous rattling, clicking and whistling sounds, which often change places.

Treatment.—Several of the remedies named under the head of acute bronchitis will be found useful in this form of the disease, especially *Bryonia, Sulphur, Phosphorus, Pulsatilla,* and *Arsenicum.*

Bryonia: Give this remedy morning and noon, and *Sulphur* before tea and at bed-time, if the disease has not been of long standing, and is the result of an acute attack; and if these remedies do not relieve the symptoms, omit *Bryonia* and give *Sulphur* and *Pulsatilla,* in the same manner. *Bryonia* is especially indicated for morning coughs and expectoration, with pains in the sides, shortness of breath, and cough after eating and drinking, with vomiting of food, and when there is an aggravation from taking cold.

Dose, see page 7.

Sulphur: Give a dose night and morning when there is a dry cough at night, without or with a copious expectoration of thick whitish or yellowish mucus during the day, cough and raising at night, stitches in the sides, a feeling of tightness of the chest, and when the symptoms are aggravated by every change of weather. *Pulsatilla* often follows *Sulphur* to advantage, especially in the case of females.

Phosphorus may be given three times a day when the cough is excited by walking in the open air, laughing, talking, or drinking; also for a dry cough, from tickling in the throat or chest; and also when there is a free expectoration of salt, sour, or sweet mucus or matter.

Stannum: Give this remedy night and morning, when there is a profuse, greenish, or yellowish expectoration, of a disagreeable, sweetish taste, or of a putrid taste and offensive smell.

Calcarea carb. may be given night and morning, when there is, in the early stage of the disease, a dry cough in the evening, or in bed, especially if the cough is caused by a sensation of tickling, as if from feather dust, or even breathing through feathers. Also when there is a profuse yellowish, perhaps offensive expectoration in the morning, or during the whole day, with difficulty of breathing.

Lycopodium: Give a dose night and morning, when there is a short hacking cough from tickling in the throat or windpipe; when deep breathing causes coughing; also when the cough is loose, with a profuse thick whitish, yellowish, grayish, or greenish colored expectoration, of a saltish taste, and there is soreness of the chest and shortness of breath.

Give *Lachesis* when the cough is worse after sleeping, and is aggravated by pressing on the windpipe.

Give *Sepia* night and morning, when the cough causes nausea and vomiting, and is dry and spasmodic; also when there is a copious yellow, green, salt, or putrid mucous expectoration morning or evening.

Give *Drosera* if, early in the disease, there is a dry hoarse cough, and if it fails, give *Spongia* or *Hepar sulph.*

Give *Silicea* when there is a profuse watery expectoration which is not relieved by other remedies. Pure air and sunlight are all-important in all chronic affections of the air passages, and of the lungs. If the patient can well avoid it, he should not occupy a room, even during the night, where the sun has not shone during the day, for the atmosphere will be unwholesome for him. He should frequently draw in a full breath, and gently thump the walls of his chest with his hand or fist; and let an assistant vibrate the chest, by pressing wi.h the hand suddenly at any point where there is pain, soreness, or uneasiness. The patient should not be starved on miserable superfine flour bread, but should have good brown bread, which contains the dark nutritious portion of the grain.

For much valuable information, which is all-important to patients snffering from this affection, consult the work on the "Avoidable Causes of Disease."

HOOPING-COUGH.

This is an epidemic and contagious disease, and is generally confined to children; but adults, who have never had it, are liable to contract it, on exposure. Individuals rarely suffer from this disease the second time. The symptoms, at the commencement, are similar to those of mild bronchitis, or cold on the chest. There are generally more or less fever, some difficulty of breathing, and cough. The fever often gradually abates after a few days, but the cough becomes more troublesome, and begins to recur in paroxysms.

At the end of ten days or two weeks the characteristic symptoms make their appearance. Paroxysms of rapid coughing occur, which interrupt inspiration until the lungs seem to be exhausted of air, the upper portion of the windpipe is spasmodically contracted, the face becomes swollen and livid, and the patient seems on the point of suffocation, when the coughing ceases, the spasm gradually relaxes, and the air enters the larynx with a long crowing or hooping sound. In severe cases the blood sometimes starts from the mouth and nose during the paroxysms. The latter may return often, every half hour or hour, or not more frequently than two or three times a day. The disease generally reaches its height in about six weeks from the commencement of the cough, and terminates at the end of six weeks more, unless its duration is prolonged by colds, or an attack of bronchitis. During the winter or spring it is liable to be thus prolonged until warm weather. When the crude, nauseating and debilitating drugging of allopathy is avoided, and homœopathic remedies are carefully administered, there is very little danger in this disease; in fact, although the disease is very distressing, the lungs are generally developed and made stronger by the involuntary training which they receive.

Treatment.—As at the commencement of the disease there is generally more or less fever, give *Aconite* once in two hours, until the fever is lessened. If at the end of two or three days the fever has abated give *Belladonna* once in two hours for the cough; but if feverish symptoms still persist give *Aconite* alternately with *Belladonna*, at intervals of two hours. These remedies may be continued when the patient is awake, until the hooping commences, unless the cough should become moist, with vomiting of mucus or food, or a diarrhœa should occur, in which case give *Pulsatilla* once in two hours. *Carbo veg.* will sometimes be of service during his stage if there is a convulsive cough in the evening, or before midnight.

Dose, see page 7.

When the hooping commences, if the patient has been taking *Belladonna*, let him omit it, and give him *Cuprum* after every paroxysm of coughing; if there is fever, headache, or symptoms of convulsions, give a dose of *Belladonna* two or three times a day, in addition to the *Cuprum*, but not within half an hour of the doses of the latter remedy. If, at the end of four or five days, *Cuprum* makes no impression on the severity or frequency of the paroxysms, omit it, and give one dose of *Drosera*, and repeat it once in twenty-four hours, until there is some improvement, but as soon as there is a perceptible change for the better, do not repeat the remedy as long as the patient improves, but if improvement ceases repeat the dose.

If the above remedies do not lessen the severity of the disease give *Veratrum* after every paroxysm, especially if there is vomiting and great debility. In obstinate cases give *Tartar emetic* after every paroxysm, and if it does not relieve the symptoms, give a dose of *Sulphur* every night, and *Belladonna* once in two hours during the day, until the patient is well.

The neck, shoulders, arms, and legs, should be well clothed, and the feet kept dry with good thick-soled shoes.

PLEURISY.

The pleura is the smooth membrane which covers the external surface of the lungs and lines the walls of the chest, and inflammation of this membrane is called pleurisy.

Symptoms.—A sharp, cutting pain in the side, usually a short distance below the nipple, but sometimes lower, occasionally at the lower margin of the ribs, which restrains every attempt at full inspiration, and renders the breath short and often catching, is frequently the first symptom; sometimes chills and fever precede the pain; if not, they may accompany or they soon follow the attack. There is generally a short, dry, hacking cough. Even without treatment the pain generally grows less at the end of two or three days, but the difficulty of breathing often increases, owing to the filling up of the pleura, which is a closed sac, with the watery portion of the blood and lymph, which are poured out on its surface when this membrane is inflamed. Without treatment the fever generally grows less at the end of four or five days, and sometimes is quite moderate; perhaps the patient has little the forepart of the day even when the effusion is increasing, with increased oppression of breathing. If at the end of two or three days you apply your ear to the walls of the chest on the diseased side, when the patient is sitting up, you will not hear, over the middle and lower portion of the chest, the gentle murmur caused by the passage of air through the bronchiæ as the patient breathes, which you will hear on the well side, and if you percuss or strike the chest with the end of your fingers you will find dullness on the diseased side, when compared with the well side, caused by the accumulation of fluid in the pleural sac. If the patient recovers, the fluid is gradually absorbed, but the lymph which is poured out on the surfaces of the pleura is not absorbed, and as the two surfaces covered with this lymph come in contact as the fluid disappears they unite and form adhesions, but the latter do not usually seriously interfere with breathing after a few weeks or months. The patient generally recovers, but he may die, or the disease may pass into a chronic form, and the whole side of the chest become filled with fluid, and the walls of the chest may even become distended, the spaces between the ribs pressed out, and the heart crowded out of place. There will be absence of respiration and dullness on percussion over the whole side.

Sometimes we have what physicians call latent pleurisy, where there is no pain, and but little fever or cough, but general debility, and slowly increasing shortness of breath and oppression. This form of the disease can only be detected by applying the ear and by percussing the chest.

False pleurisy, which is nothing more than a rheumatic or neuralgic pain in the chest, often bears a very great resemblance to the genuine disease; but there is in such cases, generally no chills or fever, and no effusion of fluid follows, and there is usually no cough. If in such cases you rub hard with the ends of your fingers on the spaces between the ribs over the seat of the pain, it will almost always increase the suffering to a far greater extent than in pleurisy.

Treatment of Acute Pleurisy.—Wring a large towel from cold water and place it over the diseased side, extending from the breast bone to near the spine, cover the wet cloth with five or six thicknesses of dry flannel, and pin a dry towel around the body over the whole so as to exclude the air. Wet the towel once in six or eight hours.

Aconite: Give a dose of this remedy every hour in all cases where there are any chills, heat of skin or fever ; even if there is but little fever this remedy should be given. As soon as the skin inclines to become moist lengthen the intervals between the doses to two hours. Continue this remedy for twenty-four hours, then give a dose of *Bryonia* once in six hours, and if there is much fever or heat of skin, give a dose of *Aconite* every hour between the doses of *Bryonia* ; but if the skin is moist, and there is but little heat about the body, give the *Aconite* but once in two hours. Continue the above remedies until the fever is gone, or nearly so ; then give *Sulphur* once in two hours during the afternoon and night and *Bryonia* at intervals of two hours during the latter part of the night and forenoon, whenever the patient is awake. Continue these remedies until the patient is entirely relieved from all cough, soreness and shortness of breath. The above remedies will rarely fail to cure this disease ; but in case of failure consult what is said as to the treatment of chronic pleurisy below

Dose of the remedies, see page 7.

Treatment of Chronic and Latent Pleurisy.—Commence the treatment with *Bryonia* once in two hours during the forenoon, and *Sulphur* once in two hours during the afternoon and evening, and continue these remedies as long as there is any improvement. If at the end of three or four days the patient is not better, omit the *Bryonia* and give *Arnica* during the forenoon once in two hours, continuing the *Sulphur* during the afternoon and night when the patient is awake. Continue these remedies as long as there is improvement. When there seems to be no change for the better omit the above remedies and give *Arsenicum* once in two hours; if the patient improves, lengthen the intervals to four hours. *Hepar sulph.* or *Sulphur.* may in some cases be required after *Arsenicum.* If the above treatment fails, as it rarely will, to cure chronic pleurisy, send for a homœopathic physician, and not for an allopathist, for, according to my experience, this disease can very generally be cured by the use of homœopathic remedies, carefully and perseveringly administered, provided an opening is not made to draw off the fluid, for the fluid is almost always simply serum or water containing shreds of lymph, and can be absorbed; whereas, if an opening is made, more or less air is quite sure to be admitted, when the whole cavity of the pleura will be converted into one vast suppurating or maturating surface, and the discharge will be quite sure to wear the patient out with symptoms of hectic fever. After the fluid has been absorbed in cases of chronic pleurisy, the side of the chest affected is liable to become contracted, from the lung being bound down by lymph, which has been organized on its surface during the long compression by the fluid, but the patient may live and enjoy good health with the use of only one lung.

Treatment of False Pleurisy (Pleurodynia).—Give *Nux vom.* once in two hours. If this remedy fails, give *Arnica,* one dose, and if at the end of twelve hours the disease is not relieved, give *Bryonia* once in four hours. In the case of nervous females give *Pulsatilla* instead of *Nux vom.*, and if it does not relieve the symptoms, give *Arnica* alternately with it, two hours apart.

The diet in cases of pleurisy should be light during the febrile stage, nothing but gruel, rice, barley water, and the like.

INFLAMMATION OF THE LUNGS (PNEUMONIA).

This disease consists of inflammation of the air cells and substance of the lungs. There is almost always more or less inflammation of the bronchia, and sometimes of the pleura.

Symptoms.—Chills followed by fever generally precede, accompany, or soon follow the local symptoms. In persons of full habit, the fever is intense, skin hot, face flushed, with red eyes and more or less headache. The pain in the chest is usually either beneath the breast bone or shoulder blade, and is sometimes intense, but in other instances, dull or aching; in some cases there is simply a deep-seated feeling of heat and weight rather than pain. There is more or less cough, which aggravates the pain; at first it is dry, and the patient raises nothing more than a little transparent mucus, but in the course of a day or two the expectoration becomes tenacious or sticky, and tinged with blood, and it gradually changes to a rusty color from the presence of blood. Respiration becomes hurried, the pulse frequent, the urine scanty and high-colored, the tongue furred, and the appetite poor. There is sometimes nausea and vomiting, and in some instances jaundice. In mild cases the disease may decline on the third or fourth day, the skin becoming cool and moist, the expectoration less bloody and sticky, and more free and opaque, as in the declining stage of bronchitis. In severer cases when the disease is not checked by treatment, the symptoms increase on the third or fourth day, the breathing becomes quicker, the cough more frequent, the pulse weaker and increased in frequency, the tongue loaded or dry, and the skin hot or cool, and partially perspiring. In some cases there is delirium or stupor, which, in aged persons, is an alarming symptom. If the disease is not cut short within the first two or three days, the portion of lung diseased, which at first was simply congested, becomes indurated so as to resemble liver, and it will usually require from one to two weeks, for the cure of the fever and symptoms. If you apply your ear to the chest, over the seat of the disease during the first day or two, when the lung is simply congested, you may hear a fine crackling sound like that caused by the rubbing of hair between the fingers; two or three days later, when the lung is indurated, this sound will be absent, and you will hear nothing when the patient breathes, except perhaps a whistling sound as the air passes through the bronchiæ; but if you ask the patient to speak while your ear is applied over the diseased part, you will hear the vibrations of the voice much more distinctly than over the well lung at a corresponding point; sometimes it will seem almost as though the patient were speaking from the diseased spot. If you percuss with the ends of your fingers, a finger of the opposite hand laid smoothly on the walls of the chest, you will find after the disease has continued three or four days, more or less dullness when compared with the well side. If the patient recovers, these signs gradually disappear, the expectoration becomes whitish or yellowish, and less sticky, the fever abates, perhaps with a profuse perspiration, or a free flow of urine, and the tongue cleans off. A degree of frequency of the pulse and breathing with some cough and expectoration, often linger some days, but gradually abate. If the disease tends to a fatal termination, the strength fails, the pulse becomes frequent, small, or irregular, the difficulty of breathing increases, the countenance becomes pale or livid, the skin cold, and covered with a cold clammy sweat, and expectoration ceases; rattling in the throat and perhaps stupor precede death.

Typhoid Pneumonia.—Inflammation of the lungs sometimes occurs in connection with typhoid fever. In such cases there is unusual prostration of strength early, the pulse is small and weak, the face dusky, and the extremities cool; the teeth are covered with sordes or dark crusts of dried mucus, and the tongue is dry and dark; there is often muttering delirium, and sometimes diarrhœa.

Pleuro-Pneumonia.—Sometimes we have both the lung and pleura inflamed at the same time. In such cases we generally have both the sharp catching pain of pleurisy, followed by effusion of serum, or a watery fluid, into the sac; and the dull heavy oppression of inflammation of the lung, followed by the signs of induration of the lung named above, together with the bloody or rusty expectoration of pneumonia.

Treatment of the Inflammation of the Lungs.—Aconite: In all cases where there are chills or fever, give a dose of this remedy every hour, and continue it for twelve hours; if, at the end of that time, the fever is not relieved, and the patient is troubled with cough, give *Belladonna* alternately with *Aconite*, at intervals of one hour. These remedies, if given at the commencement of the disease, will often cut it short or lessen its severity, within two or three days.

Dose, see page 7.

Bryonia: If, at the end of two or three days, the symptoms are not relieved, and the expectoration becomes streaked with blood, or rusty, the breathing hurried, with increase of oppression, give a dose of this remedy once in six hours, and *Aconite* every hour between the doses of *Bryonia*, and omit the *Belladonna*. Continue these remedies as long as the extremities are warm, and the body hot and dry. It may be necessary to continue them for four or five days.

Phosphorus: If, as the fever abates, the cough remains troublesome; or if, after continuing *Bryonia* as directed above, for several days, the symptoms seem to be getting worse, the breathing becomes more frequent and difficult, and the cough troublesome, omit the above remedies, and give a dose of *Phosphorus* once in two hours. Persevere with this remedy several days. But if alarming symptoms occur, such as cold extremities, rattling in the throat, or great oppression, omit the *Phosphorus*, and give a dose of *Sulphur* every hour, until there is some improvement, then lengthen the intervals between the doses.

Sulphur is generally the most important remedy during the declining stage of the disease, and may be given once in four hours.

In cases of typhoid pneumonia, give *Aconite* and *Bryonia* as directed above, the latter once in six hours, and *Aconite* every hour between, until the commencement of manifest typhoid symptoms, such as coolness of the extremities, small pulse, dusky countenance, and sordes or dark crusts of dried mucus on the teeth, with dry and dark tongue, then omit the *Aconite* and give *Bryonia* once in two hours during the forenoon and *Phosphorus* once in two hours during the afternoon and evening. If after a few days great debility and delirium ensue, omit the *Bryonia* and give *Rhus tox.* in its stead, continuing the *Phosphorus*. If the above remedies fail, and the pulse becomes very small or irregular, and the extremities covered with a cold clammy sweat, with great oppression, give *Arsenicum* every hour.

In cases of pleuro-pneumonia, give *Aconite* every hour at the commencement of the disease; at the end of twenty-four hours give a dose of *Bryonia* once in six hours and *Aconite* every hour or two between the doses of *Bryonia*, until the fever is in a great measure relieved, then omit the *Aconite* and give *Sulphur* during the afternoon and evening, and *Bryonia* during the forenoon.

In all cases you can apply a wet cloth, well covered with dry flannel, to the side of the chest diseased, as directed under the head of pleurisy, and if it fails to afford any relief, apply cloths, wrung from warm water, in the same manner—only change hot cloths at least every hour. The diet should be light and consist of gruel, rice-water, arrow-root, etc. In typhoid cases, milk and water may be added to the above articles. You had better do nothing than send for an allopathic physician, for experience has shown that more patients die when this disease is treated by bloodletting and tartar emetic, or calomel and opium in large doses, than die without any treatment. I would much rather risk any intelligent layman with simply this book, and a domestic case, than to trust a physician of any other school in this disease; but in all severe cases, if a homœopathic physician can be had, send for him

ASTHMA.

The symptoms in this disease are caused by a spasmodic contraction of the air-tubes or bronchiæ, which lessens their calibre, and prevents the free passage of air to the air-cells. An attack may be excited, in those who are subject to it, by strong odors, dust, close rooms, sudden changes or particular conditions of the atmosphere, derangements of the stomach, and mental emotions. If the paroxysm is severe the patient is compelled to sit up with the body bent forward, the arms resting on the knees, a chair or table. The chest is contracted with the feeling of a tight cord around it, or a heavy weight upon it, the face has an expression of great anxiety and distress, the veins are distended, and there is often a free perspiration, but no fever before or after it. If the patient holds his breath as long as he can he can then draw it in without difficulty, but the spasm soon returns as strong as ever. There is heard, upon the application of the ear to the chest, various whistling and wheezing sounds. The attack may last but a short time, or for several days. The spasm often partially relaxes and returns, again and again, before it entirely ceases. Those who are troubled with severe paroxysms of asthma, are seldom entirely free from shortness of breath in the intervals. The disease frequently terminates with a free watery discharge or expectoration. Asthma is occasionally caused by disease of the heart. It is sometimes inherited. Children who are affected with it, but do not inherit it, often overcome the tendency to the disease at puberty. Those who are subject to this disease are very liable to have a return of a paroxysm when they take cold. The asthma, although a very distressing, and apparently alarming, disease in its attacks, is seldom fatal when uncomplicated with organic disease of the heart, or with other organic diseases. Notwithstanding frequent and severe paroxysms, patients often live to old age, nor are they more subject to consumption than others, yet they are not exempt.

Treatment.—We should not only endeavor to relieve the paroxysms but also strive to prevent their return by the persevering use of homœopathic remedies in the intervals between them.

If the paroxysm has been caused by getting cold or exposure, or sudden atmospherical changes, give *Aconite* once in two hours, and continue it as long as there is any improvement, then *Ipecac* once in two hours. If these remedies fail to relieve the paroxysm, give *Arsenicum* once in two hours.

If the disease occurs in a nervous person, a child, or hysterical female, or is caused by mental emotions, give *Belladonna* every hour; if there is any fever which is not relieved by this remedy, give *Aconite* alternately with it, at intervals of one hour. *Ipecac* may be required if the above remedies fail, or *Pulsatilla* if there is much expectoration. Give *Pulsatilla* also when the disease occurs after a suppression of the menses from any cause.

If this affection is connected with disease of the heart, give *Lachesis* every hour, and if it does not relieve, give *Arsenicum*. *Lachesis* will also be found useful in other cases, especially in aged persons.

To prevent a return of the paroxysms, and overcome the predisposition to them, give *Sulphur* and *Nux vom.*, alternately, at intervals of forty-eight hours. If they fail or lose their effect, *Pulsatilla* and *Arsenicum* may follow, and be given in the same manner.

HUMID ASTHMA.

This disease commences suddenly, with a paroxysm of oppressed breathing, with cough, generally in the evening, and is soon followed by the expectoration of a profuse, thin, frothy liquid, sometimes to the extent of a pint or more. The paroxysm lasts from a few moments to several hours. This variety of asthma generally occurs in persons of a relaxed habit who have a languid circulation.

Treatment.—Give *Arsenicum* every half hour during the paroxysm, and if it does not soon relieve the symptoms, give *Lachesis*.

To prevent a return of the paroxysms give *Arsenicum* every night for one week, and *Lachesis* the next week, and so continue; and follow these remedies with *Phosphorus*, if necessary.

SPITTING OF BLOOD—HEMORRHAGE FROM THE LUNGS.

A patient may spit blood without its coming from the lungs; it may descend from the back part of the nostrils into the throat, or it may come from the throat itself, and even from the mouth. Hemorrhage from the lungs is generally preceded by a sensation of weight, fullness, tightness, soreness, heat, and oppression, over a part or the whole of the chest, with more or less frequency of pulse, flushing of the cheeks, and sometimes even chills and fever. A dry cough often precedes the attack. In other cases the hemorrhage commences without any premonitory symptoms. The patient may feel a slight tickling in the windpipe or in the bronchia, which causes an inclination to cough, when the blood follows. Sometimes the first sensation the patient has is a warm feeling in the windpipe, which gradually ascends toward the throat, with a salt, sweetish taste, when he simply hawks and raises blood. The blood is generally liquid, florid, and more or less frothy, owing to the admixture of air in the air passages. When it is thrown off very rapidly in large quantities it is less frothy. The quantity discharged varies from a few drops to several pints; although generally it is not large. Sometimes when the bleeding is rapid it is attended with vomiting, and you may suppose, at first sight, that the blood comes from the stomach, but the disturbed respiration, inclination to cough, and rattling in the air passages, will generally enable you to form a correct opinion. Patients may have a single attack and never have a return, but not unfrequently it returns at uncertain intervals, varying from a few hours to days, months, or years. Hemorrhage from the lungs may be caused by external violence, severe exertion in speaking, singing, coughing, violent muscular exertion, tight lacing, very cold or hot air, and disease of the heart or lungs. It is frequently caused by tubercles in the lungs, and is not an uncommon symptom during the progress of consumption.

Treatment.—If the hemorrhage has been caused by mechanical injuries, speaking, singing, or violent muscular exertion, give a dose of *Arnica* every fifteen minutes, until it ceases; then give a dose once in four hours, to prevent a return. If any fever follows give *Aconite* every hour between the doses of *Arnica*.

Dose, see page 7.

Aconite: Give this remedy in all cases when the hemorrhage has been preceded by a sensation of fullness, heat, oppression of the chest, or palpitation of the heart, and when the flow of blood is copious. In the latter case give *Ipecac* alternately with *Aconite*, at intervals of fifteen minutes; as soon as the bleeding ceases lengthen the intervals to one hour. If the patient has been troubled with a severe, dry cough before the attack, give these remedies; and they are especially useful to relieve any febrile symptoms which may follow the attack.

Pulsatilla may be given every half hour when, with females, the hemorrhage is connected with a suppression of the menses, and also in other cases when the blood is dark and clotted, from escaping slowly and remaining a long time in the air passages.

China: When the hemorrhage occurs in weak and exhausted subjects, and when it is so profuse as to cause great exhaustion and faintness, give *China* Repeat the dose every fifteen minutes until the symptoms are relieved, then two or three times a day, until the debility is relieved.

To prevent a return of the hemorrhage, if the patient is not suffering from consumption, give a dose of *Nux vom.* at night, and *Arsenicum* in the morning for one week; then lengthen the intervals between these remedies, gradually, to three or four days. If any fever or inflammation follows the attack, you need not commence with these remedies until such symptoms have been removed by *Aconite, Ipecac*, and *Bryonia*, and perhaps *Phosphorus*.

During the attack raise the head and shoulders nearly half way to a sitting posture, apply cloths wrung from cold water over the chest, and over them dry flannel; let the patient avoid speaking or moving, and the use of hot drinks. The diet should be light for several days; nothing more than boiled rice, cracker, or toast, gruel, toast water, &c., taken cold.

CONSUMPTION (PHTHISIS PULMONALIS).

A predisposition to this disease is often inherited from one or both parents; sometimes it passes over one generation, and appears in the grandchildren; but by proper care and measures during childhood and early life, a tendency to this disease can almost always be eradicated, and even in adult life, the disease can be prevented; and well-established facts abundantly prove that it is a curable disease, and that patients sometimes recover from every stage, even when hectic fever, night sweats, and purulent expectoration, have occurred. But, perhaps, in a majority of cases, this disease does not depend on hereditary transmission, but is developed by bad management during childhood and youth, and pernicious habits in after-life. Among the most frequent causes will be found the following: repelled eruptions by external applications; seclusion from sunlight, to which children and females are subjected by indoor confinement, and by the means of blinds and curtains; our abominable school system, which cruelly confines, even young children, from the sunlight, during six of the best hours of the day; indolent and inactive habits of young girls and ladies; tight-lacing; self-pollution in the young of both sexes; and improper diet, particularly the use of superfine flour, which does not contain the nourishing materials, and especially the oil, phosphorus, and other mineral ingredients, which the young absolutely require. But there are so many errors in the habits of the American people, which tend to develop this disease, that it would require a volume in which to point them out clearly, and show how to avoid them. Such a treatise is in print, and accessible to all. If you have symptoms of consumption, or fear this disease yourself, or if you would train up your children so that they will not die from it, especially if they inherit from either parent a tendency to this disease, obtain and carefully read the author's work on the "Avoidable Causes of Disease," and you will there obtain the information you need. You will find the table of contents of that work, and where you can obtain it, at the end of this volume.

Symptoms.—The immediate cause of the symptoms, is a deposition in the lungs of a substance called tubercle, which somewhat resembles cheese. This is deposited in masses, varying in size from that of a mustard-seed to the diameter of one or two inches. In some cases the lungs are studded with fine tubercles of the size of a millet-seed, without any large masses, and this is one of the worst forms of the disease, and most difficult to detect. Tubercular masses are found more frequently in the upper portion of the lungs, beneath the collar-bone, than in the lower portions.

It is rare that both sides are equally affected, and the disease occurs most frequently on the left side, but not unfrequently on the right. There is a tendency in tubercles to soften, and sooner or later this process is apt to take place; when it does the softened tubercle gives rise to irritation and inflammation of the adjoining lung, which results in ulceration with the formation of matter or pus, and an abscess is thus formed containing softened tubercle and matter. At length an opening is formed by ulceration into some of the neighboring air tubes or bronchiæ, and the contents of the abscess are discharged by coughing and raising. When tubercle is first deposited in the lungs, before it begins to soften, it often causes a dry hacking cough, with some shortness of breath; when it begins to soften and excite irritation of the lung, it causes chills, fever, and night sweats, or symptoms of hectic fever, and an increase of the cough. These symptoms increase until the abscess breaks and its contents are discharged, when they often abate temporarily, or until other tubercular masses begin to go through the same process, when they return again. If there is a very extensive deposition of tubercles in the lungs, a constant softening of different masses may keep up symptoms of hectic fever, night sweats, and profuse expectoration, until at last diarrhœa or dropsical symptoms ensue and the patient is worn out and dies; or perhaps he may be cut off prematurely by hemorrhage, acute inflammation of the lungs, bronchiæ or larynx, or perforation of the pleura from ulceration, which may allow air to enter and fill the sac, and cause the lung to collapse. This accident when it occurs produces sudden and great difficulty of breathing, and generally hastens the fatal termination. But if the tubercular masses are not too extensive, by a change of habits and proper medication, we may often prevent a deposition of more tubercles, and those already existing may soften and be discharged and the patient recover; or softening may be prevented, and portions of the tubercle be absorbed and carried out of the system through the kidneys, skin, bowels or air passages, and the patient recover, there remaining nothing more than the earthy part of the tubercle, which may be found after death of a chalky consistency. Such remains of tubercles may exist for many years and cause little or no trouble. It is not always easy to detect with certainty the existence of tubercles in the lungs, especially if they are very small; but when, as often happens, large masses are situated near the summit of the lung beneath the collar-bone, it is less difficult. In examining the chest for signs of disease, always compare the two sides at corresponding points If the upper portion of one of the lungs is indurated, or more or less filled up with tuberculous matter, there will be some dullness on percussion on that side, compared with the other. If before softening, you apply your ear beneath the collarbone on the diseased side, you will hear the respiratory murmur less distinctly on that than on the healthy side; and often there is a slight roughness, and even in some cases, jerking, as the air passes through the air passages in the part diseased, and there is a prolongation of the sound as the air passes out in expiration. If you ask the patient to count aloud when your ear is applied, you will hear the vibrations of the voice and feel the jars more distinctly on the diseased side, than on the healthy, from the fact that the solid portion of a lung conveys sound and impulse more distinctly than the spongy structure of the healthy lung. When a tuberculous mass has softened and begins to discharge through the bronchiæ, if the ear is applied over the part, a gurgling sound is often heard as the air enters the cavity, sometimes a cavernous sound, as if blowing into an empty vessel, is heard. When the cavity is nearly or quite empty, if the ear is applied while the patient speaks, it will sound as if the voice came directly from the part; and there will be less dullness on percussion than before the discharge of the contents of the abscess. It is only in a few well-marked cases that the unpractised ear is able to detect this disease with much certainty by an examination of the chest. If you find a patient with a short hacking cough, or a more severe cough, with some frequency of breathing, and the pulse beats constantly one hundred a minute, or more frequently, and these symptoms have been gradually coming on for several weeks or months, you have reason to fear the existence of this disease. The occurrence of hemorrhage during the existence of such symptoms, will be another suspicious circumstance. The average duration of tubercular consumption is from one to three years, although patients sometimes die within from three to four months, whereas in other instances, they have been known to linger for twenty or thirty years. This disease is most frequent between the ages of fifteen and thirty, although it sometimes occurs during childhood, and not unfrequently after the thirtieth year. It is more common with females than with males, and, as a general rule, it commences earlier with the former than with the latter, and runs a more rapid course.

Treatment.—The first and great object of treatment should be to check the further deposition of tuberculous matter. In a domestic work like this, little more can be done than to throw out a few hints. If the consumptive patient would obtain all the information he needs, let him read the author's work on the "Avoidable Causes of Disease," to which reference has been already made.

Sunlight: Let the naked body be exposed to the sunshine in a comfortable temperature, in a room or in the open air, for at least one half-hour every pleasant day; at the same time rub the body all over with the dry hand or a dry towel, and gently percuss or strike over the chest and shoulders with the palm of the hand or fist. Also let the patient work in the sunlight, and sit in it—excepting when the weather is very hot—also let him ride and walk in the sunshine all he is able to; and let him never sit in a room where the sun does not shine, nor sleep in a room where it has not shone all day, if it can possibly be avoided. I am satisfied that sunlight is all-important for consumptive patients.

Air and Exercise: The patient should live in the open air during daylight, whether the weather be cold or warm, wet or dry—always well protected by proper clothing. Active employment out-doors, such as will busy the body and satisfy the mind, is always best; next to this, horseback riding, riding in an open carriage, over rough roads, ball-playing, skating, &c., and walking and dancing, will do very well. The patient should never over-exert himself, but should, every day, without fail, exercise to the full extent of his ability. He must always stand, sit, and ride erect, and never stoop over: and he should frequently throw back his shoulders, put his hands upon his hips, and draw in a full breath, and then contract the upper portion of the windpipe, and allow it to escape as slowly as possible, but still forcing it out with the abdominal and chest muscles. After doing this for a few times, draw in a full breath, and expel it gently, but somewhat rapidly, to the utmost extent, once or twice. If the the patient is already so debilitated as not to be able to leave his room, or sit up, let an assistant commence by exercising his arms and legs, bend and extend them, turn them from side to side, and rotate them; as the patient gains strength let him resist slightly, and so continue until he is able to exercise himself.

Diet.—Let the chief articles of food be milk and bread, the the latter made from canel and shorts, or the second and third runnings, which contain, in excess, the mineral ingredients, and the oil which such patients require; cream and baked potatoes, fat beef and fat mutton, if the stomach will digest them; and moderately of fruits and vegetables.

If possible, as soon as a patient nas reason to fear from his symptoms, the commencement of this disease, he should consult a skilful homœopathic physician, and be sure and consult one who has the time and patience to spend an hour or two in making a thorough physical examination of the chest, and in making careful inquiries into the history of the case; for if the physician does not do this he cannot make a prescription which will be likely to benefit the patient. Everything depends on the selection of the right remedy, and then holding on to it until it has had time to exert its curative action.

Lycopodium: This remedy is perhaps more frequently required in the early stage than any other, especially when there is a short dry cough, caused by a tickling in the chest or in the lower part of the windpipe, and when there is a dry cough day and night, with wheezing, and if deep breathing causes irritation and cough. Also later in the disease, when there is a loose cough, with a sore or raw sensation in the chest, and a salt, grayish, white, or yellowish expectoration. Give a dose every night until improvement commences, and then give a dose once a week and continue it as long as there is any improvement.

Dose of this or other remedies, see page 7.

Sulphur is the chief remedy in all cases where patients have been troubled with chronic eruptive diseases; and if such eruptions have disappeared on the appearance of disease of the lungs, this will be another indication for *Sulphur*. Also give it when there is a short dry cough with soreness, and a sensation of fullness of the chest, and aggravation of the symptoms in cold damp weather. This remedy will sometimes be found useful late in the disease, when there is a copious, thick, whitish, or yellowish expectoration. When *Sulphur* seems indicated, give one dose every night for three nights, and then omit it for a week, and if at the end of that time there is any improvement, give nothing as long as it lasts, after which *Sulphur* may be repeated again. If there is no change for the better, give some other remedy; generally *Calcarea carb.* should follow *Sulphur*.

Calcarea carb. is especially adapted to young persons who have been subject to bleeding from the nose, and young females who have been troubled with profuse menstruation; also when the patient is of a full habit, and there is a suppression of the menses. It is also indicated at any age when there is a violent dry cough, with tickling as if from feather dust in the air passages. It often follows *Sulphur* to advantage, when the expectoration becomes profuse and whitish, or yellow, during the softening of tuberculous masses. Give a dose every night. *Lycopodium* is often required after *Calcarea carb.*

Phosphorus: Give this remedy early in the disease, when there is a short dry cough from tickling in the chest, which is aggravated by laughing, talking, or walking in the open air, and still later in the disease, when there is a loose cough and a sore feeling in the chest, tightness, shortness of breath, saltish, purulent expectoration morning and evening, hectic fever, night sweats, and a debilitating diarrhœa. Give a dose every night.

Avoid changing your remedies as long as there is any improvement, even though it is slow. If you change frequently you will get no benefit from any remedy. If acute inflammation of the lungs, pleurisy, bronchitis, laryngitis, hemorrhage, or diarrhœa, occurs during the progress of consumption, consult the section on that disease, and give the remedies as there directed, but as soon as the acute symptoms are removed, return to the proper remedy for this disease. In addition to the above remedies, if they fail to cure, you can consult those under the head of chronic bronchitis.

DISEASES OF THE HEART.

It is more difficult to detèct, with certainty, affections of the heart, than almost any other class of diseases, and even physicians of long experience are sometimes mistaken.

Pericarditis.—Inflammation of the smooth membrane which covers the external surface of the heart, and then surrounds the heart, except at its base, in the form of a sack—sometimes denominated the heart-case, is called pericarditis. This disease more frequently results from acute rheumatism affecting this membrane, than from any other cause, although it may arise from exposure, sudden changes of temperature, and other causes of acute diseases.

It sometimes occurs during recovery from scarlet fever and erysipelas. It is more common in early than in advanced life, and men are more subject to it than women.

Symptoms.—The attack usually commences with chills, followed by fever; but sometimes there is a great faintness, instead of chills, followed by fever. The pulse, at the commencement of the fever, may be full and strong, and beating from 110 to 120 in a minute, but as the disease advances it often becomes very irregular, beating rapidly for a few strokes, then slowly; and sometimes it is intermittent. In dangerous cases it becomes very small, so as scarcely to be felt, even when the heart is acting violently. There may be little or no pain, but simply a feeling of tightness, weight, burning, or pressure, in the region of the heart. In other cases there are sharp pains, which may extend through to the left shoulder, and even down the left arm. There is difficulty of breathing or speaking, and the patient is often compelled to sit up with his body leaning forward. Respiration is frequent, palpitation of the heart is often violent, and sometimes there is hiccough; these symptoms are often worse during the night, and occur in paroxysms. In severe cases there is great restlessness, with an anxious countenance, headache, disturbed sleep, frightful dreams, perhaps delirium, and great prostration. If the ear is applied over the heart, at the very commencement there can sometimes be heard a friction sound, caused by the rubbing of two roughened surfaces of membrane together; but this is of short duration, for in the course of a day or two a watery fluid is effused into the sac, which separates its two inflamed surfaces. When the quantity of fluid becomes considerable, the sounds of the heart become diminished and apparently distant, in consequence of the intervening fluid. If the hand is applied over the heart, its impulse often seems to be lessened, and sometimes there is an undulatory or wave-like motion felt, which may even be visible to the eye, caused by the action of the heart in the fluid. Sometimes, on applying the ear over the heart, there is a kind of churning sound heard. If the patient recovers, as the fluid in the pericardium is absorbed, so that the two surfaces of the membrane come together, covered as they are by more or less lymph which was poured out with the serum or watery fluid, the friction sound may again be heard, but generally for a temporary period, for the two surfaces soon adhere, unless they have been very long separated, and such adhesions are frequently found after patients have died from other diseases. Pericarditis sometimes terminates fatally within forty-eight hours, but more frequently, when patients die, it is not until the end of from five to ten days, sometimes several weeks. If the patient recovers, the disease generally begins to yield within a few days, the effused fluid is gradually absorbed, and the symptoms disappear. The prognosis is generally favorable when the disease is promptly treated by the use of homœopathic remedies.

Symptoms of Chronic Pericarditis.—This form of the disease may result from the acute. There may be dull pain in the region of the heart, which may extend to the left shoulder, or arm, or but little or no pain, simply oppression, tightness, or weight, with shortness of breath, perhaps difficulty of lying down, and frequent feeble and often irregular pulse. There is dullness on percussion, and absence of the respiratory sounds to a greater distance than during health, owing to the distension of the pericardium, with fluid and other signs, similar to those which have been described as occurring in the acute disease; sometimes there is fullness in the region of the heart. The face is usually pale and puffy, the lips purplish ; swelling of the extremities, and symptoms of hectic fever may ensue. The disease may not confine the patient to his bed, or even to his house, and he may be better for days and months, and finally recover or die. Death often occurs suddenly in such cases.

Treatment of Pericarditis.—*Aconite* is the most important remedy in all acute cases, where there are any chills, faintness, or fever, and this remedy should be given every hour, and it is very important that it be not discontinued so long as there is the slightest fever, or heat of skin, even over the body, for you must bear in mind that there is a tendency in this disease, to great debility, coldness of the extremities, and small pulse, even while the inflammation is unchecked. If any other remedy seems to be indicated, it is better to give it alternately with *Aconite* than to discontinue that remedy. Read under the head of *Bryonia*.

Dose of this or other remedies, see page 7.

Bryonia: After continuing *Aconite* for from twelve or twenty-four hours, until the febrile symptoms are somewhat ameliorated, give a dose of *Bryonia* once in four hours, and *Aconite* every hour between the doses. Not only is *Bryonia* useful when the disease is caused by exposure and sudden atmospheric changes, but it is especially useful when the disease has a rheumatic origin. The above remedies should generally be continued several days, especially if the patient gets no worse, until the heat, even over the body, has been entirely relieved, when *Sulphur* should follow, either alone or alternately with *Bryonia*, at intervals of two hours. But if, instead of improving, the symptoms get worse, *Arsenicum* will generally be required.

Arsenicum may be given when, notwithstanding the use of the above remedies, the patient becomes very weak, the pulse small, frequent or irregular, the extremities cold, and if there is great tightness, weight, and difficulty of breathing, and inability to lie down, with great anxiety of countenance.

Belladonna: When at the commencement of the disease the pains are shooting and darting, extending through to the shoulder, perhaps down the arm, give this remedy alternately with *Aconite*, at intervals of one half-hour until the pains are somewhat relieved, then give *Bryonia* and *Aconite*, as directed under the head of *Bryonia.* In case there is violent headache, great restlessness, or delirium, a few doses of this remedy may be given at any time

In cases where this disease is complicated with rheumatism, if *Aconite* and *Bryonia* fail to relieve the symptoms, give *Rhus tox.* instead of *Bryonia.*

Treatment of Chronic Pericarditis.—If an acute attack lingers, and threatens to become chronic, and the above remedies do not relieve the symptoms, give *Cannabis* once in two hours during the forenoon, and *Sulphur* once in four hours during the afternoon and evening. If, under such circumstances, the disease is associated with rheumatism, give *Rhus tox.* and *Sulphur* in the same manner. The above remedies are also useful in the chronic form of the disease. If they do not cure in either the acute or chronic form of the disease, give *Arsenicum* once in six hours.

General Measures.—At the commencement of an attack of acute pericarditis, apply over the heart a towel wrung from cold water, and over that four or five thicknesses of dry flannel; confine the whole to its place by a bandage around the body; wet the towel once in six hours. If, notwithstanding this application and the use of the remedies, the symptoms get worse, omit the cold cloths, and make hot applications—cloths wrung from hot water. The diet should be light at first, but if symptoms of great prostration ensue, give milk-and-water, mutton or chicken broth, or let the patient chew beef-steak.

ENDOCARDITIS.

(INFLAMMATION OF THE LINING MEMBRANE OF THE HEART.)

Rheumatism is by far the most frequent cause of this affection, although it may arise from exposure and other causes of acute diseases.

The general symptoms are very similar to those of pericarditis. Chills, followed by fever, uneasiness and oppression, a frequent, and at length a small and perhaps irregular pulse, great debility, faintness, and in severe cases, paleness and lividity of the surface, cold sweats and extreme anxiety, with, in desperate cases, symptoms of impending suffocation, are among the symptoms of this disease. There is generally little or no pain. On applying the ear over the heart we hear a sound somewhat similar to that caused by the passage of wind out of a bellows, therefore it is called the bellows murmur. It is generally soft at the commencement of the disease, but may become more or less rough. When we hear this sound in connection with the above symptoms, especially fever or rheumatism, we may be reasonably certain that the patient is suffering from the disease under consideration. But it will be well to bear in mind that in case of nervous and debilitated females especially, when the blood is thin and watery, and the face pale, we may have a similar sound without any disease of the heart, and without fever.

Inflammation of the substance of the heart itself is very rare, except when it accompanies inflammation of its lining or external membranes, and there are no symptoms by which it can be detected if it exists.

Treatment of Endocarditis.—The treatment is very similar to that which has been recommended for pericarditis; make the same external applications, and follow the same directions as to diet. At the commencement of the disease give *Aconite* and *Belladonna* alternately at intervals of one hour. If the symptoms are not soon relieved give *Bryonia* once in four hours and *Aconite* every hour between. If the disease has been caused by rheumatism, and the above remedies do not relieve it within two days, give *Rhus tox.*, once in two hours. If there is much fever remaining, give a dose of *Aconite* between the doses of *Rhus*. If the patient is a female, and has never been troubled with rheumatism, after giving *Aconite* every hour for twelve hours, give *Pulsatilla* once in two hours. *Arsenicum* should generally follow the above remedies as soon as the acute symptoms are relieved. Give a dose once in four hours. If great prostration ensues at any time, with symptoms of threatening suffocation, small or irregular pulse and cold extremities, give *Arsenicum* every hour, and if at the end of twelve hours there is no improvement, give *Lachesis* at intervals of one hour, and beef-tea, or mutton-broth, and milk and-water for drink; let the patient if able, chew beef-steak, and swallow all but the fibrous parts.

CHRONIC VALVULAR DISEASE OF THE HEART.

HYPERTROPHY AND DILATATION.

From slow or chronic inflammation, the valves of the heart sometimes become thickened, indurated, and in some instances even bony, especially during advanced life. When such a change takes place, more or less mechanical obstruction is offered to the circulation of the blood through the heart. If the progress of the disease can be arrested before the obstruction becomes too great, the patient may continue to enjoy good health to old age; but if the degeneration increases, it gives rise to a train of symptoms which sooner or later terminates in death; among which are the following: enlargement of the heart, dilatation of this organ, cough, spitting of blood, difficulty of breathing, congestion and inflammation of the lungs, dropsy of the chest, pale or livid face, swelling of the extremities, hemorrhage from different organs, nausea and vomiting, bilious derangements, drowsiness, and even apoplexy. When the disease is on the left side of the heart, the pulse is apt to be small, weak, and irregular, and sometimes it is jerking, being at first quick and strong, but rapidly receding as it were from the fingers, caused by the backward current of the blood through the imperfectly closed valves of the aorta. Disease of the valves of the right side of the heart has very little effect on the pulse. If we apply the ear over the heart we generally hear a sound similar to the bellows murmur, described under the head of endocarditis, but generally rougher and harsher, sometimes like the sound of a rasp or file. The sound, when heard most distinctly at the apex of the heart, which lies about one inch to the right and a little below the left nipple, often resembles the whispered word "who." If it is heard most distinctly above the base of the heart and in the direction of the large arteries which pass from the heart, if near the upper portion and toward the right side of the breast-bone, in the direction of the aorta, or large artery which comes off from the heart and through which the blood passes to every part of the system, the sound often resembles the whispered letter R; whereas if the sound is most distinctly heard near the upper portion of the breast-bone, toward the left, in the direction of the pulmonary artery which conveys the blood to the lungs, it often resembles the whispered letter S. We not unfrequently hear a sound over the heart very closely resembling a valvular murmur, which is simply a friction sound, and results from inflammation of the pericardium; but this sound is often heard distinctly over the entire heart, although sometimes it is much more circumscribed than the sounds which result from valvular disease, and occasionally cannot be heard over a space larger than a single square inch, and it is more superficial, and increased by pressing the ear firmly against the chest; still this sound is not unfrequently mistaken for that of valvular disease, even by physicians.

We occasionally have enlargement or hypertrophy of the heart. This affection may be caused by valvular disease, or it may exist without such disease; the same is true of dilatation of the heart. In hypertrophy the impulse, or stroke which is felt on applying the hand or ear over the heart during its pulsations, is much stronger than in health, and may be felt over a somewhat larger extent of the chest, but the sounds of the heart are generally less distinct than when there is dilatation. On the contrary, when there is dilatation, although the impulse is felt over a large space, it is soft and neither forcible nor heaving; and the sounds of the heart are loud and clear, and heard over a larger portion of the chest than in hypertrophy. But it requires a nice ear and much experience to detect with much certainty these chronic diseases of the heart, for we may have nervous affections so perfectly simulating them that physicians are often deceived. I have known patients who were told by more than one physician that they had incurable disease of the heart, and that they were liable to die any moment, when there was no disease. Nervous palpitation, and nervous pains about the heart, are often quite as severe as occur in any case of organic disease. In nervous females especially, when the countenance is pale and the blood is watery, we often have bellows murmurs, similar to those of organic disease, but generally less constant, and without roughness. Bear in mind that organic disease of the heart is exceedingly rare in young persons, except when caused by rheumatism, and even then, if recent, it is simply rheumatic inflammation, which can generally be cured. If mental emotions seriously increase the symptoms, the disease is generally simply nervous, especially if such emotions produce a greater effect on the symptoms than active exercise.

Treatment.—The remedies recommended for pericarditis and endocarditis, are the chief remedies for the various organic affections just described. If the disease has been caused by rheumatism, *Bryonia* and *Rhus tox.* are often useful, long after the active rheumatic symptoms have disappeared. *Sulphur* may follow the above remedies, and be continued as long as there is any improvement; afterward give *Arsenicum.*

When there is violent palpitation with strong impulse, give *Nux vomica* at night and *Arsenicum* in the morning; and even when the impulse is feeble, or you fear valvular disease, these are valuable remedies; *Pulsatilla* and *Phosphorus* may be given in the same manner. *Lachesis* and *Belladonna* are also valuable remedies. If dropsical symptoms occur, give *Arsenicum* once in six hours, and if it fails to relieve, give *Apis mel.* once in two hours and consult the section on dropsy: but the use of the remedies named above, especially *Arsenicum*, will tend to prevent such symptoms.

For palpitation of the heart in nervous or hysterical individuals, if a female, give *Pulsatilla*, if a male, give *Nux vomica;* if one does not relieve give the other, in either case. Give a dose every hour until the symptoms are relieved, and then once a day to prevent a return. *Chamomilla*, *Belladonna*, and *Coffea*, are often useful. If the palpitation is caused by fright, give *Opium* or *Coffea;* if by fear, and the above remedies do not relieve, give *Veratrum*. If caused by sudden joy, give *Aconite* or *Coffea*. If by chagrin, give *Chamomilla*, *Ignatia*, or *Nux vomica*. If it occurs after the loss of blood, or other fluids, such as results in diarrhœa, leucorrhœa, and seminal emissions, give *China* two or three times a day.

ANGINA PECTORIS.

This is a nervous or neuralgic disease. It rarely attacks individuals under forty years of age, and it is more frequent with men than women. The indolent, corpulent, intemperate, gouty, and rheumatic subjects are more liable to it than others.

Symptoms.—This disease is characterized by severe paroxysms of pain, generally shooting pains, in the region of the heart, extending through toward the back and into the left shoulder, sometimes down the arm, with a sensation of numbness, and lasting from fifteen minutes to an hour. At first the paroxysms may only return at intervals of months, but gradually, if not checked by treatment, they are apt to become more frequent, perhaps occurring two or three times a day, or after the slightest exertion or mental excitement. They frequently occur after the first sleep at night. There is generally oppression of breathing and palpitation of the heart, with sometimes a strong and full pulse; in other cases it is weak and irregular. The paroxysms differ much in severity in different cases; and even the pains are sometimes dull and aching, with a sensation of numbness, instead of sharp and acute. The paroxysms sometimes end in fainting, or in convulsions.

Treatment.—During the attack if the patient is of a full habit, and even if he is not, give *Aconite,* and if in fifteen minutes the symptoms are not relieved, give *Belladonna.* If these remedies do not relieve the symptoms soon, give *Nux vomica.*

To prevent a return of the paroxysms give *Nux vomica* at night and *Arsenicum* in the morning; at the end of a month lengthen the intervals between the doses to two or three days. If the paroxysms occur at night, after sleeping, give *Lachesis* at night instead of *Nux vomica. Pulsatilla* and *Ignatia* will sometimes be found useful in obstinate cases.

The patient must not use tobacco when troubled with this disease, or any affection of the heart, if he wishes to recover. Nor should he use tea or coffee. The diet should be light, easily digested and nourishing, but plain.

INTERMITTENT PULSE.

Persons otherwise in the enjoyment of pretty good health, sometimes find that their pulse intermits, or skips a beat occasionally, and are often very much alarmed. This irregularity of the pulse is perhaps more frequently caused by indigestion or dyspepsia than by any other cause, and is rarely an alarming symptom, but it should be enough so to induce a man to quit tobacco if he is using it, and also green tea.

Treatment.—Give *Nux vomica* at night and *Natrum muriaticum* in the morning. Be careful in regard to diet, and direct regular exercise. Gradually lengthen the intervals between the doses of the above remedies to three or four days.

FAINTING OR SWOONING (SYNCOPE).

This affection is characterized by a loss of consciousness, diminution, and perhaps in some instances a temporary cessation of the heart's action, with a more or less complete suspension of respiration. It sometimes occurs suddenly, in other instances it is preceded by clouded or deranged vision, mental confusion, nausea, sinking at the stomach, weak pulse, and paleness. Such symptoms sometimes pass off without loss of consciousness, but in other instances they increase until the fainting becomes complete, when the countenance is deadly pale and sunken, the surface of the body cool, the pulse absent or nearly so at the wrist, the breathing suspended, and consciousness gone. In some instances the urine and contents of the bowels pass off involuntarily. The duration of this state may be but for a few seconds or minutes, but in rare instances it may extend to hours, and even days, and yet the patient recover. Death occasionally results, especially when the fainting occurs from the loss of blood, or after an acute disease, or when there is organic disease of the heart. This disease may be caused by the loss of blood, debilitating discharges, nauseating medicines, tobacco, and other narcotics, depressing mental emotions, unpleasant sights, severe pain, drinking cold water when the body is hot, and by suddenly assuming the sitting or erect posture when the body has been debilitated by disease, the loss of blood or other fluids.

Treatment.—Always immediately place the patient in a horizontal position, with his head as low or even lower than the body. If you leave the patient sitting up, or even with a pillow under his head he may die. If he is sitting in a chair, tip him right over back in his chair, or lay him on the floor if no bed or lounge is at hand. Remove everything tight from around the neck and body. Dash a handful of cold water over the face, neck, and chest, wipe it off and dash on more, rub the limbs with your hands and slap the surface of the skin with the open hand. Let the patient smell of *Camphor*, and give a drop of it in a few drops of water. Admit fresh air freely. If the fainting results from a loss of blood, or from the loss of other fluids, give *China* two or three times a day until strength is restored. *Carbo veg.* and *Nux vomica* are also useful in such cases. When caused by fright, fear, grief, or other mental emotions, and *Camphor* does not relieve the symptoms, give *Ignatia* or *Coffea.* If, when the disease has been caused by mental emotions, there is faintness during every attempt to raise the head, give *Opium* once in six hours, afterwards *Aconite,* if it is needed. If it is caused by violent pain, give *Aconite* or *Chamomilla.*

GOITRE—BRONCHOCELE.

This is an enlargement of the thyroid gland, which causes a swelling on the lower part of the neck, in front, just above the breastbone. The gland lies upon both sides of the trachea or windpipe; the two sides connecting by a thin portion, or bridge, extending over the latter organ. The enlargement may involve the whole gland, or it may be confined to one side, or even to the connecting portion in front of the windpipe. The cause or causes of this disease are unknown.

Treatment.—Give a dose of *Spongia* every night, and continue it for two or three months; rub hard and press the swelling frequently. If the above does not cure it, obtain at a Homœopathic Pharmacy, or at a Druggist's, one grain of Iodine and two grains of Iodide of Potassa, and dissolve them in one ounce of water, and give one drop of the solution in water, or on sugar, night and morning. Also obtain one drachm of Iodide of Potassa, and dissolve it in a pint of water, and every night wet a few thicknesses of cotton or linen cloth in it, and lay over the swelling, then cover well with dry flannel. Dr. E. R. Ellis, of Detroit, formerly a student of the author's, reports having cured several cases of Goitre by means of mechanical pressure. For this purpose an elastic band or rubber, of from one-half to two and a half inches in width, is passed around the neck and over the swelling, and gradually tightened, but only to a degree that will neither render it uncomfortable nor cause fulness of the head.

CHAPTER V.

DISEASES OF THE DIGESTIVE ORGANS.

Diseases of the mouth, teeth, and throat, will be considered first, with the exception of the thrush, which will be left for the chapter on diseases of children.

CANKER OF THE MOUTH (CANCRUM ORIS).

With many individuals, while in comparative good health, occasionally a slight roughness and soreness will appear on the inside of the cheeks, on the gums, or on or beneath the tongue, followed by a small ulcer or two in the course of twenty-four hours. This is a slight disease, and of little consequence. A dose of *Mercurius viv.* two or three times a day will generally suffice to cure it soon; and the alternate use of *Mercurius viv.* and *Sulphur*, once or twice a week will tend to prevent a return of the ulcers. But the disease denominated cancrum oris, is a much more formidable and troublesome affection. It generally attacks children or young persons, and most frequently those who are ill-fed and live in damp and dark habitations. It is therefore found among the rich who feed their children on the miserable bread which superfine flour makes, and keep them in dark-curtained or shaded rooms; and also among the poor, such as lack proper food, and live in dark cellars and hovels.

Symptoms.—The mucous membrane covering the sides of the tongue, and inside of the cheeks, becomes red and inflamed, and afterwards covered with large ulcers, which may extend so as to cover both sides of the tongue, from near the tip to its roots, and also the inside of the cheeks. The tongue becomes swollen, showing upon its sides indentations caused by the teeth; there is a profuse secretion of saliva or spittle, the breath is offensive, and eating and swallowing difficult; gradual emaciation ensues. This disease may last for weeks or months if not properly treated, and even cause death.

Treatment.—First of all the child requires fresh air and sunlight, and next suitable food, milk thickened with coarse flour (the second and third runnings), a thin pudding made of the same, beef-tea, mashed potatoes, and, as soon as the patient can chew it, beef or mutton.

Mercurius viv.: This is perhaps the most important remedy, and a dose may be given once in six hours.

Nux vom.: If *Mercurius* fails, in the course of a few days, to cause an improvement of the symptoms, give *Nux vom.* alternately with it three hours apart; and these remedies should be continued at least ten days or two weeks, unless the symptoms get worse under their use.

Arsenicum may follow the above remedies if necessary, or it may take the place of them at the commencement of the treatment, when there is much burning pain and the breath is very offensive. Give a dose once in six hours, and continue it as long as any improvement follows. *Carbo veg.* may be given after *Arsenicum* if necessary. *Hepar sulph.* is sometimes useful, especially if the patient has ever been salivated, or taken large doses of calomel or blue pills. If the above remedies do not cure the disease, get at a druggist's one grain of *Iodine* and two grains of *Iodide of potassium*, put both into an ounce bottle of water and drop three drops of the solution thus formed, into a glass of water and give a teaspoonful from the glass to the patient once in six hours.

Washes are of very little use, and aside from washing the mouth frequently with tepid water, it is better to shun them.

NURSING SORE MOUTH.

A peculiar form of sore mouth frequently attacks females, either during nursing, or during the latter months of pregnancy. It commences with bright redness of the edges, upper and under surface of the tongue, and inner surface of the cheeks, which gradually extends to the throat, with a burning, smarting, and sore sensation. All hot or stimulating substances, salt, and acids, taken into the mouth, aggravate the sufferings. After a few days, small whitish vesicles or pimples make their appearance on the edges of the tongue or beneath it, which may after a time degenerate into ulcers. If the disease is not checked, it gradually extends to the stomach, and there is burning at the stomach and tenderness, with perhaps nausea and vomiting; and at last the same burning sensation extends to the bowels, and exhausting diarrhœa takes the place of the costiveness which existed while the disease was confined to the stomach. The blood becomes watery and the countenance pale, a hoarse loose cough sometimes sets in, and the vital powers are gradually exhausted, and the patient dies if not rescued by treatment.

Treatment.—At the commencement of the disease, while it is confined to the mouth, give *Belladonna* once in two hours, but if it involves the mouth and stomach, before there is diarrhœa, give *Belladonna* alternately with *Nux vomica* two hours apart. These remedies will rarely fail to relieve at this stage. The disease is one of debility, therefore give meat and a nourishing diet.

If ulcers make their appearance, and the above remedies do not relieve them, give *Mercurius viv.* once in two hours.

If the burning extends to the bowels, and a diarrhœa ensues, give *Mercurius;* if at the end of two or three days there is no relief, give *Sulphur* once in two hours, and continue it as long as there is any improvement. If these remedies fail to relieve, give *Arsenicum* once in two hours. If there is acid vomiting with diarrhœa, *Pulsatilla* is sometimes useful. When there is great debility with diarrhœa, *China* alternately with *Arsenicum* two hours apart, will often benefit the patient. Call on a homœopathic physician.

Weaning the child will generally cure the disease if it is not delayed too long; but it can generally be cured by homœopathic remedies without weaning, but not always without too great a risk.

SALIVATION.

(MERCURIAL INFLAMMATION OF THE MOUTH.)

This disease may be caused by calomel, blue pills, or any of the preparations of mercury, when they are given in large doses. It may also be caused by rubbing mercurial ointment on the external surface of the body.

Symptoms.—Metallic or coppery taste, increased flow of saliva, swelling of the gums, and soreness when pressed, and tenderness of the teeth when striking them together, are among the first symptoms. Then follows stiffness about the jaws, and the teeth feel elongated, and the gums, palate, tongue, glands beneath the ears and jaws, become swollen and painful. There is frequently toothache, pains in the jaws, ulcers on the inner surface of the cheeks, or on the lips, throat, and gums. The teeth become loose, and sometimes there is sloughing and exposure of the jaw.

Treatment.—Give *Hepar sulph.* once in three or four hours. If there is much pain give *Belladonna* alternately with it two hours apart. *Sulphur* may follow the above remedies, and may be given two or three times a day. This remedy and *Hepar sulph.* are the most important remedies to cure the chronic effects which often follow the abuse of mercury. For this purpose give one every night for a week, then the other, and change every week. *Nitric acid* is also a valuable remedy to counteract the poisonous action of mercury. It may be given once in six hours. It may be given instead of *Hepar* at the commencement of the attack if no improvement follows the use of the latter remedy.

GANGRENOUS INFLAMMATION OF THE MOUTH.

This is not a very frequent disease, and generally, but not always, occurs during childhood, and when the system is debilitated by bad air, unwholesome food, or by some febrile or inflammatory disease, such as typhoid fever, measles, inflammation of the lungs, dysentery, &c.

Symptoms.—It attacks the inside of the cheeks, lips, or gums. If the cheek or lip is attacked, the first symptom generally noticed is a white swelling on the external surface of the cheek, generally near the angle of the mouth, or on the lip, which looks as though the part had been varnished. If when this swelling is noticed the inside of the cheek or lip is examined, there will be found a grayish or ash-colored spot opposite the swelling, which is the beginning of gangrene. If this disease is not checked soon, the mortification extends more or less rapidly through the cheek or lip, until a dark spot appears upon the external surface, which spreads rapidly until much of the cheek is destroyed, or the patient dies. If the disease commences on the gums it is generally between the lower front teeth, although it may commence at other points, over the upper or lower jaw, and the ash-colored spot appears on the gums, preceded by slight swelling, and the disease soon penetrates the bony structure, and if the patient lives, portions of the jawbone, and more or less of the teeth, die, and after a time are separated from the living structure, often causing much deformity. The disease is not painful, and there is very little soreness. There is sometimes slight febrile excitement as the gangrene progresses, and diarrhœa is apt to supervene, followed by great debility, cold extremities, and death.

Treatment.—My experience has satisfied me that it will not generally do to rely entirely on internal remedies, in the treatment of this disease. We must apply locally a homœopathic remedy of sufficient strength to change the diseased action in the part, or serious deformity, if not death, will be very likely to result. Touch the gray or ash-colored spot on the inside of the cheek or lip, or on the gums, with a stick of *Nitrate of silver*, bring it in contact with the entire dead surface, and touch lightly the healthy surface for the eighth of an inch around the diseased part; then let the patient rinse his mouth with warm water. Repeat the application if necessary once at the end of twenty-four hours. *Sulphate of copper* or *Blue vitriol*, will do quite as well as *Nitrate of silver*. Dissolve a piece as large as a small pea in a teaspoonful of warm water in a cup, and with a feather wash the diseased mucous membrane twice a day, until the progress of the disease is checked.

Give at the same time internally, the following remedies.

Alternate *Carbo veg.* and *China* two hours apart. If, notwithstanding the above remedies, the disease is not soon checked, especially if diarrhœa commences, give *Arsenicum* instead of *Carbo veg.*

The diet should be as nourishing as the stomach will bear, similar to that which was directed under the head of canker of the mouth; especially milk and beef-tea.

INFLAMMATION OF THE TONGUE (GLOSSITIS).

There are two forms of inflammation of the tongue, one superficial, and the other deep-seated. It is not uncommon, especially in children and young persons, to have an inflammation of the mucous membrane of the upper surface, edges, and end of the tongue, with intense redness, great soreness, and a profuse flow of saliva. Little white points or vesicles soon make their appearance, which form ulcers after a day or two. The disease is attended with a high fever, which is often mistaken for an attack of typhoid fever.

Nux vom. is the chief remedy for the disease described above, and the fever which attends it. Give it dissolved in water once in two hours, and a dose of *Mercurius* night and morning. If at the end of two days the disease is not almost cured give *Arsenicum* night and morning instead of *Mercurius*, and continue the *Nux vomica*.

Inflammation of the substance of the tongue is a rare, but more serious disease. It may be caused by mechanical injuries, the sting of insects, chemical agents, exposure, &c. The disease may involve but a part, or the whole of the tongue; generally if it commences in a part, the whole organ soon becomes red, swollen, and painful, and sometimes so much enlarged as to fill the entire mouth, and project beyond the teeth and lips. It may even press backwards so as to seriously obstruct respiration, and cause danger of suffocation. Speaking and swallowing become difficult, the tongue becomes dry upon the surface, or moist and covered with a thick fur. Gangrene occasionally results; sometimes matter forms, but generally the disease is cured without either. The inflammation is attended with a high fever during its first stage; but later if respiration is obstructed, or the disease tends to gangrene, the pulse becomes small and irregular and the extremities cold.

Treatment.—If the disease has arisen from a mechanical injury, *Arnica* may be given internally and applied to the organ. One drop of the tincture in a glass of water, of which give a tablespoonful for a dose; but for a wash, one half a teaspoonful of the tincture may be put into a teacupful of water.

Aconite: This remedy may be given alternately with *Arnica* when the fever is high, or the skin hot and the pulse full.

Mercurius viv. is generally the most important remedy when the disease has neither been caused by mechanical injuries nor by taking mercury in large doses. If there is much fever, give it alternately with *Aconite*, one hour apart; and if at the end of twelve hours the patient is not better, give *Belladonna* alternately with *Mercurius viv.* instead of *Aconite.*

If the above remedies do not check the disease, but the tongue becomes dark, black, or greenish, give *Lachesis* every hour, and if it does not relieve the symptoms soon, give *Arsenicum* alternately with it one hour apart. If symptoms of suffocation occur, and they are not promptly relieved by your remedies, send immediately for a physician; if you cannot get a homœopathic physician, send for an allopathist, for it may be necessary to make an incision lengthwise on both sides of the upper surface of the tongue, so as to allow it to bleed freely, to gain time for the action of your remedies, in a very severe and sudden attack, but the remedies will rarely fail to relieve, without a resort to this severe measure.

MUMPS (PAROTITIS).

This is an inflammation of the parotid glands, which lie immediately beneath and in front of the lower part of the ears, and are among the glands which secrete the saliva. The disease is generally caused by contagion, and the same gland is rarely affected twice, but if the gland on one side only is attacked, that on the other will be liable to contract the disease on subsequent exposure.

Symptoms.—The swelling is usually preceded by a slight fever, or at least such a fever generally accompanies the inflammation. There is soreness and stiffness in the region of the swelling, with more or less difficulty of chewing and swallowing. On the fourth day the disease begins to subside, and during or after the abatement of the inflammation, it is not uncommon to have the breasts in females, or the testicles in males, become swollen and painful, and even serious inflammation of these organs may ensue.

Treatment.—Great care is requisite that the patient be not exposed to sudden changes of temperature, or to damp and cold weather, during the continuance of the mumps, and for several days after the disease has abated. It is also best to avoid active exercise, and all stimulating drinks, during the same period.

Mercurius viv. is the chief remedy, and a dose may be repeated once in two or three hours; and if there is much pain or headache, *Belladonna* may be given alternately with *Mercurius*, two hours apart. If, at the end of three or four days, the fever and swelling do not abate, omit the above remedies, and give *Carbo veg.* once in four hours.

Make no application over the swollen gland with the exception of a dry warm handkerchief, a piece of flannel, or of cotton batting. The diet should be light and free from stimulating condiments. No animal food should be allowed.

If, at the time, or after the disease abates, the breasts become painful and inflamed, give *Belladonna* once in two hours. If the testicles become swollen and painful, give *Pulsatilla* once in two hours; and if, at the end of twelve hours, it fails to relieve the symptoms, give *Nux vom.* once in two hours. Make warm applications, and if simple hot dry cloths do not relieve, use a warm hot poultice—beans boiled soft and mashed up do well.

TOOTHACHE (ODONTALGIA).

The pain may be caused by inflammation of the nervous pulp within the teeth, or by inflammation of the socket, after the death of the nerve; or, again, the disease may be simply neuralgic, or rheumatic, involving the nerve of one tooth or of several, and even the nerves of the jaw.

The nerve of a sound tooth sometimes, but very rarely, becomes inflamed; generally the inflammation is caused by the decay of the tooth and exposure of the nerve to the air, heat, cold, or pressure in eating. If the inflammation is not relieved, it goes on to suppuration, and matter or pus is formed, which escapes at the end of the fangs and causes inflammation of the socket. Or if the nerve of a tooth is dead, inflammation may commence in the socket and pus form there. The inflammation soon extends to the gums, and even to the cheek and lip, and they become swollen and red; the pain is severe and throbbing. The pressure caused by the accumulation of pus in the socket, either produces a loosening of the tooth which allows the matter to escape by its side between it and the gum, or it causes an absorption of the bony process over the end of the fang, which allows the pus to form an abscess at that point, where it breaks spontaneously, if not lanced, and is called a gumboil. The whole duration of the disease is usually from four to seven or eight days, and the suffering is often intense; the entire face sometimes becoming very much swollen. This disease is denominated alveolar abscess, or ague in the face, and may arise more than once from the same tooth, if it is allowed to remain in the jaw; unless, as often happens, pus continues to be secreted in the socket, and, by escaping, keeps up for years a fistulous opening—a very disagreeable and filthy disease, and one which, as a general rule, can only be cured by the removal of the offending tooth or fang.

The nerve of a tooth may become sufficiently irritated to cause severe pain, which may abate spontaneously in a few minutes or hours, and this may occur repeatedly without continuing, at any one time, until the formation of matter.

It is not uncommon to have a slow inflammation in the sockets of decayed fangs and teeth, which may last for months and cause severe pain in the jaws, face, and even in the temples, without resulting in suppuration or the formation of pus. The pain in such cases is often in sound teeth, and not at all in the one which causes the mischief, and ignorant practitioners not unfrequently extract the sound teeth, which of course affords no relief. If in any case you fail to get relieved from pain in the teeth, jaws, face, or head, by the use of homœopathic remedies, and you think of having a tooth extracted, and the pain is in a sound tooth, or, if in a decayed tooth and you are not satisfied which defective tooth is the cause of the suffering, strike all the decayed teeth and fangs in your mouth with the end of a heavy pencil, key, or some other metallic body, and if you find one more sensitive than the rest have that extracted without any regard to the apparent seat of the pain.

Treatment of Toothache.—First, the preventive treatment. This disease is generally caused by the decay of the teeth; and the early decay of the teeth among Americans, is caused by the violation of the laws of physical development in the management and education of children. The proper consideration of such causes would require a volume. In the author's work on the "Avoidable Causes of Disease" you will find the needed information. Consult the chapters on the conditions requisite for physical development, use and abuse of the digestive organs, children, and education. To prevent your teeth from decaying keep them clean by frequently washing them with water. If the least appearance of decay manifests itself, do not delay a single day, but apply to a good dentist, and have the cavity carefully filled with gold. Do not wait until the tooth begins to ache, for it is generally too late, then, or at least the operation at this late hour will be found very uncertain at best. If your teeth are already badly decayed, and you have useless old shells and fangs, have them extracted, for they tend to contaminate others, and injure the general health. If tartar collects and separates the gums from the teeth apply to a dentist and have it removed occasionally, or it may crowd out the teeth.

In all cases of toothache which results from acute inflammation of the nerve of the tooth, or of the socket, it is very desirable to check the disease before the commencement of suppuration, for if matter once forms, we can do little more than palliate the symptoms until it is discharged; fortunately we can generally cure the disease promptly, if the remedies are applied early.

Aconite is an important remedy in all cases where there is heat about the face and head, fever, and great nervous excitement.

This remedy may be given internally, and when the pain is in a decayed tooth, a part of a drop of the tincture on a little cotton or lint, may be gently pressed into the cavity. *Aconite* will require to be given alternately with some other remedy in case there are fever, heat, and swelling, if it fails to relieve the pain when given alone.

Belladonna is perhaps more frequently required than any other remedy, when the pain is caused by inflammation of the nervous pulp in the tooth, or of the socket. It is also frequently useful for the slow inflammation of the socket, named above. The following are the chief indications for *Belladonna:* sharp pains which are renewed by mental labor, aggravated in the open air, and by the contact of food in chewing, or by applying anything hot. If it is caused by cold, and the face is hot and red, with burning in the head, and attended with fever, heat, and swelling, these are further indications for this remedy. In such cases it may be given alternately with *Aconite*, at intervals of one half an hour or hour. *Phosphorus* is the best remedy when there is pain from inflammation in the sockets around decayed teeth and fangs. Give a dose every hour.

Dose for any of these remedies, see page 7.

Mercurius viv.: Give this remedy when the teeth feel long and loose, and when the pains are excited by cold damp air, or by eating or drinking anything hot or cold, and when the teeth feel sore in their sockets without much pain; in the latter case repeat the remedy night and morning only. Give a dose every hour in acute cases.

Chamomilla will relieve when the pains seem intolerable, beating and stitching, especially at night, and where the pains are aggravated by drinking anything warm, especially coffee. If the pain extends to the face and ear, this remedy will often be useful. Give a dose every hour.

Nux vom. will often do better than either of the above remedies, especially in the case of coffee or whiskey drinkers, or of those who lead a sedentary life, and when the pains are worse at night, early in the morning, in the open air, or during mental labor. Give a dose every hour.

Pulsatilla, when there is a toothache with earache, and pain in the side of the head; aggravation or renewal of the pains in the evening, or at night after midnight, and in a warm room, and from eating warm substances, relief from cold water and cool fresh air. Repeat every hour or two.

Bryonia is a valuable remedy, when there are drawing pains, with looseness of the teeth, a sensation of elongation, especially during and after a meal, and when there is soreness of the gums. If the pains are of a rheumatic character, which may be suspected when the patient has recently been, or is at present, subject to rheumatic pains elsewhere, *Bryonia* is one of the most important remedies. In such cases, it will often require to be followed by *Rhus tox.* In obstinate cases, consult the sections on rheumatism and neuralgia.

For the toothache of children, *Aconite*, *Belladonna*, or *Chamomilla*, is generally required, or *Coffea*, if there is great nervous sensibility. To prevent a return, give *Mercurius viv.* every night for a week, and then give *Calcarea carb.* every night.

For toothache during pregnancy, give *Sepia*, *Calcarea carb.* or *Belladonna*. During nursing, give *China* three or four times a day, and any other remedy which may seem indicated, every hour during the pain.

SORE THROAT (ANGINA FAUCIUM)

We have simple diffused inflammation of the throat; membranous inflammation, or diphtheria, which sometimes assumes a maglignant form; and inflammation of the tonsils or quinsy.

The first variety, or simple inflammation, is the most common form of sore throat. It is seated in the mucous membrane, but sometimes extends to the cellular structure beneath. It is characterized by increased redness and fullness of the membrane, but without much swelling. The uvula or end of the palate sometimes hangs down like a bag of water, and may be paler than natural. There is soreness, irritation, or tickling, a frequent disposition to hawk and spit, a feeling of choking, and a difficulty in swallowing and speaking. There is often some deafness, arising from the extension of the inflammation to the Eustachian tube or the passage which extends from the throat to the ear. The severity of the fever will depend, in a great measure, on the severity of the local affection. The causes of simple sore throat are the usual causes of catarrhal diseases, such as sudden changes of temperature and exposure.

Treatment.—When there is much fever, or heat of surface, a few doses of *Aconite* should be given, one every hour, and this remedy alone will sometimes cure the disease, but generally either *Belladonna* or *Ignatia*, will be required after *Aconite.*

Belladonna may be given when there are sore pains, burning, spasmodic contraction, with a constant desire to swallow, and a free flow of saliva, with fever and pain in the forehead.

Ignatia.—Give this remedy when there are burning and sore pains when swallowing, and a sensation as if a lump or crumb were in the throat, causing a constant inclination to swallow. Give a dose of either this remedy or *Belladonna* every hour.

Mercurius viv. may follow either of the above remedies when there is a profuse flow of saliva, difficult swallowing, especially of drinks, or on empty swallowing, and when there is a chill toward evening, and an aggravation at night, or in the open air. Repeat the doses once in two hours.

Lachesis will often be found useful in case the above remedies fail, especially if there are a burning and dry throat with a constant inclination to swallow, and a sensation as if a lump were sticking in the throat; aggravation in the afternoon, morning, and especially after sleeping, also from contact—relief from eating.

Chamomilla may be given when there are tickling and cough, especially useful in the case of women and children.

Continue a remedy as long as there is any improvement, but if no change is effected, at the end of from twelve to twenty-four hours, select some other remedy.

Dose of either of the above remedies, see page 7.

MEMBRANOUS SORE THROAT, OR DIPHTHERIA.

There are two forms of this disease, the one active and inflammatory, with a full pulse, hot and dry skin, the other malignant, with a low fever, small pulse, and cool extremities.

Diphtheria is characterized by the formation of a false membrane of lymph, or fibrinous matter, on the surface of the mucous membrane of the throat. The patches are of various extent, sometimes small and only here and there one, in other cases covering almost the entire throat, and sometimes extending up into the nose, or down into the air passages. In mild cases they are separate, small, and of a white or ashy color, presenting the appearance of superficial sloughs, or of ulcers, for which they are often mistaken; but in other instances they are connected, and form one uniform crust. In some cases the membrane is thin, but in others it is thick, sometimes soft, but in other instances it is dense and tough. In some of the worst, or malignant cases, the false membrane is discolored by the exudation of bloody and vitiated secretions of the throat, so as to present the appearance of mortification, and the offensive discharge and breath cause it to still more closely resemble the latter affection, but it is extremely rare, even in the most malignant form of the disease that there are actual mortification and sloughing; still they sometimes occur. The fever which attends the disease will be in keeping with the local affection. If the mucous membrane of the throat is bright red, and the patches light-colored, the fever will be active and inflammatory; whereas, if the mucous membrane is dark colored or livid, and the false membrane discolored, dark, offensive, manifesting a malignant form of local disease, the fever will be of a low typhus character, with rapid and feeble pulse, delirium, followed by stupor, sunken face, cold extremities and great exhaustion. This form of the disease is frequently epidemic, especially among those who inhabit crowded dwellings, and the poor and ill-fed classes of the community. Sometimes there are great sinking of the vital powers, prostration and death early in the disease, without the occurrence of marked symptoms of putridity.

The symptoms of diphtheria are similar to those of ordinary sore throat, excepting what we discover by an examination of the throat. If the breath is very offensive and the fever is of a typhoid character with sore throat, or if there is unusual prostration, we may suspect the existence of this false membrane, but we may have the latter without such symptoms.

There are two sources of danger, one from the malignant character of the disease, and the other from the extension of the false membrane to the air passages, when it causes symptoms similar to those of the worst form of croup. Hoarseness, a hoarse cough, and paroxysms of difficult breathing, should lead you to fear the extension of the disease to the larynx and trachea. When such symptoms occur, in addition to what is said in this section, consult the sections on laryngitis and croup.

Treatment.—If the fever is high, the skin hot, the breath not very offensive, and the patches of false membrane light colored, *Aconite* will be found of great service at the commencement of the disease. Give it alternately with *Mercurius prot.* at intervals of one hour.

Mercurius prot. is generally the most important remedy when the disease is not of a malignant character, and even when it is, it will often be of great service at the commencement of the attack. If the fever is very high and the skin hot, give *Aconite* alternately with it; but if the fever is less active, *Belladonna* may be given one hour and *Mercurius prot.* the next. You will not expect as immediate relief as in cases of simple sore throat, and after you have carefully selected a remedy, you should not change it for another sooner than twenty-four or forty-eight hours, unless the patient is manifestly getting worse. *Mercurius prot.* may require to be given for four or five days, or even longer in some cases, but if at the end of two or three days no impression is made on the symptoms, it will be better to omit the *Mercurius prot.* and give in its place *Mercurius viv.*

Dose of either of the remedies named, see page 7.

Lachesis: When the acute symptoms are somewhat releived, and the fever is less active, this remedy may be given either alone or alternately with *Mercurius*, at intervals of one hour, especially if there is a sensation as if a foreign body were sticking in the throat, and the symptoms are worse after sleeping. If sudden and alarming prostration ensues, either at the commencement of the disease, or during its progress, with cold extremities and small pulse, give either six globules or a drop of the *Tincture of camphor* every ten minutes, until the prostration is relieved.

If croupy symptoms occur, or the patient begins to be troubled with a hoarse or a squeaking cough, and paroxysms of difficult breathing come on, especially after midnight, give *Lachesis* every hour, and if it does not soon afford relief, alternate it with *Hepar sulph.* at intervals of one hour, and apply large towels wrung from hot water, over the throat, neck, and chest, as hot as the patient can bear without burning or blistering the skin, and apply dry flannels over the wet cloths. Change the wet towels every ten or fifteen minutes, when there is much difficulty of breathing; at other times once an hour.

In the putrid or malignant form of diphtheria other remedies will often be required, but *Merc. prot.*, *Mercurius viv.*, and *Lachesis*, are generally very useful during the earlier stages of the disease, and *Lachesis* at a later period. Then at the commencement of such cases, when the breath is offensive, the extremities cool, and there is great debility, give *Mercurius prot.* every hour alternately with *Rhus. tox.*, and if, at the end of two or three days, the symptoms are getting worse, omit the *Mercurius* and give *Lachesis* alternately with *Rhus tox.*

Arsenicum: If, notwithstanding the use of the above remedies, the symptoms get steadily worse, the breath more offensive, the throat dark and putrid, the extremities cool, omit the *Mercurius* and give *Arsenicum* alternately with *Lachesis*, at intervals of one hour.

Carbo veg. may be substituted for *Lachesis* if the pulse becomes small or irregular, and the extremities cold.

China: This remedy may be given night and morning after the disease is cured, for the debility which it causes.

General Direction, Diet, &c.—A dry, light, and airy room is very important, in this as in almost all other diseases. The patient may wash the mouth and gargle the throat with a tea made by pouring boiling water on dried apples. The diet in all cases of of inflammation of the throat, except when there is a decided malignant tendency, must be light, consisting of rice water, arrow-root, thin flour gruel, soft boiled rice, or soft toast, if the patient can swallow it without difficulty; to which may be added in malignant cases, especially when there is great prostration of strength, milk, thin custard, and beef-tea; as the patient recovers, mutton-broth, and even beef or mutton, if the patient can chew and swallow it. The diet must very gradually be made more nutritious.

QUINSY (INFLAMMATION OF THE TONSILS).

We have superficial inflammation of the tonsils in the varieties of sore throat we have been considering; but the disease now under consideration, consists in a phlegmonous or deep-seated inflammation of the body of the tonsil itself. The following are the symptoms of this disease: A sense of fullness in the throat, pain and difficulty of swallowing, heat and dryness of the throat, and shooting pains in the ear. The voice has a croaking sound, and on examination we find one or both tonsils projecting, and the surrounding parts more or less swollen and covered with mucus. In severe cases the swelling may be so great as to almost close the throat, and even to impede respiration. The fever attending this disease is generally active and inflammatory, with hot skin and full pulse. If the inflammation is violent, and not soon relieved, but continues active several days, it generally terminates in an abscess; but if less active, it may continue several days and abate without the formation of matter. The distress caused by large abscesses in the tonsils is very great; the formation of pus is often announced by throbbing in the part, and slight chills. Those who have once had this disease are more liable to be attacked than others. The causes are sudden changes of temperature, exposure, especially of the neck, &c.

Treatment.—*Aconite* and *Belladonna* are the principal remedies at the commencement of the disease, if the fever is high, the skin hot, and the pulse full, especially if there are pricking or shooting, pains during the act of swallowing, with spasmodic contraction, and if the throat presents a bright red appearance, with swelling of the palate, uvula, tonsils, and of the glands of the neck. Give a dose of *Aconite* every hour for six hours, and if, at the end of that period, there is no improvement, alternate it with *Belladonna* at intervals of one hour.

Dose of this or other remedies, see page 7.

Ignatia may be given instead of *Belladonna*, at the commencement, or follow that remedy, when there is a sensation of a crumb or lump in the throat when not swallowing; burning and excoriation when swallowing, and shooting pains which extend to the cheeks and ears, are also indications for this remedy.

Mercurius viv. often follows the above remedies to advantage, especially when there is a profuse secretion of saliva, and empty swallowing is more painful than that of liquids. Give a dose once in two hours.

Lachesis may be given once in two hours, if the disease threatens to go on to the formation of an abscess, notwithstanding the use of the above remedies, or at the commencement before giving them, when the pain is aggravated by the slightest external pressure, when the symptoms are worse after sleeping, and when there is a sensation of a lump or crumb in the throat.

A cloth wrung from cold water may be applied over the neck, and several thicknesses of dry flannel over that. Wet the cloth once in six hours. If there is no relief at the end of twenty-four hours, wring cloths from hot water and apply, and change often. Steaming the throat over hot water, may be useful in obstinate cases. No animal food or food in substance should be allowed until the inflammation is subdued, simply rice-water, gruel, arrowroot, &c.

CHRONIC ENLARGEMENT OF THE TONSILS.

This is a very common disease, especially in young persons of a scrofulous habit. *Calcarea carb.* is the principal remedy. Give a dose every night for one month, then give *Sulphur* for one week, and follow it by *Calcarea carb.* *Sepia* and *Hepar sulph.* may be given in the same manner afterward if necessary. If the symptoms are aggravated by taking cold, a few doses of *Aconite*, *Belladonna*, or *Ignatia*, will be required.

FOLLICULAR INFLAMMATION OF THE THROAT.

There is sometimes a chronic inflammation and enlargement of the follicles of the tonsils and throat, which results in the secretion of a cheesy matter, until those sacks are so far distended and enlarged, as to allow these little accretions to be hawked and raised up with the secretions of the throat. These masses vary from the size of a pin's head to that of a pea, and are often mistaken for tubercles from the lungs, but may always be distinguished by the peculiarly nauseous odor which arises when they are crushed between the fingers. Tubercles are nearly odorless.

Lachesis is the chief remedy for this disease, and a dose may be given every night. After this symptom is in a great measure relieved, give *Silicea* every night, and afterward *Calcarea carb.*, to preveut a return of the disease.

CELLULAR INFLAMMATION OF THE THROAT.

Inflammation and suppuration sometimes take place in the cellular tissue, back of the throat, between it and the bones of the spine. When there is a deep-seated pain in the throat, tenderness upon pressure from without, stiffness of the neck, great difficulty in swallowing, suppression of the voice and difficulty of breathing, carefully examine the back part of the throat, for you will have reason to fear the existence of this disease. If you find the parts are much swollen, and the symptoms have been of several days' duration, and you have reason to fear that an abscess has formed, especially if the pain is throbbing, and the patient has chills, send for a physician, for the abscess should be lanced early, otherwise it may burst suddenly, and, by overwhelming the air passages, may cause suffocation, a result which I have known to occur in one instance. But if the disease is promptly and early treated, an abscess can generally be prevented. This is a rare disease.

Treatment —The chief remedies are *Aconite* and *Belladonna*, to be given as directed in simple sore throat. If the symptoms are not very acute, or even if they are, after they are somewhat relieved, *Mercurius viv.* and *Pulsatilla* will be preferable, and may be given in alternation, at intervals of one or two hours. If, notwithstanding the above remedies, the disease threatens to go on to the formation of an abscess, give *Lachesis* every hour.

If an abscess forms, an incision should be made for the escape of the pus, as near the centre of the back of the throat as possible, so as to avoid arterial branches; but you had better send for a physician, and not make the attempt to lance it yourself.

INFLAMMATION OF THE GULLET OR PASSAGE TO THE STOMACH (ŒSOPHAGITIS).

This is a rare affection unless caused directly by irritating substances, yet it sometimes occurs. A sense of heat and pain, increased by swallowing, frequently referred to the lower part of the throat, or else to the upper part of the stomach, is one of the first symptoms, no matter what part of the tube is affected. Swallowing is difficult, and sometimes impossible; hiccough is a frequent symptom. There is usually little or no fever. Sometimes the membranous inflammation of diphtheria extends down this passage. In some instances ulcers and even an abscess result, but rarely. This disease is sometimes chronic. It may be caused by very hot or corrosive substances, mechanical injuries, exposure, &c.

Treatment.—If the disease has been caused by mechanical injuries, or by burns, put one drop of *Arnica* into a glass of water, and give a spoonful every hour or two.

Belladonna, when the disease arises from cold or exposure, is the chief remedy. Give a dose once in two hours. If *Belladonna* fails to relieve, give *Arsenicum* alternately with it. *Sulphur* may follow the above remedies. This remedy and *Arsenicum* are also useful when the disease becomes chronic.

STRICTURE OF THE ŒSOPHAGUS OR GULLET.

Stricture of the passage occasionally occurs. It may be of the upper, or quite as frequently of the lower portion of the tube. It may be but slight, simply sufficient to cause the patient to choke readily on attempting to swallow large pieces of meat or bread, or it may gradually increase so as to entirely obstruct the passage.

Treatment.—Give *Nux vomica* at night and *Sulphur* in the morning for one month; then give *Arsenicum* in the morning for a month; then *Silicea.* If the patient becomes choked by meat, or other food, it is sometimes necessary to crowd it down into the stomach by the aid of a probang, or a small sponge fastened securely on the end of a long slender piece of whale-bone.

SPASM OF THE ŒSOPHAGUS OR GULLET.

Spasm of the passage may be distinguished from permanent stricture by its coming on suddenly, and by the ability to swallow readily at times, when the spasm is not on. The food is arrested, and is often rejected immediately if the spasm is at the upper part of the œsophagus: if it is lower down, it may remain for some time and then rise by regurgitation. Occasionally after the food has been a short time in contact with the stricture, the latter gives way, and the food passes into the stomach.

Treatment.—*Belladonna* is one of the best remedies for this difficulty, and may be given three or four times a day. *Nux vomica* may follow *Belladonna* and be given every night. Continue the above remedies several weeks, and if they do not entirely cure the disease give *Cuprum* every night.

INFLAMMATION OF THE STOMACH.

(GASTRITIS)

This disease is generally caused by substances taken into the stomach, either improper articles, or such as are wholesome in excessive quantities. It is often a very rapid disease, sometimes terminating fatally in a few hours, or within two or three days; or it may extend two or three weeks, and even become chronic; or the patient may recover. Acid and corrosive poisons, when taken into the stomach, cause this disease.

Symptoms.—Intense pain in the region of the stomach, with a peculiar feeling of distress extending up under the breast-bone, and to the sides, beneath the short ribs. There is frequently a burning sensation, sometimes extending up the œsophagus or gullet. Pressure, swallowing, and breathing, aggravate the suffering; vomiting is very common and very distressing, and alternates with nausea and retching. At first the contents of the stomach and bilious matters are thrown up; afterward simply mucus, perhaps mixed with blood. There are excessive thirst, and a craving for cold drinks, which are rejected the moment they are taken, and but increase the sufferings of the patient. There are heat and fullness in the region of the stomach. The countenance, in severe cases, is pale, sunken, and altered, and there is great prostration of strength, with a frequent and small pulse, and cold extremities. In less severe cases, the countenance, early in the disease, may be flushed, and the skin hot, dry, and harsh. If the inflammation does not extend to the bowels they are generally costive; the urine is scanty and high colored; the edges of the tongue are generally red, and the centre covered with a thick, flaky fur.

Chronic inflammation of the stomach not unfrequently follows the acute form of the disease, or it may come on gradually without any severe attack. It may be caused by an indigestible and irritating diet, acrid medicines, ice water, alcoholic drinks, and exposure. The local symptoms differ but little from those of the acute variety, except in degree, and in being more variable. There is pain or uneasiness more or less constant, which is generally increased by eating. Hot liquids, tea or water, usually aggravate or induce pain; whereas, in dyspepsia, they generally relieve the sufferings temporarily. There is tenderness on pressure at the pit of the stomach, and sometimes a gnawing sensation. Great faintness at the pit of the stomach, or a gone feeling, is not uncommon. There may be loss of appetite, a variable appetite, or an unnatural craving for food, even for the most inappropriate articles. Various sympathetic symptoms frequently occur, such as headache, confusion of thought, sleeplessness, and distressing dreams; derangements of sight, hearing, and of sensation; a hard, sounding spasmodic cough; irritation of the urinary passages and of the genital apparatus; a scaly and dry pimply eruption on the skin. In inveterate cases, there is emaciation, with an inability to pinch up the skin, owing to its being drawn tight over the muscles. There is sometimes hectic fever.

Treatment of the Acute Form of the Disease.—If the inflammation has been caused by a poisonous substance, consult the section on poisons, and follow the directions there given, until the poisonous substance is either evacuated from the stomach, or properly antidoted, then follow the directions in this section; only if *Arsenic* has caused the disease, do not give *Arsenicum.*

Aconite should generally be given at the commencement of all acute attacks of this disease; even if the pulse is small and frequent, and the surface of the body cool, it will be well to give a few doses of this remedy every half hour or hour. If in such cases there is excessive nausea, alternate it with *Veratrum* at intervals of one half hour. If at the end of a few hours the prostration and coldness are increasing, omit the *Aconite* aad give *Arsenicum* alternately with *Veratrum*, in the same manner, until there is a manifest improvement, then lengthen the intervals to one or two hours.

Dose of these or other remedies, see page 7.

If the vomiting is frequent, either give the medicine dry, or dissolve it in a very small quantity of water, and give the patient but a few drops of the liquid at a time for a dose.

In all cases, if symptoms of great prostration come on, either at the commencement of the disease or later, with burning pain and excessive nausea, *Veratrum* and *Arsenicum* are our main remedies. But in case there is high febrile excitement at the commencement, or if the attack is not very severe, other remedies will often do better. In such cases *Aconite* will require to be continued longer, or until the acute febrile symptoms are relieved; and if there is incessant vomiting, with pain in the stomach, anxiety, restlessness and difficulty of breathing, *Ipecac* may be given alternately with it. *Belladonna* may follow *Aconite* if there are cerebral or head symptoms, such as pain in the head, delirium, or stupor, and may be given alternately with *Ipecac*, or if *Ipecac* fails to relieve the nausea and vomiting, alternately with *Veratrum*.

Bryonia: If the disease has been caused by cold drinks, taken when the patient was hot and in a perspiration, and there is a feeling of weight or load at the pit of the stomach, give this remedy. *Bryonia* will also be found useful when the disease continues several days, with slow fever which is not relieved by other remedies. Give a dose once in from one to two hours.

If the vomiting is excessive and long continued, and the patient very thirsty, keep the stomach empty, but give injections of rice-water, arrow-root, or corn-starch, two or three times a day, not to move the bowels, but to relieve the thirst and supply the system with fluids and nourishment. In all cases nothing more than boiled water, thin arrow root, rice-water, or toast-water, should be used until the inflammation is subdued, and then gradually make these warm drinks thicker, and very slowly return to a more substantial diet. You cannot be too careful. Warm applications over the stomach sometimes afford some relief. At the very commencement, if there is great nausea, but not free vomiting, and you have reason to suppose that indigestible or improper food remains in the stomach, let the patient drink freely of warm water (all he can) until he vomits. Aid by tickling the throat with the finger, if necessary.

Treatment of Chronic Inflammation of the Stomach.—Give *Arsenicum* night and morning when there are acrid and bitter eructations, dry or red tongue, great thirst, nausea, burning pains in the pit of the stomach, and great sensitiveness on pressure. If there is much nausea or vomiting, which *Arsenicum* does not relieve, give an occasional dose of *Veratrum*.

Nux. vom. may precede or follow *Arsenicum* when there are bitter eructations, nausea, and vomiting of food, tension and pressure in the region of the stomach, constipation, headache, confusion of mind, restlessness or peevishness; give a dose before every meal until the symptoms are in a great measure relieved, then give a dose at night, and a dose of *Sulphur* in the morning. If *Nux vom.* fails to relieve the above symptoms, especially if the patient is a female, give *Pulsatilla* in the same manner.

If the symptoms are relieved by eating, give *Lachesis* before every meal; and if other remedies fail to entirely remove the symptoms, give *Carbo veg* night and morning.

A warm bath every day, or once in two days, is a very important auxiliary. Stimulants must be avoided, and the diet unirritating, but more nourishing than in the acute form of the disease. A milk diet often does well when it agrees with the patient.

NEURALGIA OF THE STOMACH (GASTRALGIA)

This affection is frequently confounded with spasms of the stomach, and in fact the two diseases sometimes coexist. Neuralgia of the stomach is often connected with a general neuralgic predisposition; in other cases with either rheumatic or a gouty diathesis. It frequently attacks patients recovering from acute diseases, and those exhausted by profuse discharges. Nursing females are very subject to it. Mental emotions, and improper articles of food, may cause an attack of this disease. The pain is usually acute and severe, sometimes occurring in shocks, like electric shocks, causing the patient to start suddenly. The pain may leave altogether for a time, then return suddenly; it may be relieved by pressure, but not always. The pain is less constant than in chronic inflammation of the stomach, and the appetite is often unimpaired. Hot drinks generally temporarily relieve the suffering in this affection, whereas, they aggravate it in cases of chronic inflammation.

Treatment.—*Nux vomica* is one of the most important remedies for this disease, especially when the pains are severe like an electric shock, or the attack has been caused by improper diet, and the pains are worse after a meal, at night or in the morning. In such cases, if *Nux Vomica* fails to relieve, give *Pulsatilla*. Give a dose of either every hour.

Dose of the above or other remedies, see page 7.

Belladonna: Give this remedy when there are violent lancinating or cutting pains in the pit of the stomach, and also if the pains are brought on by eating or drinking.

In the case of weak and exhausted persons, *China* is the most important remedy, especially to prevent a return of the paroxysms. For this purpose give a dose three or four times a day. If nursing females have this disease, *Belladonna* or *Nux vomica* may be given during the paroxysms of pain, and *Pulsatilla* may be given at night and *China* in the morning during the intervals, to prevent a return of the symptoms. Also, consult the general directions under the head of neuralgia and follow them.

If the patient is subject to gout or rheumatism, *Bryonia* will often be found useful, and if this fails *Nux vomica* or *Pulsatilla* will generally be required, *Nux vom.* in the case of men, and *Pulsatilla* for women. If one fails give the other. Also consult the sections on rheumatism and gout.

SPASMS OF THE STOMACH,

OR CRAMP IN THE STOMACH.

This disease is characterized by paroxysms of pain, stricture, and spasmodic contraction in the region of the stomach. In the intervals between the spasms the patient may be free, or nearly free from pain. The stomach sometimes feels as if it were gathered in a ball, and in some instances as if drawn backward. Pressure often affords partial relief, and the patient generally bends forward. The spasms may be slight, or so severe as to cause screams from the most resolute individual. The pulse and skin may remain natural in moderate cases, but when the spasm is very violent, the pulse sometimes becomes small and fluttering, and the skin covered with a cold clammy sweat, and even death sometimes ensues, but very rarely. When the disease has been caused by offending matters in the stomach, there is often nausea and vomiting between the paroxysms. Spasms of the stomach are frequently caused by indigestible food, such as unripe fruit, boiled cabbage, lobsters, clams, &c.; even cheese and honey will cause the disease in some individuals. Gout, rheumatism, spinal irritation, intemperance, or the use of tobacco, may cause this affection. Hysterical females are very subject to it. When a predisposition exists, the least irregularity of diet, or unusual mental emotion, may induce an attack.

Treatment.—*Nux vomica* is perhaps more frequently indicated than any other remedy, especially when the disease attacks the intemperate, coffee-drinkers, or tobacco-users; also when the attack occurs after eating. This remedy may be selected when there are contractive cramp-like pains in the stomach, with pressure as of a load or weight, and a sensation as if the clothes were too tight over the stomach. Repeat the remedy every hour.

Dose, see page 7.

Pulsatilla may be given if *Nux vomica* aggravates the symptoms, or fails to relieve. It may be given at the commencement if there are heartburn and acrid vomiting, especially if the patient is a female. If the above remedies fail, give *Ignatia* every half hour.

Chamomilla will be found useful for spasms of the stomach, particularly for persons who are addicted to the use of coffee, when *Nux vom.* fails to relieve such cases, and also in the case of children, when the stomach is distended with air or gas.

Give *Bryonia* if the patient is subject to rheumatism or gout, especially if there is a sensation of weight or load at the pit of the stomach between the spasms, and *Nux vom.* fails to relieve the symptoms.

Carlo veg.: If the above remedies fail to afford relief, or only partially relieve the suffering, give this remedy once in six hours. *Carbo veg.* is especially useful to prevent a return of the spasms. For this purpose give a dose morning and noon, one half an hour before eating, and a dose of either *Nux vom.* or *Pulsatilla*, before tea and at bedtime. To eradicate a predisposition to this disease, continue the above remedies for four weeks, then give *Sulphur* every night, or if the patient is young and of full habit, and apt to bleed from the nose, or a female, and subject to frequent and profuse menstrual discharges, give *Calcarea carb.* every night.

The patient should shun all articles which excite attacks of the disease, and live on plain, easily digested food, spend his time in the fresh air and sunlight, and take regular active exercise.

WATERBRASH (PYROSIS).

This is a paroxysmal disease, commencing with a spasmodic sensation in the stomach, accompanied by an irritation of the mucous membrane, resulting in a profuse watery secretion, which either flows from the stomach and mouth in a constant stream, or is removed by eructations; after which the pain and spasm gradually abate. The attacks more frequently occur in the morning or forenoon, when the stomach is empty, but they may happen at any time, and are very apt to be repeated. Very little is known in regard to the causes of this disease. It generally attacks those whose digestive organs are debilitated.

Treatment.—*Bryonia* is more frequently required than any other remedy, and it will generally cure the disease. Give a dose during the attack, and before every meal, one half hour before eating. Give *Nux vom.* in the case of drunkards or those accustomed to high living.

If the water which is discharged is sour or acrid, give *Pulsatilla* before every meal. If the disease is not entirely cured by the above remedies, give *Carbo veg.* every night for a few weeks, then omit it and give *Calcarea carb.* once or twice a week.

HEARTBURN, SOUR STOMACH, ERUCTATIONS.

These are generally symptoms of deranged or weak digestion, and in addition to what is said below, consult the section on dyspepsia. If the food we eat instead of being digested, decomposes in the stomach, it gives rise to acidity and heartburn. Sometimes there is an excessive secretion of acid by the stomach itself, causing a burning sensation, which may extend up the œsophagus or gullet. In either case the patient may be troubled by sour eructations and even vomiting. Such symptoms are very common during pregnancy. Occasionally there are offensive eructations, resembling in smell, rotten eggs; such frequently precede a diarrhœa, when the latter is caused by undigested food. Sometimes the eructations are bitter.

Treatment. - Shun all alkalies, for they simply neutralize the acid in the stomach for the time being, and they weaken the digestive organs, and thereby increase the evil.

Nux vomica: Give this remedy night and morning, and at any time when the patient is suffering from heartburn, sour or bitter eructations, especially if the bowels are costive. If it fails to relieve, give *Pulsatilla* in the same manner

Dose of this or other remedies named, see page 7.

Pulsatilla: Give this remedy for heartburn, sour stomach, or sour eructations, especially if the bowels are loose: also for eructations smelling like rotten eggs, and if it fails to relieve, give *Chamomilla.* Give a dose night and morning, and one when the patient is suffering.

Give *Bryonia* for bitter eructations, if *Nux vom.* fails to relieve. It is sometimes useful for heartburn, if the stomach feels distended, and there is either headache or pains in the limbs.

As soon as the symptoms are somewhat relieved by the above remedies, give a dose of *Calcarea carb.* every night for two weeks; then give *Hepar sulph.* for a week or two. *Carbo veg.* may follow the above remedies, if there is any disposition to a return of the symptoms. As to diet, consult the section on dyspepsia.

HICCOUGH.

This symptom is generally connected either with derangement of the digestive organs, or with an irritation of the stomach. It is caused by a spasmodic contraction of the midriff or diaphragm. In severe cases, even the muscles of the abdomen, and other muscles of the chest, may be involved in the involuntary action, causing a shaking of the whole trunk.

Treatment.—*Nux. vom.* is generally the most important remedy. Give a dose every half hour, until this symptom abates, then give it every night to prevent a return. *Ignatia* is next in importance, and may be given if *Nux. vom.* fails. *Belladonna* will sometimes be required, and may be given as directed for *Nux vom.*

SEA-SICKNESS.

This disease is the same as that which is produced by riding backward in a close carriage, or by whirling around. The disease is evidently produced by the impressions made on the brain by the unusual motion; and that the impressions made through the organs of sight have much to do with causing this disease, is evident, from the fact that the symptoms are materially relieved, if the eyes are closed.. The symptoms are lessened, although not generally entirely relieved, by keeping the horizontal position. The sick stomach is often preceded and accompanied by dizziness, and even headache; and these symptoms sometimes remain for several days after landing from the ship or carriage.

Treatment.—If an individual is liable to this affection, a dose of *Nux vomica* taken a few hours previous to going on board a ship, or into a carriage, will often prevent the disease. This remedy will sometimes check the symptoms if taken at the commencement of the dizziness or headache, and it will generally relieve the latter symptoms if they continue after leaving the ship or carriage.

While seasick take *Ipecac* alternately with *Nux vom.*, one hour apart, and if they fail, take *Arsenicum* once in two hours. In obstinate cases, omit other remedies for a time, and take *Sulphur* once in six hours.

Dose, see page 7.

NAUSEA AND VOMITING,

Sickness of the stomach and vomiting may be sympathetic, arising from irritation of the brain, as in sea-sickness, inflammation of the brain, concussion of the brain from a fall or blow, dizziness and threatening symptoms of apoplexy, sick-headache, offensive odors, disgusting sights, &c., or from sympathy with the womb, as during pregnancy, or when there are ulcerations on, or displacement of, this organ. In all such cases consult the section on the disease from which the patient may be suffering. Also when it occurs during fevers, inflammation of the stomach, and other diseases, do the same.

Sickness of the stomach and vomiting may arise from an irritation of the stomach, which does not amount to inflammation. This may be supposed to be the case when there is no fever, frequency of pulse or pain, or evidence of disease in other parts. It may arise from overloading the stomach, and intemperance; also from the debility of this organ, which results from the want of active exercise, masturbation, and from over mental exertion. In all such cases the patient should shun the causes which produce the symptoms.

Treatment.—Give *Ipecac* for sickness of the stomach, caused by overeating, and if it does not soon relieve, let the patient drink freely of tepid water until he either vomits freely or the nausea is relieved; then give another dose of *Ipecac.* If *Ipecac* fails to relieve, give *Veratrum.* If the stomach is sour give *Pulsatilla* instead of *Veratrum.*

Give *Nux vomica* if the patient is intemperate, also if the disease results from over mental exertion or from lack of exercise. In obstinate cases give *Sulphur* every night for a week, then *Arsenicum* or *Carbo veg.* may be of service. As to diet, consult the section on dyspepsia.

VOMITING OF BLOOD (HÆMATEMESIS).

This affection may result from mechanical injuries, over-exertion, rupture of the vessels of the stomach from chronic ulceration or violent vomiting. It sometimes results from a sudden suppression of the menses, and in other cases suppression of the discharge from bleeding piles.

Treatment.—If the disease has been caused by mechanical injuries, or by over-exertion, give *Arnica* alternately with *Ipecac,* at intervals of half an hour.

If the blood is of a bright red color, and there is fullness and uneasiness of the stomach, and the patient is of a full habit, and the affection has not been caused by a mechanical injury, give *Aconite* alternately with *Ipecac,* at intervals of half an hour. If suppression of the menses is the cause, give *Pulsatilla* every hour, and follow it with *Nux vomica* if necessary. If caused by a suppression of the discharge from bleeding piles, give *Nux vomica* every hour, and a dose of *Sulphur* at night.

Give *Arsenicum* if the patient has been suffering from chronic inflammation of the stomach, and there is burning pain or soreness. In such cases *Carbo veg.* may follow *Arsenicum*, or be given alternately with it at intervals of two or three hours. In any case if the patient loses a large quantity of blood, and becomes faint, give *China* every half hour until the latter symptom is relieved. Quiet and rest of mind and body are essential.

Let the diet be light and unirritating for some days; all drinks should be cold; and a cloth wrung from cold water and placed over the stomach during the attack of hemorrhage will be useful.

DYSPEPSIA OR INDIGESTION.

This affection is often confounded with chronic inflammation of the stomach, but it is very important to distinguish between these two diseases, as in one case the stomach is simply weakened and unable to perform its functions from this cause; whereas, in the other it is owing to undue excitement that this organ fails. The following are among the causes of this disease: Sedentary habits; intense and protracted study, or absorbing mental emotions, by calling off the nervous energy from the stomach, cause this disease; also errors of diet, a change from an active to a sedentary or inactive mode of life, over-eating, the use of alcoholic liquors, high-seasoned food, spices, tea, coffee, and narcotics. Beyond all question the use of tobacco is one of the most fruitful causes of the prevalence of this disease among Americans. Let every dyspeptic who uses this poisonous weed read the chapter on tobacco, in the author's work on the "Avoidable Causes of Disease," and let every parent who cares for the health, morals and lives of his sons, place that work in their hands if possible, before they have commenced its use, as prevention is far better than cure.

Symptoms of Dyspepsia.—A feeling of vague uneasiness in the region of the stomach, which does not amount to pain, but is often worse than pain, is one of the most prominent symptoms.

This symptom often extends to the chest, sides, and even shoulders, and upper parts of the arm, especially on the left side. The uneasiness is often greatest when the stomach is empty, and is frequently changed after eating to a feeling of fullness, distension, and weight. Patients frequently strike themselves over the stomach and sides, so as to change the sensation. Sometimes there is a slight sensation of heat, or burning and gnawing pain, which arises from irritation of the stomach. Not unfrequently there are spasmodic or neuralgic pains and distension from flatulency. The appetite may be impaired or wanting, craving or perverted. There is frequently a gone or sinking sensation at the pit of the stomach, especially when the disease has been caused by the use of tea. Eructations of wind, and regurgitations of sour, bitter, acrid, oily, or offensive liquids, are common symptoms; there may be water-brash or vomiting. Heaviness of the head, dizziness, headache, perverted visions; ringing in the ears, pains between the shoulders, and in various parts of the body, not unfrequently occur; also stricture or uneasiness about the throat, and irritation of the throat and larynx, with a frequent inclination to clear the throat, and a sensation of coldness between the shoulders, are not uncommon symptoms. The patient is apt to be low-spirited, irritable, anxious, fretful and apprehensive. Not unfrequently patients imagine themselves affected with consumption or disease of the heart, and the frequent occurrence of palpitation and irregularity of the pulse, tend to confirm them in their impressions. Unpleasant dreams disturb the sleep; the bowels are generally constipated; the surface of the body dry and of unequal temperature. The feet and hands may be cold or hot, and sometimes there is a profuse perspiration. The urine may be almost colorless, or scanty and high colored. The symptoms above enumerated are not all present in every case.

As has been stated, it is important to distinguish this disease from chronic inflammation of the stomach, for the two affections require very different treatment. In cases of chronic inflammation, the pain is generally more severe, and there is greater tenderness, on pressure, over the stomach; vomiting is more common, and the pulse more frequent, than in dyspepsia. The tongue, especially its edges, is often red, which is seldom the case in dyspepsia. When there is mucus, blood, or dark matter, like coffee grounds, thrown up by vomiting, inflammation may be inferred; and the same is true when hot or stimulating drinks increase the uneasiness in the stomach, for such drinks generally relieve the dyspeptic, and food is more acceptable to the latter. Diarrhœa is more frequent in cases of chronic inflammation, than in dyspepsia, and the same is true of febrile excitement.

Treatment.—As in this disease the gastric juice is either lessened in quantity or deteriorated in quality, which allows the food to be decomposed instead of being digested, it is all-important that the patient abstain entirely from drinking with his meals, so as not to dilute the gastric juice. The patient should also abstain from drinking for one hour before eating, and for at least two or three hours after eating. He may gratify his thirst at other periods. We can only expect to permanently cure this or any other chronic disease, by removing the cause; therefore the reader will do well to consult the chapters on the use and abuse of the digestive organs, the conditions requisite for physical development and preservation, excessive labor, and amusements, in the author's work on the "Avoidable Causes of Disease," and he will there find information more valuable to him than all the medicine in the world. In this connection there is space for only a few hints. The patient should avoid all substances which are of difficult digestion, or which disagree with him, and he must not be constantly trying different articles of food. As a general rule, he should avoid all vegetables with the exception of well-boiled rice, Irish and sweet potatoes, and these should be cooked dry and mealy. Sweet peaches and ripe blackberries may be used with moderation. Good fresh milk can generally be taken, unless it disagrees with the patient. Sweet cream and good fresh butter, *cold*, may be used moderately with stale brown bread, rice, or potatoes. Also tender mutton, beef, venison, turkeys, chickens, partridges, and some of the smaller birds, if kept some time before being cooked, may be used; and even soft boiled eggs are often allowable. Salt may be used moderately, but all other condiments should be avoided. Among the above articles the patient will find all he needs, and he must confine himself strictly to the above list, and above all things shun the use of stimulating drinks, for if they afford temporary relief, they are sure to weaken the stomach still more. Cold water is the best drink, or milk and hot water, only moderately sweetened, weak cocoa, and at most, weak black tea, drank a couple of hours before eating. He should eat at regular hours, never more frequently than three times a day, and eat slowly, and masticate or chew his food well. If the disease has been caused by sedentary habits, severe study, or mental anxiety, active exercise in the open air and sunlight are all-important.

Nux vom.: When this disease occurs in persons of sedentary habits, or those who have been given to free indulgence in the use of stimulants or condiments, or are subject to costive bowels, with or without piles, a dose of this remedy every night will often afford great relief. If there is a gnawing sensation in the stomach, craving or aversion to food, bitter eructations, headache, drowsiness, and mental depression, these are still further indications for *Nux vom.* A dose may be given every night for a week, then omit for two or three days, after which give a single dose of *Sulphur*, then omit all medicine for one week, after which give *Nux vom.* again, and follow it by *Sulphur* in the same manner, and continue these remedies as long as there is any improvement.

Dose of the above or other remedies, see page 7.

Pulsatilla is especially suitable for females, and it is also useful for males when there is great acidity of the stomach or acid eructations, and when there is little or no thirst. A dose may be given every night for a week, then after omitting the remedy for two days, give a dose of *Hepar sulph.* and wait a week; then give these two remedies in the same manner again, and continue them as long as there is any improvement.

China may be given every night if the disease has been caused by the loss of blood, or secretions from the blood; also if the patient is constantly troubled with flatulency or wind.

If the above remedies do not entirely relieve the symptoms give a dose of *Calcarea carb.* once a week. Consult a homœopathic physician, if one is accessible.

CHOLERA MORBUS.

This disease is characterized by vomiting and purging. It may commence suddenly without premonitory symptoms, or it may be preceded for hours and even days by a feeling of weight or uneasiness of the stomach, with or without the same sensation in the bowels, and with a coated tongue. Long-continued hot weather, especially with cold nights, predisposes the system to this disease. It may also be caused by overeating, improper food, and by poisonous substances taken into the stomach. There may be severe spasmodic pains in the stomach, and colic pains in the bowels, or there may be very little pain. At first, simply the contents of the stomach and lower bowel are discharged, but bilious matter, green or yellow, and more or less acrid, soon makes its appearance. If the disease is not soon relieved, the pulse becomes feeble, the countenance pale and shrunken, the skin cool and damp, the urine scanty, and sometimes painful cramps appear in the muscles of the abdomen and extremities. If the disease is neglected, alarming symptoms may ensue, such as brown, blackish, or bloody discharges, great thirst and burning in the stomach and bowels, small, frequent, and irregular pulse, short and frequent respiration, cold extremities, sunken eyes, cold sweat, hiccough and distention of the abdomen, with perhaps a cessation of the vomiting; and, if not relieved by treatment, the patient may sink and die within a period of from twelve or twenty-four hours to two or three days, often retaining his mental faculties until the last. In some severe cases, the discharges are colorless or whitish, almost like those in Asiatic Cholera. In some cases a diarrhœa follows the attack, and in some instances a gastric or typhoid fever seems to result. Cholera morbus is rarely fatal in persons of a good constitution, especially under homœopathic treatment, as the disease is generally soon relieved by our remedies. When the difficulty has been caused by offending matters taken into the stomach, as soon as they are evacuated the patient is often relieved, even without medicine, but in other instances the symptoms continue unabated. Vomiting and purging are not unfrequent attendants upon other diseases, such as bilious fever, inflammation of the stomach, bowels, and liver, but such cases may be distinguished from the disease under consideration by the presence of fever, headache, tenderness and soreness of the stomach and bowels; whereas, in cholera morbus there is no fever, especially at the commencement of the disease.

It is not always so easy to distinguish cholera morbus from the effects caused by various irritating poisons such as *Arsenic*, *Tartar emetic*, *Corrosive sublimate*, *or Calomel*. If this disease is not prevailing, and the attack is sudden, without premonitory symptoms, and has not been caused by any irregularity in diet, such as over eating or drinking, or the use of unusual articles, it is well to bear in mind the possibility of the disease having been caused by the accidental or intentional use of a poisonous substance. In all cases where you have the least reason to suspect that the disease has been caused by a poison, carefully save all the discharges, give the homœopathic remedy or remedies as directed below, and send immediately for a physician. If you know that the disease has been caused by a poison, consult the section on poisons, and send for a physician.

Treatment of Cholera Morbus.—When there are premonitory symptoms of this disease, such as a coated and yellow tongue, weight and uneasiness, or pain in the stomach or bowels, give a dose of *Chamomilla* every hour until the symptoms are relieved. It may still be useful after vomiting and diarrhœa have commenced, if there is great pain.

Dose of this or other remedies, see page 7.

Ipecac: Give this remedy every half hour, if there is great nausea and vomiting, with profuse watery diarrhœa, especially if the disease has been caused by overloading the stomach, or by indigestible substances. If there is severe pain in the bowels, give it alternately with *Chamomilla*, one half hour apart. If the disease has been caused by cold or acid drinks, acid and unripe fruits, or if there is great acidity of the stomach, give *Pulsatilla* and *Ipecac*, alternately, one half hour or hour apart, according to the severity of the symptoms.

Veratrum: This is by far the most important remedy in very severe cases of this disease; and in lighter cases, when the above remedies fail to relieve them, within a few hours, give *Veratrum* every half hour, when the evacuations are very profuse, with or without pain, especially if there are cramps in the calves of the legs, hollow and sunken eyes, and cold extremities. It may be given alternately with *Arsenicum*, in severe cases.

Arsenicum: Give this remedy every half hour, if *Veratrum* fails to check the progress of the disease, and the eyes become sunken, the extremities cold, and there are great thirst and a burning sensation at the pit of the stomach. If, during the progress of the disease, there is very intense pain in the bowels, a dose or two of *Colocynth* will often relieve it.

China may be given night and morning, after the symptoms are relieved, for the debility which remains.

Diet, &c.—During the continuance of the disease, nothing should be taken into the stomach but rice-water, arrow-root, toast-water, and boiled water, and the like unirritating drinks. When there is much pain, cloths may be wrung from warm water, and applied over the stomach and bowels.

ASIATIC OR EPIDEMIC CHOLERA.

An attack of this disease is generally, but not always, preceded by certain premonitory symptoms, such as a furred tongue, poor appetite, impaired digestion, thirst, uneasiness, distention, and weight of the stomach and bowels, with general weakness. A profuse, watery, *painless* diarrhœa, with rumbling in the bowels, generally precedes the attack of fully-developed cholera, for from a few hours to several days. This diarrhœa is attended with so little suffering, that patients are exceedingly liable to neglect it until attacked by cholera. If a watery diarrhœa is attended with pain, there is far less danger of an attack of cholera, than when it is painless. During the prevalence of an epidemic, overeating or irregularities of diet, exposure, mental excitement or fatigue, may induce an attack, or it may come on without any exciting cause. A feeling of weakness, and sometimes chills, copious sweats, feebleness of the pulse, disordered vision, dizziness, and ringing in the ears, are symptoms which frequently occur about the commencement of the attack; or without any premonitory symptoms except the painless diarrhœa, and occasionally even without this, the patient is seized with violent vomiting and purging, with severe pains in the abdomen, neuralgic or cutting sharp pains in different parts of the body, and cramps in the muscles, especially of the arms and lower extremities. The passages from the bowels soon become thin, watery, and whitish, resembling thin gruel or rice-water, which, when allowed to stand, separates into a colorless fluid and a white, insoluble matter, which settles in the bottom of the vessel. In some instances the passages are brown, and in mild cases, when the disease is abating, they are sometimes tinged with bile. The matter vomited may be white and glairy, or similar to the stools. The evacuations are often very copious, and apparently without much effort, and rapidly exhaust the system of its fluids. The features become shrunken, the extremities cold, the pulse small, and the fingers and toes often distorted by cramps in the muscles of the arms and legs. If the disease is not arrested, the pulse becomes very feeble, and almost imperceptible at the wrist, the skin begins to assume a leaden or dark purple color on the face and extremities, and is shrunken and inelastic, and on the hands and feet wrinkled and shrivelled as if long soaked in water. The eyes are deeply sunken in their sockets, and surrounded by a livid circle. The urine is scanty and sometimes suppressed, the thirst intense, with a constant desire for cold drinks, and also for fresh air. The respiration is short, hurried, and oppressed, and there are great restlessness and extreme prostration of strength. The patient often complains of great heat over the entire body, when the surface is very cold to the touch. There is more or less dullness of the mental faculties, although the mind is generally free from any derangement. The patient usually gives himself very little uneasiness about the result of his disease.

We have now followed the symptoms up to the beginning of the collapse, when if the patient is not relieved, the pulse becomes imperceptible, the voice feeble, the breath cold, the respiration very feeble, and the urine suppressed. The vomiting and purging may continue or cease some time before death. The cramps may abate some time before the patient dies or not until after respiration ceases. Sometimes stupor precedes the fatal termination, in other instances the patient is conscious to the last. Death may occur within from four to twelve hours from the commencement of the attack, but more frequently not sooner than from one to three days. The patient may recover from any stage, even from the collapse; the appearance of bile in the passages is generally a favorable sign. If the patient has been very much reduced by the evacuations when reaction becomes established, more or less febrile excitement is apt to ensue. This is generally of a typhoid character, and during its continuance there is a great tendency to congestion of the brain, giving rise to headache, delirium, convulsions and stupor. A fatal collapse sometimes occurs without vomiting, and in some instances vomiting occurs without diarrhœa. Occasionally, but very rarely, the collapse almost immediately follows the attack. The cholera is an epidemic disease, and nothing is known in regard to the poison which causes it. The intemperate and those who use alcoholic and fermented drinks even moderately, are more liable to have the disease than others; but while the temperate should never commence the use of such drinks during the prevalence of the disease with any thoughts of thereby preventing it, as they will be far more likely to contract it if they do, the intemperate and those who have been accustomed to their use should simply use them more moderately, but not break off entirely until the epidemic is over, as the sudden change may cause an attack.

Preventive Treatment.—Eat temperately of vegetable and animal food, if you have been in the habit of using both; simply shun indigestible food, unripe fruits and crude vegetables, small beer, cider, ice-water, ice-cream, &c. Follow the following directions and you need have very little fear of being attacked during the prevalence of any epidemic of cholera. Avoid excessive physical or mental labor, and all undue mental excitement. Take *Veratrum, Cuprum,* and *Sulphur*, in the order they are named, at bedtime, two days apart; and after taking each of them twice, lengthen the intervals between the remedies to three or four days; and then continue them to the end of the epidemic. Take four globules of either for a dose.

Treatment of the Painless Diarrhœa which precedes Cholera.—Never neglect such a diarrhœa during the prevalence of cholera, for a single hour, but resort immediately to the use of homœopathic remedies, which, if carefully selected and promptly administered, will rarely, if ever, fail to cure the diarrhœa, and thereby prevent the cholera; so that very few homœopathic patients can ever have this disease, except through gross neglect. Take no other than homœopathic remedies, either for this diarrhœa or for the cholera. It is all-important that you shun all allopathic nostrums and quack medicines, for a single dose of a remedy which contains any of the preparations of opium, will often so far paralyze the system that it will be impossible to get a sufficiently prompt action from our remedies, to save the life of the patient. All experience shows that from one fourth to one half of all the patients who take opium, in any form, during a well-marked attack of cholera, will die, in spite of any known treatment.

Arsenicum is perhaps more frequently required for this diarrhœa, than any other remedy, especially when the passages are very profuse and watery, with or without much pain, and if there is great thirst, give a dose every hour. If there is any nausea or sick stomach, or if the diarrhœa is very painful, with profuse evacuations, give *Veratrum* alternately with *Arsenicum,* at intervals of half an hour.

Phosphorus: If the passages are light colored and nearly painless, with moderate thirst, give a dose of this remedy once an hour, but if it does not relieve the symptoms within a few hours, give *Arsenicum.*

China may be given once in two hours, in obstinate cases, when the passages are painless and watery, and there are rumbling and distention of the bowels with wind. Relief will be more certain and speedy, if the patient keeps quiet, and covers himself up well in bed.

Treatment of Cholera.—At the commencement of the attack, if there are great weakness, or chilly sensations, copious sweats, and feeble pulse, disordered vision or dizziness, give either six globules, or a drop of the *Spirits of camphor*, every five or ten minutes, until such symptoms are relieved; at the same time cover the patient up in bed, and apply hot dry flannels to his feet, so as to get him into a gentle perspiration if possible. This course will often check the disease in an hour or two, but if it should not, give

Veratrum: This is the chief remedy at the commencement of the attack, after *Camphor*, especially when there are profuse vomiting and purging, coldness, blueness, cramps, and rice-water passages. Repeat the dose once in fifteen minutes.

Dose of this or any other remedy, see page 7.

Cuprum may be given alternately with *Veratrum*, at intervals of fifteen minutes, if, notwithstanding the use of that remedy, the patient begins to be troubled with cramps in the extremities, and distortion of the fingers and toes.

Arsenicum: If, in the course of three or four hours, there is no improvement (and even sooner if the patient seems to be getting rapidly worse), omit the *Cuprum* and give *Arsenicum* alternately with *Veratrum* at intervals of fifteen minutes or half an hour, and persevere with these remedies until the patient is either relieved or symptoms of collapse approach, such as very small pulse, livid surface, and cold perspiration on the extremities. If such symptoms appear, omit the *Veratrum* and give a few doses of *Camphor*, as directed for the commencement of the disease, and then give *Carbo veg.* alternately with *Arsenicum*, at intervals of half an hour, until either reaction ensues or the patient dies.

External Applications, Diet, &c.—At the commencement of the disease, cover the patient up warm in bed, and apply warm flannels or bottles of hot water, or a warm iron, or brick, to the feet; but if the patient is in the stage of collapse, and the surface is bathed with a profuse cold perspiration, do not apply external heat, as it will only make him uncomfortable, and increase the exhausting perspiration. In this stage, rub the surface, especially the extremities, freely with the dry hand, or a dry warm piece of flannel, or a coarse towel—the bare hand is the best. During the active stage of the disease, nothing but the most simple drinks, such as rice-water, arrow-root, corn-starch, and toast-water, should be allowed, and even such liquids only in small quantities at a time.

When the vomiting and purging cease, the above drinks may be made thicker and more nourishing, and when the appetite seems to demand it, thin puddings of arrow-root, rice, or corn-starch may be allowed, and after a day or two more, toast, cracker and meat. Food in substance, like toast, rice, or meat, should never be given more than three times a day, to a patient while recovering from this or any other disease, as the stomach needs seasons of rest.

INFLAMMATION OF THE BOWELS (PERITONITIS).

There are two forms of inflammation of the bowels; one in which the disease involves the smooth membrane which lines the internal surface of the abdominal walls, and the external surface of the intestines, and sometimes extends to their muscular coat; the other consists of inflammation of the mucous membrane or internal lining of the intestines. The former will be considered in this section, the latter under the head of "Inflammation of the Mucous Membrane of the Bowels, or Small Intestines"

Symptoms.—Either after, or without preceding or accompanying chills, languor, and loss of appetite, the patient is seized with acute or sharp pain in the abdomen, generally in the lower part, sometimes on one side only. It may be circumscribed, or extend over a large portion of the abdomen, according to the extent of the disease. The pain is aggravated by movement, coughing, sneezing, sighing, &c. Pressure causes great distress, and even the weight of the bedclothes often increases the suffering, and the patient lies with his knees drawn up so as to relax the muscles over the parts diseased. The abdomen is hot und hard, and, as the disease advances, distended by gas; the bowels are generally constipated, or soon become so, but sometimes they are regular, and nausea and vomiting are not uncommon; the skin is dry and hot, the pulse rapid, small, and hard. The countenance indicates great distress and depression, the cheeks are pale, the eyes sunken, and the tongue and lips are dry. The frequency of the pulse varies from eighty to one hundred and thirty in a minute.

The disease may be caused by exposure to cold, mechanical injuries, irregularities of diet, the breaking of abscesses, or by the perforation of the intestinal tube from ulceration, and the escape of the contents of the bowels into the abdominal cavity. In one instance of the latter kind, in a child, on examination after death we found that the ulceration and perforation were caused by an accumulation of magnesia which had been administered months before; and I have good reason to think that the use of this drug, and prepared chalk, is not an unfrequent cause of this accident, and thereby of fatal inflammation of the bowels, for an examination in another instance of perforation rendered it quite manifest that it arose from the same cause. When this disease results from perforation of the intestine it almost always terminates fatally; only in rare instances, under the most favorable circumstances, can the patient be expected to recover. Therefore, let every one beware of giving or taking either crude magnesia or prepared chalk.

Peritonitis, or the form of inflammation of the bowels under consideration, when not caused by perforation of the intestine, or the bursting of an abscess, can generally be cured by homœopathic treatment, provided always that the bowels are allowed to remain constipated until the symptoms are entirely relieved. If the disease is attended by a low or malignant form of fever, denoted by an early prostration of the vital powers, cold extremities, small irregular pulse, sordes or crusts on the teeth, and delirium, there is more danger of a fatal termination.

Treatment.—The first and most important point is, to let the bowels alone, and never attempt to obtain a passage even by injections, as the motion of the intestines and of the patient, necessary for an evacuation, is sure to increase the severity of the disease. Wring a large towel from cold water and apply over the abdomen, over that put four or five thicknesses of dry flannel large enough to cover entirely the wet cloth; then pin a dry towel around the body and over the flannel so as to confine the whole to its place. Wet the towel once in six or eight hours. Later in the disease, if the above and proper remedies fail to relieve promptly, cloths wrung from hot water and changed every fifteen minutes or half an hour, or an oil-meal or ground flaxseed poultice, will often do better.

Aconite: This is generally the most important remedy in the treatment of this diesase, and it should be continued as long as there is much heat of skin, even over the bowels and body. If the attack is severe, give a dose of this remedy every hour until there is some improvement, then lengthen the intervals to three hours. If the pain is very severe or sharp, and the skin hot, and *Aconite* alone does not relieve, once in four hours omit it, and give a dose of *Belladonna* in its stead.

Dose of this, or either of the following remedies, see page 7.

Bryonia: This is a very important remedy as soon as the severity of the febrile symptoms has been somewhat relieved by the use of *Aconite*, or the latter remedy and *Belladonna*—usually required at the end of twenty-four or forty-eight hours. Even earlier it will be found useful; if there is a tendency to a low or malignant form of fever, or if the extremities are cold and the pulse small, give this remedy once in four hours, and *Aconite* every hour between, if fever still continues, bnt if it has abated, give it alone.

Veratrum: If there is excessive nausea or vomiting, *Veratrum* may be given alternately with *Aconite*, one hour apart, until this symptom is relieved.

Arsenicum: If, notwithstanding the above remedies, alarming symptoms make their appearance, such as cold extremities, small or irregular pulse, great prostration of strength, distended bowels, and if the teeth are covered with crusts of dark dried mucus, and the tongue is dark and dry, give a dose of *Arsenicum* once in two hours.

A formidable and sometimes a malignant form of this disease occasionally occurs in the case of females after child-birth. The remedies already named are often the proper remedies in such cases; bnt *Arnica* given once in three or four hours during the confinement, will tend to prevent such attacks, and *Aconite*, *Belladonna*, or *Bryonia*, will generally relieve them, if applied early, unless the disease is prevailing as an epidemic, and is of a malignant character. When this is the case, the above remedies may still be useful at the commencement of the disease, but *Rhus tox.* and *Arsenicum* will be required at a later stage, in case the other remedies fail to relieve the symptoms. These may be given alternately, at intervals of two hours.

If in any case there is irritation of the neck of the bladder, with frequent and painful passage of urine, *Cantharides* is the remedy, and an occasional dose may be administered for this symptom; and if it fails to afford relief, give *Apis mel.*

Acute inflammation of the bowels sometimes, instead of being cured, assumes a chronic form, or the inflammation may come on so gradually as not to manifest acute symptoms. For this form of the disease, give *Sulphur* night and morning for a week, then omit and give *Lachesis* in the same manner. These remedies may be continued as long as there is any improvement, when *Arsenicum* may be given night and morning.

Diet.—During an attack of acute inflammation of the bowels, nothing but rice-water, arrow-root, corn-starch, toast-water, or weak gruel should be allowed.

INFLAMMATION OF THE MUCOUS MEMBRANE OF THE SMALL INTESTINES (ENTERITIS).

This disease may be caused by exposure to sudden changes of temperature, but more frequently by excesses in eating or drinking, or by improper articles taken into the stomach. Like inflammation of the stomach, it not unfrequently occurs during the course of febrile diseases, especially during typhoid fever. It may also be caused by a change of water.

Symptoms.—This disease generally begins with uneasiness in the bowels, followed by griping pains, which gradually become more severe, especially about the navel and a few inches below, and at the sides, and there is almost always more or less tenderness on pressure. Diarrhœa usually soon follows, and the stools follow the attacks of griping pain, and consist of watery and natural discharges, mixed with bile, mucus, and undigested food, sometimes tinged with blood; occasionally they are green or clay-colored. Chills and fever either precede, accompany, or soon follow the local symptoms; the pulse is frequent and full, the skin dry, and the tongue somewhat furred. There is generally little or no headache. This disease is often mild and attended with but little pain, but in other instances the pains are very severe, the bowels very tender and distended, with flatulence, and the discharges offensive. Sometimes the inflammation ascends to the stomach, and vomiting occurs, with great thirst and tenderness of the stomach on pressure. The liver, in some cases, becomes involved, causing yellowness of the skin and eyes. If the disease continues, the tongue becomes red and dry, and the pulse frequent and feeble, and the patient either sinks or slowly recovers.

An acute attack not unfrequently terminates in chronic inflammation, or the disease may be so gradually developed as not to manifest any acute symptoms. Diarrhœa is a general attendant on the chronic form of the disease, and in fact many of our most obstinate cases of diarrhœa are caused by this affection. There may be but two or three passages in twenty-four hours, or they may be very frequent. They are sometimes scanty, but in other instances profuse. The evacuations are similar to those of the acute form of the disease; sometimes portions of false membrane are discharged, and in some instances of a tubular form, resembling portions of the intestine, but lacking the smooth external surface of the latter. In advanced stages of the disease, the evacuations are sometimes mingled with pus or matter.

If there is pain, it is generally partially relieved after the discharges. The abdomen may be distended or very flat, the appetite craving or moderate. The pulse is generally increased in frequency, the tongue slightly furred, and in the advanced stage often smooth and red, and the skin dry and harsh, with more or less rapid diminution of strength and emaciation. The spirits are often depressed, and cases of insanity have sometimes had their origin from chronic inflammation of the mucous membrane of the bowels. Towards the close of fatal cases, hectic fever usually occurs, and the patient becomes much emaciated. The duration of the disease is exceedingly variable, in light cases it may last years.

Treatment.—In acute cases, when there are thirst, hot skin, and full pulse, *Aconite* should be given—a dose every hour, until the febrile symptoms are relieved.

Dose of this or other remedies, see page 7.

Mercurius viv. If, at the commencement of the disease, there are severe griping pains, causing a weak or faint sensation, or if the passages from the bowels contain mucus, give a dose of this remedy once in two hours; and if there is much fever, give a dose of *Aconite* between the doses of *Mercurius viv.* These two remedies alone will very frequently cure the disease; but in some instances, if the pain is severe at the end of twelve or twenty-four hours, the *Aconite* may be omitted, and *Colocynth* may be given alternately with *Mercurius viv.* If the symptoms improve, lengthen the intervals between the doses to two or three hours.

Pulsatilla: If the disease has been caused by green fruit, acids, or other errors of diet, and the passages are watery, without much mucus, and not attended by much pain, give this remedy once an hour, but if it does not soon relieve, give

Arsenicum: This is a very important remedy after *Pulsatilla*; or at the commencement, especially when there are great thirst, burning in the bowels, or profuse, watery, brownish, or yellowish evacuations, containing shreds of mucus. In severe cases, give a dose every hour.

Bryonia will often be of service during hot weather, if the passages are watery and contain mucus, with or without pain, especially if the tongue inclines to be dry, and the bowels are tender. *Arsenicum* may be required after *Bryonia.* Give *Chamomilla* when the pains are very severe and long continued, and *Colocynth* and *Mercurius viv.* fail to relieve them. If the disease threatens to become chronic, give *Sulphur* every night.

In the chronic form of the disease the above remedies, especially *Arsenicum* and *Sulphur*, may still be useful. Give a dose of *Sulphur* night and morning for a week, unless the symptoms improve before the end of that period; in that case, give but one dose a day, and continue it as long as the patient improves. If there is much thirst, or heat in the bowels, and the passages are watery, give *Arsenicum* night and morning after *Sulphur*, but if there is but little thirst or pain, give *Phosphorus* instead of *Arsenicum.*

If the passages contain pus or matter, give *Lachesis* night and morning for one week, and *Silicea* the next week. If diarrhœa alternates with costiveness, give *Nux vomica* at night while the bowels are constipated, and one of the above remedies when they are loose. If the passages are painless, and contain undigested food, and the patient is troubled with flatulency, give a dose of *China* one hour before every meal.

Diet, &c.—During an acute attack, if the disease is attended with fever, soreness in the bowels, and diarrhœa, the patient should retain the horizontal position, and eat neither food in substance nor animal food, but simply use rice-water, arrow-root, barley-water, toast-water, and the top or thin part of oat-meal or corn-meal gruel. As the disease abates and the appetite returns, make the above drinks thicker, and very cautiously return to a more nutritious diet. In chronic cases, milk may be added to the above articles. A warm bath daily, especially in chronic cases, will be found of great service.

DYSENTERY, OR INFLAMMATION OF THE LARGE INTESTINE.

This disease may be caused by unripe and acid fruits, indigestable food, cathartics, exposure to cold night air after a hot day, and sudden changes of temperature. It is not contagious, but it sometimes prevails as an epidemic. Dysentery may be either acute or chronic, and of every grade of severity, from the lightest without fever, to the most severe form, with a high grade of febrile excitement.

Symptoms.—Sometimes chills and fever precede the local symptoms, in other cases they either accompany them or soon follow, if the attack is at all severe. Griping and cutting pains in the abdomen, irregular in their recurrence and position, followed by discharges from the bowels, which generally afford partial relief, are the first prominent symptoms. The first two or three passages may be composed simply of the contents of the bowels; in other cases they are of a dysenteric character from the commencement, without any of the natural discharges. Weight, uneasiness of the bowels, and sometimes burning, soon follow the paroxysms of griping pain, together with a frequent inclination to go to stool, evacuating simply a small quantity of mucus each time.

A straining or forcing-down sensation, called tenesmus, soon follows and becomes one of the most distressing symptoms of the disease. Sometimes the bowels protrude, owing to the severity of the straining, and the discharges are often followed by burning and cutting pains in the anus or passage. The discharges are seldom less than a dozen in twenty-four hours, and in bad cases they may be as frequent as once in five or ten minutes. The evacuations generally consist of transparent or whitish mucus, or mucus mixed with blood, sometimes of nearly clear blood. As the disease advances, portions of thicker mucus, or shreds of membranous matter often mixed with bile, and sometimes with lumps of the natural discharge, make their appearance. At first there is very little smell to the evacuations, but after a time there is exhaled a peculiar fleshy odor. The bladder often sympathizes with the intestine, and there are frequent and painful passages of urine. The bowels are tender on pressure, the urine scanty, and the pulse is frequent. In a majority of cases the disease abates within a week or ten days, but if the symptoms are not relieved within that period, they are apt to become aggravated, the pain and st aining increase, the discharges are more frequent, and the abdomen more tender; the pulse smaller and more rapid, the tongue brownish and dry; and after a few days the coating peels off, leaving the surface smooth, glassy, and sometimes gashed. In protracted cases pus or matter is often discharged, and the stools become more copious and offensive, containing bloody water and greenish mucus. In some cases the liver is deranged, the skin and eyes yellow, and vomiting is frequently present. The disease sometimes assumes a typhoid or even typhus form when it is attended with great danger. In such cases, while the body is hot, the limbs are cool, the pulse small and frequent, the tongue is brown or black; crusts or sordes appear on the teeth, very offensive and copious brown or black stools make their appearance, and occasionally there are free discharges of altered blood. There is great prostration of strength in such cases, and sometimes dark spots appear, from an effusion of blood in and beneath the skin.

The following are among the favorable signs: Gradual abatement of the fever, pain, straining, and frequency of the stools, with the appearance of free natural discharges. When improvement commences, the passage of the natural contents of the bowels over the inflamed surface of the intestine, often causes intense pain, but this generally is followed by a free evacuation from the bowels, after which the pain abates. The following are unfavorable symptoms. Sudden abatement of pain and straining, distention of the bowels with gas, cold clammy sweat, hiccough, involuntary stools, delirium, or stupor. Some of the above symptoms may be present and yet the patient recover, but they denote great danger.

Treatment.—The first, and by far the most important measure in all cases, whether severe or light, is absolute rest in the horizontal position. Perhaps in no disease is it so important that the patient constantly keep his bed, as in dysentery; and in all cases of any severity, he should not even be allowed to rise up to have a passage, but should use a bed-pan; or, what is better, fold up a sheet and place under the hips, and over that small cloths, which can be removed after the passage, without disturbing the patient; nor should he be allowed to sit up until the disease is entirely cured, otherwise the symptoms will be aggravated. The next and most important point, is proper care in regard to substances taken into the stomach. Nothing should be allowed in any case of much severity, excepting light unirritating drinks, such as rice-water, arrow-root, toast-water, barley-water, slippery-elm, or a thin gruel of farina or of oat-meal, or at most, warm milk-and-water. When the disease is cured, cautiously return to a more substantial diet. If the patient is a young child, it may continue to nurse.

Aconite: Give this remedy in all cases when there are chills or fever, and soreness of the bowels on pressure. Give a dose once an hour, for three or four hours, and if it does not relieve the symptoms, give *Mercurius viv.* alternately with it.

Dose of this, or of other remedies, see page 7.

Mercurius viv.: In cases where there are no chills or fever, this remedy may be given at the commencement of the disease, when there are frequent discharges, with straining, which does not abate with the passages, and they consist of slimy, bloody, or green mucus, with or without severe griping or cutting pains in the bowels, which are not relieved by the evacuations Give a dose once an hour. In cases attended with chills or fever, *Aconite* should either precede this remedy or be given alternately with it. Continue *Mercurius* for at least twenty-four or forty-eight hours, and longer if the patient is improving.

Mercurius cor.: If the passages at first are very bloody, containing bile and mucus, with severe colic pains and straining, and also when there is straining to pass urine, or retention of urine, this remedy may be given instead of *Mercurius viv.*; also if the latter remedy, when it seems indicated, fails to relieve the symptoms, especially when the disease occurs during the fall of the year, give a dose once in from one to two hours.

Colocynth: If, notwithstanding the use of the above remedies, the pains in the bowels are very intense, causing the patient to bend up, and there is pressure and fullness of the abdomen, omit *Mercurius*, or any other remedy you may be giving, for five or six hours, and give a dose of *Colocynth* every hour during that period.

Sulphur: This remedy is rarely of service at the commmencement of this disease, but after the acute symptoms have been relieved by other remedies, or in obstinate case, where *Mercurius viv.* or *Mercurius cor.* fails to relieve, especially if it aggravates the symptoms, *Sulphur* is the remedy. Give a dose once in two hours and lengthen the intervals between the doses as the patient improves.

The above are the most important remedies in a majority of cases; yet, in a few instances, other remedies will be required.

Bryonia may follow a few doses of *Aconite*, when the disease occurs during the hot weather of summer, especially when it is caused by the use of cold drinks. Give a dose once in two hours.

Nux vom.: This remedy is often useful during the hot weather of summer, especially when the discharges are chiefly mucus, very frequent, small, attended with pain in the abdomen, and great straining, which cease with the passages, or when the latter have a putrid smell. Give a dose once in two hours.

Arsenicum: Give this remedy, if *Nux vomica* fails to relieve, when the stools are putrid involuntary, and there is great debility, offensive breath, crusts on the teeth, or dark spots on the skin.

If there are nausea and bilious vomiting, give *Ipecac* after, or alternately with *Aconite*, especially when these symptoms occur at the commencement of the disease, during the fall of the year.

In the case of children, in addition to the above remedies, *Chamomilla* may be required if the child screams before the passages, and is very restless. When teething children are attacked with this disease, *Aconite* should always precede *Chamomilla*. Generally the globules of *Aconite* should be used, with both children and adults, especially when the fever is high and the skin hot ; but when there is but little fever, or simply a slow fever, and the disease is obstinate and does not readily yield to remedies, in the case of children or adults, drop one drop of the prime tincture of *Aconite*, or twelve globules saturated with the tincture of *Aconite*, into half a glass of water, and give a child half a teaspoonful, or an adult a teaspoonful, every hour until there is some change in the symptoms, then lengthen the intervals between the doses.

In chronic cases, if there are passages of mucus and pus, or matter, with more or less straining, give a dose of *Sulphur* night and morning, and if it fails to relieve the symptoms at the end of a week, give *Lachesis* night and morning for several days, and afterward *Phosphorus*. If the patient improves under the use of either of the above remedies, gradually lengthen the intervals between the doses to two or three days, and continue the remedy as long as there is any improvement.

DIARRHŒA.

This affection may arise from an increased action or motion of the bowels, which may be caused by mental emotions, such as fear, joy, &c., or by overeating, when the quantity of food may cause semi-liquid stools, without pain or soreness in the abdomen. Diarrhœa may depend on an irritation of the mucous membrane of the bowels, which hardly amounts to inflammation. Hot weather and atmospheric influences often predispose individuals to this affection; and when this is the case a slight irregularity of diet or exposure may bring on an attack. This affection may be caused by substances acting directly on the mucous membrane or inner surface of the intestines, such as various cathartic remedies, indigestible food, unripe fruits, acid and very cold drinks, &c. An increased secretion of bile, or bile of a perverted quality, may cause bilious stools of a dark brown, yellow, or black appearance, and sometimes of a tarry consistency. An insufficient secretion of bile may also cause a diarrhœa; the passages appearing clay colored, or of a dirty white. When the digestive organs are weak, undigested portions of food may irritate the mucous membrane and cause this affection, when undigested food will appear in the passages. Diarrhœa may arise from debility, as in the last stages of consumption, and other chronic diseases, when it sometimes alternates with the profuse sweats which depend on the same cause. Earlier in consumption it often depends on inflammation, and in some instances ulceration of the mucous membrane. This affection in children is frequently caused by sympathy with the gums in teething. The evacuations in diarrhœa may be few, not exceeding two or three daily, or they may occur every few moments; the quantity may be but little greater than during health, or very great, and has been known to amount to forty pounds in twenty-four hours. Sometimes there is pain before the passages, but in other instances they are painless. The skin is usually dry and the urine scanty; the pulse may be nearly natural, or small and irregular; and there may be little or no debility, or great sinking and prostration. This disease may last but for a few hours, or for days, months, and even years; there may be little or no danger, or in neglected cases, the patient may die from exhaustion

Treatment.—If the passages from the bowels are slimy, mucous, or bloody, with or without fever, consult the section on dysentery. If there are fever and soreness of the bowels on pressure, with little or no mucus, especially when even if there is mucus there is no straining, consult the section on inflammation of the mucous membrane of the bowels. If diarrhœa occurs during any febrile or eruptive disease, consult the section on that disease; but if the remedies there recommended fail to relieve, you can then consult this section.

Opium may be given when the diarrhœa has been caused by mental emotions, especially fright, fear, or horror. If in such cases this remedy fails to relieve at the end of six or eight hours, give *Veratrum*. If the disease has been caused by joy, give *Coffee* every hour for six hours; follow, if necessary, with *Opium*. If the diarrhœa has been caused by grief or sorrow, give *Ignatia* once in two hours for twenty-four hours, and afterward, if necessary, give *China*, especially if there is no pain. When the disease has been caused by anger, give *Chamomilla* after every passage, and if it does not relieve the symptoms within twelve or twenty-four hours, give *Colocynth*. If the patient simply has semi-liquid, but otherwise natural passages, from overeating, let him eat less, and take a dose of *Pulsatilla* before every meal.

Does of either of the remedies, see page 7.

Pulsatilla: Give this remedy when the diarrhœa has been caused by errors of diet, unripe or acid fruits, acid drinks, cold water, rhubarb, or tobacco, and especially when the discharges are bilious, yellowish, whitish or green, very offensive, and occur during the night; also, if there are nausea, sour stomach, and acid vomiting. Give a dose as often as the passages occur. After this remedy *Arsenicum* is often required.

Arsenicum may be given when the passages are very watery and profuse, when there is great thirst, extreme debility, and when eating or drinking causes passages with more or less pain. *Arsenicum* is especially useful when the diarrhœa has been caused by cold drinks or acid fruits, and when the passages are brownish; also for the watery diarrhœas of teething children, aged persons, and consumptives. In severe cases give a dose every hour, and gradually lengthen the intervals to six or eight hours as the patient improves. In chronic cases give a dose two or three times a day.

Dulcamara: Give a dose of this remedy after every passage, when the disease has been caused by a cold damp atmosphere, or getting wet. If at the end of twelve or twenty-four hours the symptoms are not in a great measure relieved, give *Mercurius viv.*

Mercurius viv. is the remedy for bilious diarrhœa, when the stools are yellow, green or whitish, or if they look like stirred eggs, and especially if there are severe griping pains in the abdomen or any straining during the passages; also when the passages are watery, if they contain shreds of mucus or slime. Give a dose every hour, and gradually lengthen the intervals between the doses as the patient improves. *Sulphur* is often required after *Mercurius* if the symptoms are not entirely relieved within two or three days.

Chamomilla: Give this remedy for bilious diarrhœa when there are severe colic pains, watery, yellowish, or greenish passages, smelling like rotten eggs or acid, and especially in the case of children where there are rumbling and distention of the abdomen, screams, and restlessness. Give a dose once in one or two hours.

Colocynth is an important remedy, not only for children but also for adults, when with or without nausea there are intense spasmodic or cutting pains in the bowels with yellowish passages. Give a dose every hour.

Veratrum: If at the commencement of a watery diarrhœa there is nausea, give a dose of this remedy every hour, and if it does not relieve at the end of twelve or twenty-four hours give *Arsenicum. Veratrum* may also follow either *Arsenicum* or *Pulsatilla* in case they fail to relieve watery diarrhœa when they seem indicated, even though there is no nausea, especially when there are cramping pains in the bowels or extremities. Give a dose every hour.

Ipecac may be given instead of *Veratrum* if there is nausea or vomiting, with pains in the bowels, and bilious, white, or green passages. Give a dose once in two hours, and if the symptoms are not relieved at the end of six hours, give either *Veratrum, Colocynth,* or *Mercurius viv.*, the one which seems most indicated.

China: Give this remedy for a painless, watery diarrhœa, especially if the evacuations are brownish or light colored and contain undigested food, and there is a disposition to a passage immediately after eating or drinking. This remedy is useful in some cases where there is pain, provided it is simply caused by wind, and the passages are undigested. Give a dose after every passage. *China* is often required in the case of children when the passages are undigested, but in sucn cases only two doses should be given a day, one at night and the other in the morning; and in chronic cases this remedy need not be repeated more frequently. If *China* fails when it seems to be indicated give either *Phosphorus* or *Arsenicum*.

Bryonia is sometimes very useful when the disease occurs during the hot weather of summer, and is apparently caused by the heat, or the use of cold water when overheated.

In chronic cases the remedies need not be repeated more frequently than two or three times in twenty-four hours, and if the above fail to cure give *Phosphorus* when there is little or no pain and the passages contain undigested food. Give *Sulphur* when there is soreness of the bowels on pressure, and also if there is much pain or any straining with the passages. *Calcarea carb.* may follow either *Phosphorus* or *Sulphur* if relief is not obtained after continuing the remedy for from five to seven days in chronic cases.

Rheum, is one of the best remedies, especially when there is severe pain, or when the passages have an acid or sour smell. Give a dose every hour.

For the diarrhœa of children, if the passages are watery, consult among the foregoing remedies what is said in regard to *Arsenicum*, *Pulsatilla*, *Ipecac*, *Veratrum* and *China*. If the passages are bilious with severe colic or pains in the bowels, consult *Chamomilla*, *Mercurius viv.*, *Pulsatilla*, and *Ipecac*. If there is nausea or vomiting with diarrhœa, consult *Ipecac* and *Veratrum;* and also consult what is said in the section on cholera morbus. Cholera infantum is but one form of cholera morbus, occurring with children. If, during the continuance of diarrhœa and vomiting, or soon after they have ceased, the child has fits of crying, starting, squinting, or is either very wakeful or sleepy, give *Belladonna* alternately with *China* two hours apart, and increase its nourishment, if the stomach will bear it.

Diet.—When attacked by diarrhœa, a patient should abstain from acid, fruits, eggs, and solid food, especially if there is much pain and soreness of the bowels, and drink rice-water, barley-water, oat-meal gruel, and moderately of milk. If the attack is not very severe, he may eat moderately of toast or soft-boiled rice.

COSTIVENESS

Costiveness is generally caused by either sedentary or inactive habits or cathartic remedies. Tailors, shoemakers, and others who follow occupations which require them to sit a great deal of the time, if they neglect general exercise, are quite sure to be troubled more or less with this affection. The disease may also be caused by neglecting to attend regularly to the calls of nature. It often results in infants from some peculiarity in the mother's milk.

Symptoms.—The evacuations become either less frequent or less free, and dryer than in health, and frequently come away in knotty lumps with much straining and painful distention of the passage. They are generally natural in color, but in some instances they are clay-colored, and in other cases blackish, and occasionally covered with bloody mucus. They sometimes accumulate in large quantities in the lower portion of the intestine, so as to cause over-distention of the part, giving rise to much irritation and causing small mucus passages with straining, resembling dysentery, except in not being accompanied by fever. If on examining the abdomen you find an unusual fullness on the left side, extending down as low as you can feel, and this distended part when you strike it with the ends of the fingers gives forth a dull sound, you have reason to think that there is an accumulation there which should be removed. In such a case give free injections of tepid water, and the remedies and take the exercises hereafter named. Constipation under homœopathic, compared with the same disease under allopathic treatment, is of comparatively little moment; and where there is no mechanical obstruction and the patient has not been in the habit of taking cathartics, we find very little difficulty in relieving the unpleasant symptoms which arise. If the bowels have been very costive for a long time they may never get so as to move every day, perhaps not more frequently than once in two or three days, which will do very well in such cases.

Treatment.—The most important measure, without which remedies will be of little use, is to make an attempt to have a passage at a regular hour every day, or every other day, and never neglect this duty. Eat brown bread, fruits, vegetables, and only moderately of meats. Never use cathartics or laxatives of any kind, nor high-seasoned food. Take active out-door exercise, walking, running, horseback-riding, &c. When lying down, night and morning, with the lower extremities straightened out, and the head and shoulders slightly elevated, place a hand upon each side of the abdomen and vibrate it sidewise for a minute or two, then commencing at the lower part of the abdomen on the left side, with the ends of the fingers, knead the abdomen directly up to the short ribs on the left side, then across to beneath the right short ribs, and down on the right side of the abdomen, then knead back over the same course. In the morning, on arising from bed, thump with the fist across the lower part of the back and hips, below the small of the back, for a minute or two. Gently vibrating and kneading the abdomen, and thumping across the hips in the erect position as directed above, will be useful in case of nursing children, as well as for adults. Costiveness generally disappears as soon as the child is weaned, and he begins to run around, unless the bowels have been weakened by cathartics or laxatives. In all cases of *recent costiveness*, where there is soreness and pain, rest is required, therefore, in such cases, omit the above exercises.

Nux vomica: Give a dose of this remedy every night if there are derangements of the stomach, distention of the abdomen, and headache, or frequent urging to stool, with no passage, or slight mucous discharges. *Nux vom.* is especially useful for patients of sedentary habits, and those troubled with piles, and also for pregnant females who are troubled with nausea and vomiting. In the latter case give this remedy at night, and a dose of *Ipecac* in the morning. *Sulphur* should generally follow *Nux vom.;* or give *Sulphur* mornings, and *Nux vom.* nights.

Dose of either of the remedies, see page 7.

Opium is an important remedy for recent cases of constipation, when there is beating and heaviness in the abdomen, or congestion of blood to the head, headache, and red face. It is often useful during pregnancy. Give a dose night and morning.

Bryonia may be given for the constipation of aged persons, and of those who are troubled with rheumatism, also when *Nux vom.* fails to relieve cases for which it seems indicated. Give a dose every morning.

If the patient is a female, and of a mild disposition, *Pulsatilla* will often succeed when *Nux vom.* fails, and it will be useful in all cases when there is acid stomach with the constipation. Give a dose every night. *Sepia* may follow *Pulsatilla* at the end of a week or two. In cases of long standing, if the above remedies fail, give a dose of *Natrum muriaticum* every night, and wet a towel in cold water every morning and apply over the bowels, and over that four or five thicknesses of dry flannel, so as to completely cover the wet towel, and confine the whole by a bandage around the body, pinned or tied tight so as to exclude the cold air. In recent cases of constipation, a remedy should be continued several days without being changed, and in chronic cases several weeks.

COLIC.

This disease is characterized by pain in the bowels, without inflammation. The pain generally occurs in paroxysms, and the bowels are usually constipated. We have two or three varieties of this disease.

1. Flatulent Colic.—This form of the disease is generally caused by undigested food in the intestinal canal, giving rise to a copious formation of gas, which produces spasms of the bowels by its irritating effects. It may be caused by cold, worms, and improper food, and is sometimes connected with a gouty, rheumatic, or hysterical diathesis. There is usually more or less rumbling, with distention of the abdomen, and eructations of wind, which almost always afford more or less relief. The pains are severe, spasmodic, twisting, pinching, cutting, or contracting, and are generally felt in the region of the navel, but may occur in other parts, or over the whole abdomen. The patient often presses his hands upon his bowels, and bends over, and turns from side to side in bed. This affection is very common with children, and

sometimes causes convulsions. Even with adults, when the attack is very severe and sudden, the countenance may be pale and shrunken, and the pulse feeble, with faintness and temporary insensibility.

2. Bilious Colic, characterized by paroxysms of severe colic pains, which usually terminate, or are attended by vomiting of yellow or green bile, which affords temporary relief. The attack is often preceded by loss of appetite, nausea, yellowness of the skin and eyes, and uneasiness in the right side, beneath the lower ribs. There is often some fever ; and tenderness on pressure over the region of the stomach and liver is not uncommon after a few hours. There are sometimes convulsive movements in different parts of the body, and occasionally partial paralysis of some portion of the upper or lower extremities. The bowels are generally costive, and whether they are or not there may be either an excess or a deficiency of bile in the discharges. If the colic and vomiting continue a long time, even the offensive contents of the bowels may be thrown up ; but this is rare, except when the symptoms are caused by a rupture, or by some other obstruction of the bowels. Bilious colic is very common during the hot weather, especially when the nights are cool, and among those exposed to the cool night air. It may also be caused by depressing mental emotions, improper food, over-eating, &c.

3. Lead Colic.—Lead miners, glaziers, plumbers, manufacturers of white lead, and painters, are subject to this affection. Persons using water, especially soft water, which has passed through or stood in lead pipes or cisterns, are liable to attacks of this disease. Many of the symptoms are similar to those of other forms of colic; but the pain generally commences less abruptly, and is at first dull and afterward increases and extends to the back and sides. The abdomen about the navel is generally retracted, but sometimes distended. The stools are usually hard, dry, and knotty, but sometimes there is diarrhœa. The tongue is flat and tremulous, the face of a dingy hue, with a dejected and anxious expression. Trembling of the hands and weakness of the wrist-joints, are not uncommon.

Treatment of Colic.—In all cases when there is vomiting, and even if there is not, examine the abdomen carefully, and see if you can find a rupture, which, if present, will be manifested by a tumor or swelling, usually situated either at the navel, in the groin, or a little above the groin. If you find such a swelling, consult the section on obstruction of the bowels; also do this in all obstinate cases of colic, especially if there are nausea and vomiting. A warm bath is one of the best measures in every form of colic. When you have not conveniences for giving a warm bath, fold a flannel blanket in one direction so that it will be wide enough to extend from the knees to the shoulders, then lay it lengthwise across the bed; fold a sheet in the same manner, but not quite as wide as the blanket, wring the sheet out of warm water, and wrap it around the body and hips, and wrap the ends of the flannel blanket as the patient lies upon it, over the wet sheet; wet the sheet again as soon as it becomes cool. This is a very good substitute for a warm bath. Cloths wrung from hot water and applied simply over the bowels, often afford some relief. In all cases where the bowels are costive, or in any case where there is no diarrhœa, copious injections of warm water will be found useful. Also let the patient drink freely of warm water, especially if there is nausea and vomiting.

Remedies for Flatulent Colic.—Give *Belladonna* when there are cutting pains through the bowels, and there is a swelling like a pad across the abdomen above the navel. This remedy is often useful in the case of children as well as in that of adults. Give a dose every half hour or hour.

Dose of either of these remedies see page 7.

Chamomilla will be required in the case of children and females, and even males, when the bowels are distended with wind and there are tearing and drawing pains, and a sensation as if the intestines were drawn up into a ball. Give a dose every half hour or hour.

Nux vom.: Give this remedy if the disease has been caused by errors of diet, especially if the bowels are costive, and the patient is a man and troubled with piles, and in other cases if there is pressure in the abdomen, as if from a stone, with rumbling and contractive pains, aggravation by walking, and relief from rest and lying down. Give a dose every hour. If at the end of four or five hours the symptoms are not relieved, give *Colocynth* and consult what is said under the head of that remedy.

Pulsatilla should be given when the disease has been caused by over-eating, or by the use of improper articles, especially if the patient is a female, or if a male, if the eructations are sour, or smell like rotten eggs, or the bowels are loose, and if the pains are worse when sitting or lying, and relieved by walking, and when the face is pale with blue margins around the eyes. Give a dose every hour, and if the patient is not relieved at the end of four or five hours, give *Colocynth* as directed under the head of bilious colic. To overcome a disposition to flatulent colic, give *Carbo veg.* nights, and *China* mornings.

Remedies for Bilious Colic.—*Colocynth* is one of the most important remedies in this form of the disease, and also for flatulent colic, when it is of a decidedly spasmodic character. It is indicated when there is a feeling as if the intestines were squeezed between stones, and when there are cutting, twisting, grasping pains in the bowels, which extend to the stomach with nausea and bilious vomiting, which afford partial relief. Give a dose every hour, and if the patient does not improve after taking the second or third dose, give two tablespoonfuls of common coffee, without milk or sugar, a half an hour from the dose of *Colocynth*, and repeat it, if necessary, two or three times. As soon as the symptoms improve, lengthen the intervals between the doses of *Colocynth* to three or four hours.

Nux vom. is next in importance to *Colocynth*, in the treatment of this affection. The indications are similar to those given under the head of flatulent colic, with the addition of bilious vomiting, which affords temporary relief, with pressure in the pit of the stomach. Repeat the dose every hour. If there is sour vomiting, *Pulsatilla* will generally do better than *Nux vom.* Consult what is said in regard to *Pulsatilla* under the head of flatulent colic.

Chamomilla will often afford relief in the case of women and children, when there is bilious vomiting or eructations, smelling like rotten eggs, with fullness at the pit of the stomach. Give a dose every hour, until there is some change, then lengthen the intervals.

Give *Veratrum* when the vomiting is frequent, with cramp-like pain in the bowels, and pressure at the pit of the stomach.

In obstinate cases, where there is great debility, severe pains, burning or a feeling of coldness in the abdomen, with nausea and vomiting, give a dose of *Arsenicum* every hour. To overcome a predisposition to this disease, give *Sulphur* and *Nux. vom.* alternately, three days apart.

Remedies for Lead Colic.—When the pain is severe, give *Belladonna* once in one or two hours, and if it fails to relieve, alternate it with *Nux vom.* at intervals of two hours; and, as soon as there is a decided improvement, lengthen the intervals between the doses. These remedies will require to be continued for several weeks. If the patient does not improve rapidly, occasionally for two or three days, omit them and give *Opium* three or four times a day.

The patient should use to a great extent a milk diet, with more or less meat and vegetables, and he must shun the cause of his disease—give up his occupation if it requires him to use lead. If there is weakness of the wrist-joints, they must be exercised freely every day. A warm bath once in two or three days will be useful.

OBSTRUCTION OF THE BOWELS, RUPTURE, &c.

The most severe and obstinate form of colic is sometimes caused by obstruction of the bowels, preventing the passage downward of their contents. Such an obstruction is sometimes caused by a rupture of the internal layers of the walls of the abdomen, and the protrusion of a portion of the intestine, forming a tumor beneath the skin, which may become strangulated at the point where it protrudes, or at some point, so as to prevent the passage of the contents of the bowels, and also the circulation of blood through the strangulated part. If this state of things is not relieved, mortification and death usually ensue. Ruptures generally occur at the navel, in the groin, or a little above the groin, extending down toward the scrotum in men and labia in females. Sometimes they occur in other parts of the abdomen. In young children the intestine frequently follows the testicle in its descent from the abdomen down into the scrotum; and, if it is not returned and retained by a proper bandage, it is liable to become strangulated. Obstruction of the bowels may also be caused by a fold or loop of the intestine being turned around upon itself, also by one portion falling into another and becoming strangulated. In other cases, gall-stones may form in the intestines; or magnesia, chalk, cherry-stones and the like, with those who are in the habit of swallowing such improper substances, may accumulate and cause obstructions. Tumors pressing upon the bowels, also the contractions which result from the healing up of extensive ulcerations of the mucous membrane, may cause obstruction. The obstruction may be complete or only partial; in the latter case the symptoms may abate in a great measure and return again and again for months and years, and the patient finally either recover or die.

Symptoms of Obstruction.—Severe colic pains, followed by vomiting, without fever or marked bilious derangement, are the first symptoms. If the obstruction is not relieved the vomiting continues until the offensive contents of the bowels are thrown up, and the bowels become more or less distended with gas, the respiration oppressed, hiccough appears, the pulse becomes small and irregular, and cold and clammy sweats appear on the surface, and death generally follows. Sometimes delirium, and in children convulsions, precede the fatal termination. The abdomen generally, as the disease progresses, gradually becomes tender, perhaps only near the point of obstruction, and there is more or less fever.

Treatment.—In all cases where there are symptoms of obstruction, the abdomen and groin should be carefully examined, to ascertain if there is a rupture, which will manifest itself by a tumor or swelling, which is liable to be more or less tender on pressure, and may be very small or quite large. If you find that the symptoms are caused by a rupture, give a dose of *Nux vom.*, and if, at the end of two hours, the symptoms are not relieved, give a dose of *Aconite*, and afterward continue these two remedies alternately, two hours apart; immediately raise the hips until they are a foot or so higher than the shoulders, then place the thighs and legs bent at nearly right angles, as when an individual is sitting, and either have the feet rest against the side of the house, or have them held by assistants, then with the fingers of one hand, press gently but steadily on the tumor, and with those of the other, endeavor to work the contents of the swelling back through the opening through which they have protruded. Remember that the part last protruded or nearest the opening must return first. With a little patience and perseverance, you will often succeed. But if you do not soon succeed, send immediately for a physician or surgeon—an allopathist if you cannot obtain a homœopathist. After the intestine has been returned, a truss should be carefully fitted, and worn constantly.

In all cases of obstruction of the bowels, copious injections of warm water should be used, and repeated from time to time, as they sometimes mechanically overcome the obstruction. Also, a warm-bath will often be found useful.

Nux vom. is an important remedy for this disease, and may be given once in two hours. If, at the end of twelve or twenty-four hours, it fails to relieve the symptoms, give a dose of *Bryonia* once in two hours. *Colocynth* is sometimes useful, repeated as directed for bilious colic. Also consult the section on bilious colic.

Opium: If, notwithstanding the use of other remedies, the patient becomes very much exhausted, or the substance vomited become very offensive, give *Opium* every hour. Dose, six globules, or one drop, dissolved in a few spoonfuls of water.

If the patient becomes very much exhausted in this disease, give him beef-tea, mutton-broth, and rice-water. These articles may be given by injection, if the stomach will not retain them.

This affection cannot always be cured, for sometimes the obstruction is of so permanent a character that the patient must die, but we cannot tell when this is the case, and there is always hope while there is life, for patients sometimes recover when we least expect it, especially when the disease has neither been aggravated by drastic cathartic remedies, nor the bowels rendered torpid by large doses of opium, administered during its early stage.

RUPTURE (HERNIA).

If this disease is attended by colic or nausea and vomiting, consult the section on obstruction of the bowels, and follow the directions you will find there for the treatment of strangulated hernia or rupture. A patient who is troubled with a rupture, should never go a single day without wearing a good truss, for if the intestine is allowed to protrude, it is liable to become strangulated at any moment, and life is always endangered by this accident. For a rupture at the navel in children, cut circular pieces of cotton cloth, from the size of a pea to that of a half dollar, and enough when stitched together to be at least half an inch in thickness; then cover the rounding surface of the pad thus formed, with adhesive plaster, and stitch the back of the pad to the centre and plastered surface of a strip of adhesive plaster about two inches wide, and long enough to extend about three quarters of the way around the body; then warm the plaster, press back the intestine, and place the pad directly over the navel, and carry the ends of the long strip snugly around the body, and put a belly-band around the whole. Change the plaster as often as it becomes loose—once in one or two weeks. For a rupture which descends toward the scrotum, in infants, make a compress of cotton cloth, about the size of a hen's egg, press back the intestine, and place it over the part where the intestine protrudes, and pin the diaper closely over the compress, and when you change the diaper, keep up gentle pressure, so as to prevent the intestine from protruding until the compress is again applied.

In addition to the above mechanical measures for the relief and cure of hernia, give to either adults or children who are troubled with this affection, a dose of *Nux vom.* every night for three weeks, then give a dose of *Silicea* every night for one week, after which give *Nux vom.* again and so continue; *Sulphur* will sometimes be of service if the above remedies fail. In the case of children the disease will generally soon be cured if the remedies named are given, and the compress is properly applied and kept on, so as to prevent the protrusion of the intestine.

PILES (HEMORRHOIDS).

This disease is frequently caused by sedentary and indolent habits, and by occupations which confine to the sitting position.

Sitting on cushions favors the development of piles by heating the parts. High-seasoned food, stimulating and fermented drinks and cathartic remedies are also among the causes which give rise to this affection.

Symptoms.—A sensation of fullness, heat, and perhaps itching is felt about the anus, caused in a great measure by the dilatation of the veins in the lower part of the intestine or rectum, and in the anus or external passage. The swelling increases until small tumors form which are sore and painful. These may be external and visible or internal, and are often of a bluish color, and when inflamed they are very sore and painful to the touch. There is frequently a discharge of blood, especially from internal piles, and such discharges often return repeatedly until a habit is established, and there is a feeling of fullness before and relief after such discharges.

Treatment.—If there are much inflammation, heat, pain, soreness, and fever, give *Aconite* once in two hours until these symptoms are relieved. If there is hemorrhage give *Nitric acid* once in two hours until it is relieved, and then give a dose every morning, and a dose of *Nux vom.* every night for two weeks, after which give *Nux vom.* at night and *Sulphur* in the morning. These two remedies may be continued for several months. If notwithstanding the above remedies hemorrhage returns, a dose of *Calcarea carb.* given night and morning for a few weeks will rarely fail to relieve this symptom, and also to benefit the piles. If the flow of blood is very profuse give a dose of Ipecac every hour until it is relieved. If there is no hemorrhage and the patient is either of sedentary habits or a high liver, give *Nux vom.* at night and *Sulphur* in the morning. With females *Pulsatilla* sometimes does better than *Nux vom.* In obstinate cases if the piles are bluish and there is burning in them, give *Carbo veg.* night and morning.

If a patient expects a permanent cure of this disease, he must shun the causes which have produced it, or he can never obtain anything more than palliative relief from the best remedies. He must shun all stimulating drinks and spices, use brown bread, and but little meat, and eat temperately, and take active out-door exercise. Lie with the face downward, and sustain the weight of the body by the elbows and toes, resting on a sofa or bed, for a few moments, and then slowly raise the hips and lower them five or six times; this tends to relieve the congestion of the veins about the anus, and if repeated two or three times a day, it is an excellent form of exercise, not only for the piles, but also for falling of the bowels, as well as for falling of the womb.

FALLING OF THE BOWELS (PROLAPSUS ANI).

This affection is characterized by the protrusion of the mucous membrane of the rectum, or lower portion of the intestine, through the anus. This accident is generally caused by straining at stool, and is much more common with children than with adults.

Treatment.—To return the protruded portion of the mucous membrane, let the child lie on his face, with the hips elevated higher than the shoulders, oil a soft piece of muslin, three or four inches square, with sweet oil, cream or lard, place it over the protruded part, hold it lightly but smoothly over the tumor with the fingers of one hand, and pass the forefinger of the other hand directly into the centre of the tumor, in the direction of the anus, carrying the muslin before the finger through the anus, until the entire protruded part has been returned; then hold the finger there for a moment or two, and afterward gently withdraw it, together with the muslin. Sometimes simply pressing the flesh on each side, over the tumor, with the hips elevated, will cause the bowel to return; this can be tried first. Patients who are much troubled with this difficulty, should be required to have their evacuations in a position halfway between sitting and standing, and should avoid straining.

Give *Ignatia* at night, and *Calcarea carb.* in the morning, and continue these remedies one month, and longer if the patient is doing well. If, at the end of a month, the disposition to this affection is not overcome, give *Nux vom.* at night, and *Sulphur* in the morning for a month, after which *Sepia* will sometimes be useful in obstinate cases. If there is a frequent inclination to go to stool, with small mucous passages, give a dose of *Mercurius viv.* once in two hours, until this symptom is relieved, then give *Sulphur* night and morning. Also take regularly, at least night and morning, the exercise directed for piles, in the last section.

ITCHING OF THE ANUS.

This may be caused by piles; in that case there is generally more or less swelling and soreness; for its relief consult the section on piles. It may be caused by pin-worms, and when this is the case there is generally a creeping and tingling sensation, and on examination the worms often can be seen, and they are frequently found on the passages from the bowels. This is a very frequent cause of itching of the anus in the case of children. For the proper remedies consult the section on worms. Itching is frequently caused around the anus, by a very fine eruption of pimples; they may be scarcely perceptible. In all cases when you are satisfied that the itching is neither caused by piles nor by worms, consult the section on lichen, and follow the directions you there find, for the treatment of that disease.

INTESTINAL WORMS.

There are three different kind of worms which have been found in the intestines of man—the pin-worm, the long round worm, and the tapeworm.

The pin-worm inhabits the very lower portion of the intestines, the rectum, and causes an intense itching, tingling and creeping sensation, which annoys the patient excessively, especially at night, and while sitting. The whole nervous system is sometimes intensely excited by them, so as to cause twitchings and convulsions. I have known the most intense headache, through the forehead, lasting almost without cessation for years, to result from the irritation caused by these worms; the headache disappeared immediately when the worm disease was cured.

Treatment for Pin-Worms.—If there is intense itching on going to bed with heat and restlessness, give a dose of *Aconite*, about one hour before retiring, and if the patient when in bed does not soon fall asleep, but remains nervous, give a dose of *Ignatia*. This variety of worms generally affects delicate children, and persons whose digestive organs are weak and easily deranged. To cure this affection permanently and prevent a return of the symptoms, it is necessary to give remedies for several weeks, and in fact months *Aconite* and *Ignatia* will do little more than palliate the symptoms for the time-being. To permanently cure the disease give a dose of *Sulphur* every morning for a week. If the symptoms are not so severe as to require *Aconite* at night, it will be better to give the *Sulphnr* at night. At the end of the week omit *Sulphur* and give *Calcarea carb.* in the same manner for a week, then omit it and give *China* for a week, then discontinue all remedies for one week, after which give in rotation a single dose of the above remedies at intervals of one week, and continue them for months, as they will benefit the general health of the patient, and tend to eradicate any constitutional predisposition on which the existence of these worms may depend. A small injection of *Sweet oil*, or of weak *Whiskey-and-water*, may be given every night until the symptoms disappear, then give it once a week for a few weeks.

The long round worm inhabits the small intestines principally, sometimes it passes up into the stomach, and occasionally up the gullet toward the mouth; when in the latter situation, it causes a strangling or choking sensation, and the patient may swallow it or throw it up. If an individual is troubled with these worms, they will occasionally be seen in the stools. They sometimes grow to the length of eight or ten inches. Many children who are comparatively healthy, are troubled with such worms, and generally without their being a source of any particular inconvenience; in fact, within my own observation, I have seen worse symptoms from the popular worm medicines, than I have ever seen from this variety of worms. We can rarely say, with any great degree of certainty, that a child or an individual is troubled with these worms, unless we see them, for we may have, from an improper diet, or weak digestive powers, all the symptoms which are supposed to denote their presence; such as picking of the nose, craving appetite, nausea, colic, pains in the bowels, hardness and distention of the abdomen, crying out in sleep, grating the teeth, twitching and convulsions.

Treatment for Long Round Worms.—Give a dose of *Cina* every morning until the symptoms are relieved; also give *Mercurius viv.* every night for one week, after which give a dose of *Sulphur* once a week for several weeks. For worm fever give *Aconite;* for convulsive symptoms, give either *Belladonna* or *Ignatia;* and for worm-colic give *Cina,* and if it does not relieve within one hour, give *Mercurius viv.*

Tapeworm.—Undoubtedly the most frequent cause of the tapeworm in man, is the use of measly pork, which contains these worms in one stage of their development. If fresh measly pork is fed to the dog, tapeworms are developed in his intestines, and if joints of the tapeworm, which contain ova or eggs, at maturity, are fed to the pig, they cause measly pork. If such pork is well cooked, there is no danger of its generating tapeworms, and there is less danger when it has been some time cured or salted. Tapeworms are quite common in dogs and various other animals, and it is supposed also, that they may sometimes be developed in the intestines of man by his swallowing their eggs, which are voided by such animals, in his food and drink, as the Hindoos, who eat no flesh, are sometimes affected by these worms; but it is undoubtedly true, that man contracts tapeworms far more frequently by eating imperfectly cooked flesh of animals, generally of the pig, which contains them in their cystic state or stage of imperfect development.

If a patient is troubled with a tapeworm, he is quite sure to pass portions of it frequently. This worm is flat, and jointed somewhat resembling gourd seeds, strung together lengthwise, and often grows to a very great length. The sight of portions of the worm in the stools, is the only sure sign of its existence, for the craving appetite, colic pains, emaciation, and other symptoms which sometimes result, may all arise from other causes; and patients may be affected with tapeworm, and yet enjoy very comfortable health, and have few symptoms.

Treatment for Tapeworm.—Bruise well a tablespoonful of pumpkin seeds, and make a strong tea from them by steeping, and drink half of it at night and the rest of it in the morning, and repeat it for three or four days, if necessary; also, take for several months, *Sulphur* and *Mercurius viv.* one week apart. If this does not cure, call on a homœopathic physician. The patient should eat no pork, nor raw or imperfectly cooked meat of any kind.

Patients troubled with any kind of worms, require a good nourishing diet, but should abstain entirely from candies, much sweet food, pies, cakes, and coffee. Children troubled with worms, require sunlight, fresh air, and active out-door exercise.

INFLAMMATION OF THE LIVER (HEPATITIS).

This disease in both the acute and chronic forms, is much more frequent in hot than in temperate and cold climates. It may be caused by exposure to cold damp air when the body is hot, also by the use of mercury, alcoholic and fermented drinks, and high living.

Symptoms of Acute Inflammation of the Liver.—This disease commences with either sharp and almost lancinating, or else dull or aching pains beneath the lower ribs on the right side · sometimes extending across toward the left side; there is also a feeling of oppression and tenderness on pressing up beneath the lower ribs, and sometimes there is pain in the right shoulder. Chills and fever either precede, accompany, or soon follow, the local symptoms, and not unfrequently there are nausea and vomiting. The bowels are generally costive, but in some cases loose; the urine is scanty and high colored, and the skin is frequently jaundiced. There are often fullness and swelling beneath the right lower ribs. If the disease is very acute, it may run a rapid course, terminating either in recovery, or the commencement of an abscess within a week. If an abscess forms, which rarely occurs, the pulse becomes more frequent, and there are chills, perspiration, feeling of weight, and throbbing in the side; it may break externally, or into the stomach, bowels, or into the air passages, and the patient may recover or die. Sometimes the patient dies before the abscess breaks; in rare instances it breaks either into the abdominal cavity, or into the pleura, and causes inflammation and death. The disease may be less acute, and last two or more weeks, and even become chronic, without the formation of an abscess.

Chronic inflammation of the liver may be the result of an acute attack, or it may come on slowly and may terminate in recovery, or the formation of an abscess; or again, the liver may become indurated and enlarged, and in other instances contracted. The symptoms are often obscure; there may be little or no pain, perhaps simply uneasiness in the region of the liver, and tenderness on pressure; and there may be some of the following symptoms: Furred tongue, bitter taste, occasional vomiting, irregular bowels, unhealthy evacuations, dry skin, yellowness of the skin, eyes, and urine, a short dry cough, depression of spirits, slight febrile excitement toward night, and emaciation. Sometimes dropsy of the abdomen and swelling of the lower extremities, result. The patient's easiest position, in either the acute or chronic form of the disease, is usually on the affected side.

Treatment of Acute Inflammation of the Liver.—Give a dose of *Aconite* every hour if there is much fever with a dry skin, or there are sharp and severe pains. Continue it until the fever is relieved. If *Aconite* alone does not relieve the sharp pains in three or four hours, omit it and give a dose of *Belladonna* in its stead, especially if there are great restlessness, sleeplessness, and headache.

Dose of either of the remedies, see page 7.

Bryonia is one of the most important remedies after *Aconite* for this disease. If in the course of twelve or twenty hours *Aconite* does not relieve the fever and pain, give a dose of *Bryonia* once in six hours, and *Aconite* every hour between the doses; especially when there are dull aching pains, fullness, soreness on pressure in the region of the liver, or beneath the right floating ribs. As soon as the fever is relieved the *Aconite* can be discontinued, and the *Bryonia* can be given alone. *Nux vomica* is often required after *Bryonia*.

Nux vomica: If notwithstanding the use of the above remedies fr three or four days, the skin and eyes become yellow, or there are great sensitiveness in the region of the liver on pressure with dull pains, bitter taste, vomiting, and high-colored urine, give a dose of *Nux vom.* once in four hours, and if this remedy fails to relieve the above symptoms at the end of twenty-four hours alternate it with *Mercurius viv.* at intervals of three hours. If the bowels are loose this will be another indication for *Mercurius viv.*

Lachesis may be given once in two hours, if you have reason to fear that an abscess is about to form, or if the severity of the disease is not relieved within five or six days after the attack. If an abscess forms which will very rarely happen, give *Silicea* three times a day, and *China* at bedtime. In all cases as soon as the symptoms are relieved give *Sulphur* night and morning. Wring a towel from cold water and lay it over the region of the liver and stomach, and cover it entirely with five or six thicknesses of dry flannel, and with a dry towel around the body confine the whole to its place; wet the towel once in eight hours; but if at the end of twenty-four hours there is no improvement apply warm cloths.

Treatment of Chronic Inflammation of the Liver.—Give a dose of *Nux vom.* every night and *Sulphur* every morning, and continue them as long as the patient improves. When the improvement ceases give *Lycopodium* every night and *Bryonia* every morning. If the patient has recently suffered from intermittent or bilious fevers, instead of the last remedies named give *Carbo veg.* at night and *China* in the morning.

JAUNDICE.

This disease is characterized by yellowness of the eyes, skin, and urine. The yellow color is caused by the yellow constituent of bile remaining in the blood; and this results either when the liver ceases to secrete bile, or when there is an obstruction in the biliary duct, so that the bile secreted cannot enter the intestine, which mechanically prevents the further secretion of this fluid.

An attack of jaundice is often preceded by depression of spirits, disordered vision, general uneasiness, especially in the region of the stomach and liver, loss of appetite, nausea, and vomiting. The eyes usually first become yellow, then the face, neck, and upper part of the chest; and more or less rapidly the entire surface, but sometimes only a part of the body assumes this hue, and generally the color is the most intense where the skin is the thinnest. At first the color is a light yellow, but if the disease continues it may become of a deep orange color, occasionally of a greenish hue, and in very bad cases almost black; sometimes there is itching of the skin. The urine undergoes about the same changes of color as the skin, and the stools in a majority of cases are of a whitish gray, or clay color, from the absence of bile. There is often some fever in connection with this disease, and there may be uneasiness, fullness, and even pain in the region of the stomach, and beneath the lower ribs on the right side. More or less drowsiness is not uncommon. This disease may last but for a few days or weeks, or for months and even years in obstinate cases. New-born infants are very subject to jaundice, which generally soon disappears. Jaundice rarely proves fatal except when complicated with or caused by organic disease of the liver, and when it occurs in a depraved state of the system, when the skin assumes a blackish or greenish hue. The first favorable sign is usually a reappearance of a healthy color to the stools and this is generally accompanied by an improvement of the general symptoms, and the patient is often much better before the color of the skin materially changes.

Treatment of Jaundice.—When this disease is accompanied by fever, fullness, soreness, or pain in the region of the liver, give *Bryonia* once in six hours. If there is headache or depression of spirits, give *Belladonna*, alternately with *Bryonia*, three hours apart, when the patient is awake. These remedies should be continued several days, and even for two or three weeks, if the general and local symptoms improve.

Dose of either of the remedies, see page 7.

Nux vom. may follow *Bryonia*, in case that remedy fails to relieve all the symptoms, and it may be given at the commencement of the attack, instead of *Bryonia*, when the disease has been caused by mental application, passion, intemperance, or the suppression of an intermittent fever. Give a dose three or four times a day. *Bryonia* will often follow this remedy, to advantage.

Mercurius viv.: Give this remedy if, notwithstanding the use of the above remedies, the skin becomes very yellow, and the region of the liver painful to the touch, swollen and hard, and when the stools are of a grayish white color. Give a dose three times a day.

China may be given, if the disease has been caused by the use of *Mercury*; also if it is connected with intermittent fever, and *Nux vom.* fails to relieve the symptoms. When the disease has in a great measure abated, give a dose of this remedy every night. *Sulphur* is useful to complete the cure. Give a dose every night. In obstinate cases, *Sulphur*, *Nitric acid*, *Hepar sulph.*, and *Lachesis*, one or more may be required.

For the jaundice of new-born infants, give *Mercurius viv.*, two doses twelve hours apart, then give a dose of *China* once a day. Dose, two or three globules.

The diet should be light and free from stimulants, and while the fever and uneasiness at the stomach remain, the patient should abstain from animal food, and eat rice, stale bread, gruel, and farina, and roasted potatoes well mashed with a little salt and cream.

PASSAGE OF GALL-STONES.

Gall-stones are earthy concretions, of a yellowish or brownish color, which form in the gall-bladder, or in the gall-duct; sometimes in the intestine near the entrance of the gall-duct. When they form in the gall-bladder, there may be but one, or several; they may be small or large enough to fill the gall-bladder. So long as they remain in the gall-bladder, they generally cause little or no inconvenience, but when they find their way into the gall-duct, and put the coats of that tube on the stretch, they produce the most intense pain and suffering, perhaps as severe as any to which the human frame is liable. The pain usually comes on suddenly, and occurs in paroxysms and is felt a little to the right of the stomach, beneath the lower ribs, and may shoot through to the back. There are sometimes nausea and vomiting, anxiety, great restlessness, faintness, and great prostration, with pale skin, small and frequent pulse. Several paroxysms may occur in an hour, and the attack usually lasts from a few hours to several days, until the stone enters the intestine, when the sufferings are immediately relieved, and the stone passes off with the discharges.

Treatment.—If the pain is the direct result of the irritation caused by the passage of a rough stone through the duct, mechanically irritating and over-distending the passage, we can hardly expect to relieve the sufferings with homœopathic remedies any more than we can expect to relieve the sufferings caused by the knife while amputating a limb, by the use of such remedies. In both cases the sufferings result from the direct action of a mechanical cause, and can only be removed by the influence of some remedy, in large doses, which is capable of lessening the general nervous susceptibility for the time-being. But it undoubtedly often happens that the paroxysms of pain are caused by a spasmodic contraction of the duct on the passing substance, and therefore these spasms can perhaps in some cases be relieved by homœopathic remedies, and as they often cease in a short time owing to the passage of the stone, it is well to give the remedies a trial.

Belladonna: Give a dose of this remedy, and if there is no change in the symptoms in half an hour repeat it. If at the end of an hour there is no change, give a dose of *Nux vom.* and repeat this at the end of another hour if necessary. In addition to the above give a tablespoonful of *Sweet oil,* and if the pain persists, repeat it once in two hours until four doses have been taken, then omit it. If the above remedies fail to relieve, you can try *Bryonia,* and give a dose every hour.

If you have conveniences, give a warm bath, and if you have not, wring large cloths from warm water and apply them over the seat of the pain. If you fail to relieve the patient, and his sufferings are very severe, and you cannot obtain the services of a homœopathic physician, you can give the patient, if an adult, either twenty-five drops of *Laudanum* or one sixth of a grain of *Morphine,* and repeat it once at the end of one or two hours, if necessary.

BILIOUSNESS.

Some persons are frequently troubled with what they call biliousness, and although it is not a scientific term, yet it is one which is generally understood. Patients who are in the habit of taking cathartics or emetics, when the period arrives for their usual "cleaning out," are sure to be troubled with biliousness.

Symptoms.—There is more or less fullness, sensation of a load or other symptoms of uneasiness in the region of the stomach. The appetite is impaired and the bowels constipated. There is languor, dull headache or sleepiness, and sometimes slight yellowness of the eyes and skin.

Treatment.—Shun emetics and cathartics, especially blue-pills and all mercurials, for patients can never be cured while continuing to take such remedies—for although they may afford palliative relief, they never fail to do harm in the end. Let the patient live light, and take a dose of *Bryonia* every morning, and a dose of *Nux vom.* every night, until the symptoms disappear.

INFLAMMATION OF THE SPLEEN (AGUE CAKE).

This disease may be caused by direct violence, great muscular exertion, various febrile diseases, and the malaria or poison which causes agues. Chronic inflammation or congestion, resulting in enlargement, is quite common in connection with intermittent and remittent fevers.

Symptoms.—Dull or sharp pain, deep beneath the lower left ribs, with more or less tenderness on external pressure, are among the first symptoms. In some instances there is very little pain, simply a feeling of weight or fullness, which is worse when the patient lies on the affected side. The attack is generally accompanied with chills and fever, and sometimes there are nausea and vomiting, cough, difficulty of breathing and hiccough. The bowels are usually constipated. The spleen often becomes enlarged so as to be felt beneath the lower left ribs, and in chronic cases it sometimes becomes very much enlarged, and nearly fills the left side of the abdomen.

Treatment.—If the disease has been caused by mechanical injuries or over muscular exertion, give *Arnica* once in two hours. If there is high febrile excitement, give a dose of *Aconite* every hour until it is lessened.

Bryonia, after either *Arnica* or *Aconite*, in acute cases, is generally the most important remedy, especially when there are sharp or dull pains, with soreness which is increased by pressure or movement. Give a dose once in three hours. As soon as the acute symptoms have been relieved, give a dose of *China* once in four hours.

China should generally follow the above remedies, and when the disease occurs in districts where intermittent and remittent fevers prevail, if the symptoms are not very acute, it may be given at the commencement of the disease. Give a dose once in six hours. If there are vomiting, burning, and great debility, give *Arsenicum* once in two hours. In chronic cases, give *China* every night for two weeks, then *Sulphur*, and afterward *Arsenicum*, each for two weeks. Wring a towel from cold water, and apply over the diseased organ, and over that four or five thicknesses of dry flannel; wet the towel once in eight hours.

CHAPTER VI.

DISEASES OF THE URINARY AND GENITAL ORGANS.

INFLAMMATION OF THE KIDNEYS (NEPHRITIS).

THIS disease may be caused by wounds, bruises, exposure to wet and cold, the application of blisters to the skin, the use of certain medicines internally, such as turpentine, Spanish flies, and alcoholic drinks. The presence of gravel or stone in the kidneys, or in the passage to the bladder, may cause this disease. Gouty individuals are very subject to it.

Symptoms.—A sharp and severe, a dull and heavy, or a burning pain, deep in the small of the back on one side, is the most prominent symptom. The pain frequently extends down in the direction of the bladder, groin, scrotum, or even the inside of the thigh. Sudden motions of the body, or heavy pressure over the kidneys, increase the sufferings. There is often a feeling of numbness extending down the thigh, and the testicle is sometimes drawn up and sore. There is generally a frequent inclination to pass urine, and it is high colored, scanty, and perhaps mixed with blood or mucus, and it may deposit a gravelly or earthy matter on standing. Sometimes there is a suppression of urine from the diseased kidney; in that case the urine discharged may be clear, coming entirely from the well kidney. If both kidneys are inflamed, and the urine is entirely suppressed, if relief is not soon obtained, stupor and death follow. Chills followed by fever attend this disease; the fever may be slight or high, and is apt to be remittent. The bowels are generally constipated, and nausea and vomiting are not uncommon, in severe cases. The inflammation may gradually abate and the patient recover, or ulceration or an abscess ensues often within a week or ten days; in that case matter or pus may appear in the urine, and the patient gradually recovers or the disease may become chronic. Sometimes the passage to the bladder may become blocked up by a stone, or from swelling from inflammation, and urine, mucus, and matter or pus, may collect in the pelvis of the kidney or commencement of the passage, and distend the part so as to form a large tumor, which may break into the colon or large intestine, and its contents be discharged by the bowels; or, in rare instances, the contents of the tumor make their way externally through the loins, in the form of an abscess, and are thus discharged. In other cases, the tumor breaks into the abdominal cavity, which causes fatal peritonitis. Inflammation of the kidneys sometimes, although rarely, terminates in gangrene or mortification; this may be suspected when there is a sudden cessation of pain, followed by cold sweat, sinking of the vital powers and death.

Chronic inflammation of the kidneys sometimes follows an acute attack, in other cases it comes on gradually, with but little pain, scanty, but frequent passages of urine, which is high-colored, and deposits an earthy sediment on cooling. If the disease continues, mucus and pus, or matter, generally appear in the urine, and if the disease is not arrested, the patient is worn out by hectic fever, night sweats, and gradual emaciation. Chronic inflammation of the kidneys is very apt to be confounded with inflammation of the bladder, which gives rise to similar mucous and purulent discharges with the urine; but on careful inquiry, you will find that the patient feels more or less pain and uneasiness in the kidneys, and that on heavy pressure there is some tenderness. We sometimes have a neuralgic affection of the kidneys, in which the pain is very severe, but it occurs in paroxysms, and is without fever.

Treatment.—In all cases which are attended with chills and fever, give a dose of *Aconite* every hour. If, at the end of twelve hours, the symptoms are not relieved, give *Cannabis* alternately with it, at intervals of one hour. If, at the end of twenty-four hours more, there is an abatement of the symptoms, continue the above remedies, but at intervals of two or three hours; but if no improvement follows, omit the *Cannabis*, and give *Cantharis* alternately with *Aconite*, at the same intervals. If there are severe shooting pains extending from the kidneys toward the bladder, and there is heat, with feelings of distention in the kidneys, with a scanty discharge of orange-yellow urine, omit the *Cannabis* or *Cantharis*, for twelve, out of every twenty-four hours, and give *Belladonna* alternately with *Aconite*. *Belladonna* is also useful for neuralgia of the kidneys.

Dose, see page 7.

As soon as the acute symptoms have been relieved by the above treatment, *Nux vom.* often becomes a valuable remedy, especially for gouty subjects, and the intemperate; also for those subject to gravel or piles. Give a dose once in two hours. This remedy is also useful for neuralgia of the kidneys. *Pulsatilla* may be given in the case of females, instead of *Nux vom.*, especially if there is a suppression of the menses.

If the disease has been caused by mechanical injuries, give *Arnica*, alternately with *Aconite*. If the disease has been caused by a blister, or by *Cantharides* or *Spanish flies*, give either six globules or drop doses of *Camphor* every hour.

For chronic inflammation of the kidneys, several of the above remedies will be found useful, but others will often be required. If at the end of five or six days, in acute cases, the patient feels chilly at times and the pain becomes throbbing, or if matter appears in the urine, omit *Aconite* and give *Hepar sulph.* once in six hours. Either *Cannabis* or *Nux vom.* may be given alternately with it, if pain and soreness linger, or if there is a frequent inclination to void urine with pain or burning.

Lycopodium: Give this remedy in chronic cases, when there is a red or yellow sediment in the urine, with or without pus or matter. Give a dose night and morning, and if it fails to relieve, give *Phosphorus*, especially if, with or without a reddish sediment, there is whitish matter or mucus in the urine.

Give *Calcarea carb.* when the urine is offensive, dark brown, or there is a whitish or light-colored earthy sediment. Give a dose night and morning. If while giving either of the last three remedies there is much pain in the kidneys, or irritation in voiding urine, you can give a dose of either *Cannabis*, *Pulsatilla*, or *Nux vom.* occasionally between the doses of the other remedy. If the above remedies fail in chronic cases, drop one drop of *Spirits of turpentine* on to some powdered sugar, rub it up well, and make ten doses of it, and give one once in six hours.

Diet, &c.—In all acute cases, the diet should be light, and *Slippery-elm tea*, or *Gum-arabic water* may be used as a drink.

BRIGHT'S DISEASE OF THE KIDNEYS.

(GRANULAR OR FATTY DEGENERATION OF THE KIDNEYS.)

This is a somewhat rare disease, and in the acute form, the symptoms resemble those of acute inflammation of the kidneys, but it is distinguished from the latter affection by the urine containing albumen, or a substance similar to the white of an egg; and often by the occurrence within a few days of symptoms of acute dropsy. To detect albumen in the urine, if it is cloudy or muddy, strain it, then heat it in a silver spoon, earthen dish, or tin cup, to the boiling point, then if there is no change in its appearance, drop in a few drops of vinegar and heat it again. If the urine contains albumen when it is thus treated, there will soon appear white curdy flakes, if the quantity is considerable, but if it is small, there will merely be a whitish cloudiness.

The chronic form of this disease is much more common than the acute. The symptoms are often very obscure at their commencement. A growing weakness, some derangement of the digestive organs, an occasional tendency to frequent passages of urine, with diminution of the quantity discharged, or some irregularity in its appearance, with perhaps obscure pains in the small of the back, are usually among the first symptoms noticed; and even these may escape notice, or at least may not cause the patient to apply to a physician until dropsical swellings appear, which usually commence in the face and extend over the whole body. There may be some tenderness over the region of the kidneys on strong pressure, and the quantity of urine discharged is found to be less than during health, and its density or weight is also diminished, and it usually contains more or less albumen. As the disease progresses the blood gradually loses its coloring matter, and the patient becomes very pale. The albumen although generally present in the urine, is not always constantly so, but its specific gravity, or weight, in equal quantity compared with healthy urine, gradually diminishes, and the countenance of the patient, from the loss of the red globules of the blood, often acquires, before death, a waxen yellowish white death-like hue. Dropsy generally attends this disease, but it is not always present; nor is the presence of albumen in the urine always positive evidence of the existence of this affection; but when the urine is scanty and contains more or less albumen, although perhaps free from it at times, and when at the same time the specific gravity or weight of the urine is steadily diminishing, until it is considerably less than during health, you may be reasonably sure that the patient is suffering from this disease; and the occurrence of dropsy. and a pale and bloodless countenance, will strengthen this opinion. Disease of the heart, especially enlargement of the heart, and also disease of the liver, are frequent complications of this affection, and patients suffering from this disease are very subject to inflammatory diseases.

Treatment.—The treatment in both the acute and chronic form of the disease is very similar to that recommended in inflammation of the kidneys. In acute cases *Aconite*, *Cannabis*, and *Cantharis* may be given as there directed; *Belladonna* will not be required. In chronic cases the last two remedies will often be useful, also *Lycopodium*, *Calcarea carb.* and especially *Spirits of turpentine.* If symptoms of dropsy occur in either case give *Apis mel.* once in four hours, and if within a few days there is no improvement, alternate it with *Arsenicum* at intervals of four hours.

DIABETES.

(EXCESSIVE SECRETION OF URINE.)

This disease is characterized by copious discharges of sweet urine of a pale yellowish or greenish yellow color, and sometimes of a faint sweetish odor. The saccharine matter resembles grape sugar. The first symptom which usually attracts the attention of the patient is the frequency of the calls to pass urine, and he generally soon notices that the quantity is increased, and sometimes he accidentally discovers that it is sweetish to the taste. The patient soon begins to be troubled with great thirst, the appetite often becomes craving, the mouth and throat dry and parched. There is a sensation of hollowness or sinking, with faintness at the pit of the stomach, and other dyspeptic symptoms with great debility and emaciation. The quantity of urine discharged usually varies from ten to twenty, and sometimes from thirty to fifty pints or more in twenty-four hours, and this often for weeks or months together. The specific gravity or weight of the urine is generally increased owing to the presence of sugar. If sugar is present in any quantity you can detect it very readily short of tasting. Add a little yeast to some of the urine and set it down in a warm place, and if there is sugar present it will begin to ferment within twenty-four hours, whereas healthy urine will not go through the same process. Albumen is also sometimes present. This disease is very slow in its progress, sometimes lasting for many years, and in many cases patients die of some other affection, such as consumption, disease of the brain, liver, or stomach. Occasionally they die early in the disease from exhaustion occasioned by the profuse secretion.

We sometimes have a profuse flow of urine without the presence of sugar, caused by various nervous affections, especially hysteria, but this form of the disease is not usually serious.

The cause of sugar being found in the urine in diabetes has been long a question with medical writers. Some have supposed that the stomach and bowels are chiefly in fault, others that the liver secretes an excessive quantity in this disease, and some of the latest writers attribute it to deficient action of the lungs, in that the sugar which is formed in the blood which comes from the liver on its arrival in the lungs fails to be decomposed by the oxygen of the air, and to disappear as in health, but passes in the general circulation to the kidneys, and is there separated from the blood.

Treatment.—General measures are perhaps more important

than medicine, although the latter may be of great service. As to diet it is necessary that it should be nutritious, but that it should contain neither sugar nor starch, therefore potatoes and fine flour in every form should be omitted. Give bran or canel bread with butter, beef or mutton, fowls and eggs, also cabbage and turnips. Let the patient drink moderately at a time, but in all about enough to relieve his thirst. Let him spend his time in the open air in taking active exercise, and follow the diréctions as to particular exercises contained in the section on consumption.

Carbo veg.: Give a dose of this remedy night and morning for two weeks; then continue it if there is any improvement, and as long as the patient continues to mend. After the above remedy has ceased to act, give *Mercurius viv.* night and morning, and continue it as long as there is any improvement. *Veratrum* can follow the above if it is needed, also *Natrum mur.*

GRAVEL—STONE—SPASMS OF THE URETER.

A fine, gravelly or gritty matter is sometimes discharged with the urine, causing much pain and irritation, and earthy concretions not unfrequently form in the kidneys, from the urine, and pass to the bladder, and are either discharged with the urine, or remain and form a nucleus around which more earthy matter collects, and forms what is denominated stone in the bladder. It sometimes happens that before the gravel-stone leaves the kidney, it becomes too large to pass readily through the ureter, or passage from the kidney to the bladder, and if it happens to be rough, as it often is, its passage causes great irritation and the most terrible spasmodic pains to which the human frame is subject. The attack usually commences suddenly during comparative health. A severe pain is felt in the region of the kidney, shooting to the groin, testicle, or thigh, and extending especially obliquely down the abdomen from the kidney to the bladder, in the direction of the passage. Sometimes the pain is felt chiefly about the hip. The pain occurs in severe paroxysms, and is often accompanied by nausea and vomiting, and sometimes by a small and feeble pulse, cold, pale surface, and profuse sweat. A frequent inclination to pass urine is another symptom which is usually present. The patient frequently changes his position without obtaining the relief which he covets. At length the stone escapes into the bladder, and the patient obtains relief immediately. Not unfrequently the symptoms return after a time, upon the entrance of another stone into the ureter, and a similar train of symptoms ensues. Occasionally the spasms may abate for a considerable time, without the escape of the stone, and return again. It is well to keep watch of the urine for the stone, as it is all-important that it pass the urethra as soon as possible after it enters the bladder, or it may become a nucleus for stone. If it does not pass, let the patient drink freely of *Slippery-elm tea* or *Gum-arabic water*, and retain the urine until the bladder is distended, and then pass it in a full stream while standing up, with the legs separated, and the body leaning forward; by so doing, it will sometimes pass. Stone in the bladder causes a frequent desire to pass urine, attended with severe pain toward the last that is passed, itching of the end of the penis, and sudden stoppage of urine while passing it, by the stone blocking up the passage.

Treatment.—In all cases where you notice a gravelly, gritty, or earthy sediment in the urine, medicine should be given so as to counteract this tendency, and thereby prevent the formation of gravel or stone in the kidney or bladder. If the sediment in the urine is red or yellowish, give *Lycopodium* every night. If it is light colored, give *Calcarea carb.* every night. If any derangement of the digestive organs occurs during the treatment, give *Nux vom.* before every meal; if it fails to relieve, give *Pulsatilla* in the same manner.

The above, together with *Cantharis* and *Cannabis*, are among the most important remedies for the irritation caused by either stone in the bladder, or in the pelvis of the kidney, before it engages in the ureter or passage to the bladder.

For spasms of the ureter, or the severe paroxysms of pain described above, caused by the passage of stone or gravel from the kidneys to the bladder, give *Belladonna* every half hour, and if, after giving four doses, no relief follows, give *Nux vom.* in the same way. Put the patient into a warm-bath if convenient; if not, wring a sheet from warm water, and wrap it around the body from below the arms to the hips, and put over the sheet, dry flannel; wet the sheet often. If the above measures afford no relief, and you cannot obtain the services of a homœopathic physician, if the patient is an adult, and the pains are very severe, give either twenty-five drops of *Laudanum*, or one sixth of a grain of *Morphine*, and if at the end of one hour, there is no relief, repeat the same dose; even a third dose may be given at the end of two hours more, if necessary. The cause of the suffering is a mechanical injury, which is being done by a rough stone passing through a small delicate passage, mechanically distending it, and tearing its delicate structures, and causing spasmodic contractions. Homœopathic remedies may sometimes, but according to my experience, not often, relieve the latter; or the stone may soon pass, and relief follow. If they fail, there is no serious objection to the use of the anodyne, as all we want is palliative relief, until the stone passes.

INFLAMMATION OF THE BLADDER (CYSTITIS).

The affection denominated strangury or dysuria, or painful urination, is but one form of this disease, and consists of inflammation of the mucous membrane, which is not of sufficient severity or extent to cause general febrile symptoms. There is a frequent desire to pass urine, with burning, cutting pains along the neck of the bladder, in the course of the passage, and at the end of the penis, similar to what we have in severer cases of cystitis. The causes are similar to those which cause the severer forms of the disease, and the treatment is similar.

Inflammation of the bladder may be caused by mechanical injuries, the introduction of instruments, stone in the bladder, overdistention from retained urine, severe labor, sexual excesses, exposure to cold while perspiring, sudden drying up of old ulcers, or other habitual discharges; the extension of inflammation to the bladder, in cases of gonorrhœa, dysentery, inflammation of the womb or bowels; also the application of blisters, and the internal use of *Cantharides*, *Spirits of turpentine*, or some other substance which acts specifically on the bladder. Gouty, rheumatic, and intemperate subjects, are very liable to this disease.

Symptoms.—Chills, followed by fever; more or less severe pain, frequently with a burning sensation in the region of the bladder, which often extends to the end of the penis in the male, and the external orifice of the urethra or urinary passage, in the female, and sometimes to the anus or passage from the bowels, and upper parts of the thighs, loins, and abdomen. The pain in the region of the bladder is generally increased by pressure on the lowest part of the abdomen; there is, in most cases, a frequent inclination to pass urine, which passes in small quantities, sometimes drop by drop, with much straining; but in some instances the urine is retained, and produces a feeling of distention and fullness in the region of the bladder. In some cases, nausea, vomiting, and distention of the abdomen, occur. The frequent and ineffectual efforts to urinate, cause great restlessness and anxiety. If the severe symptoms are not relieved within a few days, the patient begins to sink; the pulse becomes small, frequent, and irregular, the tongue dry with great thirst; the extremities cold, the bowels distended with gas; perhaps hiccough, or delirium, followed by stupor or convulsions, and the patient dies the latter part of the first, or during the second week. Death sometimes results from mortification, in which case the pain abates suddenly, sometime before this event. If the patient gets well, the symptoms gradually subside; sometimes there is a copious discharge of mucus in the urine, as the disease abates; in other instances pus or matter is discharged, which may come from an abscess in the walls of the bladder, or from ulceration of the mucous membrane. Abscesses may break into the lower bowel or vagina. At the commencement of the disease, the urine is often but little altered, perhaps rather scanty and high-colored, but as the case progresses, it becomes cloudy, or thick, from the presence of mucus or matter; sometimes bloody at any period of the disease, and sometimes offensive at a late stage. When there is great pain and tenderness at the lower part of the abdomen, and the effort to pass urine is very painful, or impossible, so as to give rise to retention of the urine, while there is little inclination to strain, the probability is that the external surface, or the muscular coat of the bladder, is chiefly affected. But when there is little or no pain in the lower part of the abdomen, but a frequent inclination to void urine, with burning and straining, we have reason to suppose the disease is principally confined to the mucous membrane or inner surface, perhaps in a great measure to the neck of the bladder.

Chronic inflammation of the bladder frequently results from the acute form of the disease, in other instances it comes on gradually, with symptoms similar to those of the acute disease, only less severe. There is a frequent inclination to pass urine, sometimes with burning or shooting pains and straining, and even spasms of the bladder. The urine contains mucus, and sometimes pus, which gives it a whitish, yellowish, or greenish appearance. The quantity of mucus is sometimes very large, and it may be so thick as to be passed with difficulty, and so irritating as to cause burning pain in the passage. Occasionally blood appears in the urine. After a time, if the disease continues, all the symptoms are aggravated, and pus or matter, in a great measure, takes the place of the mucus, and the patient is gradually worn out by the discharge, and hectic fever.

Treatment of Acute Inflammation of the Bladder.—If the disease is attended with severe symptoms of strangury, with constant inclination to pass urine with scalding, the patient may be allowed to drink freely of *Slippery-elm tea* or *Gum-arabic water*, for these drinks tend to increase the quantity of urine, and render it less acrid, and are therefore useful. But if there are pain, soreness, and a feeling of distention in the lowest part of the abdomen, and the contraction of the bladder causes great pain, when an attempt is made to pass urine, and there is neither straining to pass, nor scalding during its passage, the disease is doubtless in the muscular and external coats, and the less the patient drinks the better, as there is liable to be retention of urine in such cases; and even if there is not, the frequent contraction of the bladder to expel it, only increases the suffering.

If the disease has been caused by a blister, or by *Cantharides* given internally, give either six globules saturated with *Camphor* or one drop of the tincture of *Camphor*, every half hour until the symptoms are relieved.

Aconite: In all cases attended with fever, pain in the region of the bladder, with or without burning, scalding, and straining while passing urine, give this remedy every hour. Even if there is not much fever it will often be useful, given alternately with one of the following remedies, at intervals of one hour, especially with *Cannabis.*

Dose of these remedies, see page 7.

Cannabis should either follow *Aconite* or after a few doses of *Aconite* have been given, it should be given alternately with it, when there is mucus or blood discharged, and when there is a constant desire to pass urine, and its passage is accompanied by straining or burning; also, when there is suppression or retention of urine.

Cantharis: Give this remedy once in two hours if *Cannabis* fails to relieve the symptoms at the end of twenty-four hours, especially if there is ineffectual urging to urinate, stinging, cutting, or burning pains in the region of the bladder, and if the lower part of the abdomen is distended and tender to the touch or on pressure.

Nux vomica may be given after the fever and acute symptoms have been somewhat relieved by the above remedies, especially if there is a frequent inclination attended with violent straining to urinate, pain during and after the passage, burning pain and scanty urine. This remedy is especially useful in the case of intemperate or gouty subjects, and for those subject to piles.

Pulsatilla: Give this remedy after the acute symptoms have been somewhat relieved by other remedies, when there is a frequent discharge of bloody or slimy urine, with straining and aching or cutting pains in the region of the bladder. *Pulsatilla* is especially useful during pregnancy, and in the case of females generally, also for gouty subjects.

In case the disease is simple strangury and not attended with chills or fever, *Pulsatilla* or *Nux vomica* may be given at the commencement, but even such cases are often benefited by *Aconite,*

Cannabis, or *Cantharis*, and especially by *Camphor*. Let the diet be light, avoid all acids, and apply cloths wrung from warm water over the lower part of the abdomen, hips, and between the thighs.

Treatment of Chronic Inflammation of the Bladder.—The remedies already named, especially *Pulsatilla*, *Cannabis*, and *Nux vomica*, are often useful. Select one of these remedies and give before every meal, about half an hour before eating, and give a dose of *Sulphur* at bedtime; and continue these remedies as long as there is any improvement. Then give another remedy before meals, and *Calcarea carb* at bedtime. *Dulcamara* and *Lycopodium* are sometimes useful in chronic cases. If all remedies fail you can try one tenth of a drop of *Spirits of turpentine* two or three times a day; drop one drop on some pulverized sugar, mix it well and divide into ten powders.

If during the continuance of inflammation of the bladder, either acute or chronic, there is retention of urine, and the bladder becomes distended, give the patient a warm bath, or at least wring a sheet from warm water and wrap around the hips, thighs, and abdomen; give an injection of warm water into the bowels, give *Belladonna* internally, and if these measures fail to relieve which will rarely be the case send for a physician, even an allopathic physician if you cannot get a homeopathist, for it may be necessary to use a catheter.

RETENTION OF URINE,

OR INABILITY TO PASS WATER.

When the urine is retained, the bladder becomes over-distended, and pressing upon it causes the peculiar disagreeable pain which arises from pressing upon a distended bladder. Sometimes the bladder can be felt in the lower part of the abdomen, and percussion or striking with the ends of the fingers over it yields a dull sound. There are various causes of retention of urine. It may depend upon obstruction caused by the swelling which results from inflammation of the neck of the bladder, and in this case we have symptoms of an inflamed bladder added to those of retention. In old men it may arise from inflammation or enlargement of the prostrate gland—which in the male, surrounds the passage as it leaves the bladder. It may arise from the pressure of tumors, or of the womb during pregnancy, on the neck of the bladder; and strictures sometimes cause retention. A spasmodic contraction of the urethra or passage, especially in hysterical persons, sometimes causes this affection. Retention of urine may result from voluntarily restraining its flow until the bladder becomes over-distended, which causes paralysis of the organ. In diseases of the brain or spinal cord in low forms of fever, and even during old age, we may have retention from diminished innervation, or from the muscles losing their power of contracting for the want of due nervous energy. In such cases the retention is generally not complete; when the bladder is distended to a certain degree the patient passes a small quantity of urine voluntarily, but does not empty the bladder; if he has no control over it, and the bladder becomes distended, small discharges frequently take place from time to time; therefore we may have both retention and involuntary discharge of urine at the same time. We may have a similar state, that is, small discharges and retention, from inflammation of the bladder. Retention of urine if not relieved ends in rupture of the bladder and death, or of the urethra or passage, and its escape into the cellular structure in the neighborhood, when it causes sloughing and often death.

Treatment.—If the disease seems to be caused by inflammation, which may be suspected when there are pain and soreness in the region of the bladder with chills and fever, also when there is pain and scalding during the passage of small quantities of urine, consult the section on inflammation of the bladder. But if it is caused by paralysis of the bladder, as frequently happens during the continuance of low fevers, inflammation of the brain or spinal cord, and during old age, give *Hyoscyamus* once in three or four hours, and if it fails to relieve, give *Dulcamara* in the same manner. *Arsenicum* in obstinate cases will be found useful. *Belladonna* may be given when the brain or spinal cord is diseased; also give injections of warm water into the bowels.

When the retention is caused by a spasmodic contraction of the passage in nervous or hysterical patients, give a dose of *Pulsatilla* every hour, and if at the end of three or four hours there is no relief, give *Opium* every half hour for three hours, afterward give *Nux vom.* To overcome a disposition to this form of the disease, give *Pulsatilla* one night and *Nux vom.* the next. In cases of spasmodic retention, a warm bath, or simply a warm hip-bath, and injections of warm water into the bowels, will often relieve the retention for the time being.

If the retention occurs during pregnancy, give *Pulsatilla*, and if it fails, give *Nux vom.*, and let the patient try to pass her urine lying down on her back or side; or while on her hands and knees, and even with her hips higher than her shoulders if necessary.

If the retention is caused by inflammation and enlargement of the prostate gland, give *Aconite* alternately with *Pulsatilla* one hour apart; and a warm hip-bath for present relief. To cure the disease, give *Pulsatilla* at night and *Sulphur* in the morning.

If stricture is the cause of the retention, it must be dilated by bougies, if *Pulsatilla* at night and *Sulphur* in the morning do not relieve it. *Mercurius* and *Dulcamara* are also sometimes useful in such cases.

In no case should a patient be allowed to go longer than twenty-four hours without a passage of urine, and if he takes much drink or fluids, and perspires but little, twelve or eighteen hours is as long as it is safe to allow him to go without drawing off his urine by the means of a catheter. Any physician can perform this operation.

SUPPRESSION OF URINE (ISCHURIA RENALIS).

In this disease urine is not secreted at all; or if any is secreted only a few drops. Suppression of urine may result from inflammation of the kidneys, and perhaps from paralysis of these organs, and various other causes not well understood. It sometimes occurs when the patient is otherwise in comparatively good health, and occasionally comes on during the progress of other diseases, such as cholera, febrile and inflammatory affections. If the suppression continues for several days the blood becomes deteriorated, chills, perhaps slight fever, nausea and vomiting may ensue. The patient becomes dull and torpid, at length sleepy and perhaps delirious, and at the end of four or five days, in cases of entire suppression, stupor, and perhaps convulsions, and death occur, if the disease is not relieved. If a small quantity of urine is secreted, the patient may live for weeks, and either recover, or die from coma, as in the cases of complete suppression.

When there is suppression of urine there is generally little or no inclination to urinate; and no sensation of fullness in the region of the bladder, nor is there any fullness in the lower part of the abdomen; and if the catheter is introduced, as it always should be, no urine is obtained.

Treatment.—If there is fever, or pain and uneasiness in the small of the back, consult the section on inflammation of the kidneys.

If the disease occurs when the patient otherwise seems well, and free from fever, give *Belladonna* and *Cantharis* alternately, at intervals of two hours. If these remedies fail to relieve, give *Hyoscyamus:* if drowsiness ensues give *Opium* once in two hours, and if it fails to relieve the symptoms, or if convulsions occur, give *Nux vomica* every hour. If at the commencement there is a chill, a few doses of *Aconite* may precede the above remedies. If suppression occurs during an attack of the cholera, or during any febrile disease, give *Cantharis* alternately with the remedy which seems best indicated for the existing general disease, at intervals of one or two hours; if this remedy fails at the end of twenty-four hours give *Hyoscyamus* in its stead. A warm bath is often a useful auxiliary in the treatment of this disease. The diet should be light and contain no animal food.

INCONTINENCE OF URINE (ENURESIS).

WETTING THE BED.

A want of power to control the urine may depend upon an irritable condition of the bladder, especially of the neck of the bladder, so that the presence of even a small quantity of urine excites the organ to contract; or it may depend upon a debilitated or paralyzed condition of the passage at its commencement, so that it cannot contract sufficiently to retain the urine. This fluid itself may be so acrid as to excite an irritable state of the bladder. Involuntary discharges of urine are sometimes caused by fear and other mental emotions. Involuntary discharges during sleep are very common with children, and sometimes this symptom continues until adult age. It does not usually affect the general health, but is very uncomfortable to the patient, and annoying to housekeepers. But by far the most troublesome cases of incontinence of urine are those which are caused by complete paralysis, or loss of power in the muscular fibres which usually retain it, when the urine almost constantly dribbles away.

Treatment.—If the disease seems to be caused by an irritable state of the bladder, give *Pulsatilla* three or four times a day, and if it fails to relieve, consult the section on inflammation of the bladder and gravel.

For wetting the bed give a dose of *Pulsatilla* before tea, and at bedtime, for one week; then omit it for a week and give *Silicea* in the same manner, for a week; after that give *Pulsatilla*, and so continue, changing every week. If at the end of a month this disease is not cured, give *Belladonna* at night and *Sulphur* in the morning. *Cina* is sometimes useful for children troubled with worms. Do not allow the patient to eat or drink milk for supper, nor to drink anything after two or three o'clock in the afternoon. This is a disease which the child cannot help, and punishment should never be resorted to as a remedy, for it is cruel, and can do no good.

If the disease seems to be caused by paralysis, give *Hyoscyamus* before every meal, and *Arsenicum* at bedtime, and continue them in recent attacks, for at least one week; in chronic cases, for at least one month, and as much longer as there is any improvement. *Dulcamara*, *Belladonna*, or *Nux vom.*, can be tried, if those remedies fail.

Let the patient lie on his back or side, with his thighs drawn up on the abdomen, and two or three times a day, gently percuss or strike, with the end of the fingers, over the passage or urethra, as it emerges beneath the bones of the pelvis, and backward over the perineum, to the anus; continue this for a few minutes at a time —in paralytic cases only. Never resort to this measure when there is any pain or soreness in the bladder, or irritation in passing urine.

HEMORRHAGE WITH THE URINE.

(HEMATURIA.)

This is a rare disease, yet it sometimes occurs during the progress of malignant forms of fever and scurvy; and in other cases, where the blood seems to be partially disorganized, as in cases where dark spots appear in and beneath the skin (*perpura hemorrhagica*). It may also be caused by mechanical injuries over the kidneys or bladder, by stone or gravel in the kidneys, ureters, or bladder, and by inflammation The blood may proceed from the kidneys, ureters or passages from the kidneys to the bladder, from the bladder, or from the urethra or external passage, and it is not always easy to decide from what portion of the urinary passages it comes. If it is intimately blended with the urine, it probably comes from the kidneys.

Treatment.—If the disease has been caused by mechanical injuries, give a dose of *Arnica* every hour; if any fever results give *Aconite* alternately with *Arnica*, at intervals of one hour.

If the disease seems to be caused by inflammation of the kidneys or bladder, and is attended with pain and scalding on urinating, consult the sections on inflammation of the bladder and kidneys, also the section on gravel. *Cantharis*, *Cannabis*, *Pulsatilla*, and *Calcarea carb.*, are among your remedies in such cases.

If this affection occurs during the course of a malignant fever, or eruptive disease, or the scurvy, consult the section on the disease existing. In such cases, the remedies are generally *Pulsatilla*, *Arnica*, *Arsenicum*, or *China*.

In all other cases, give a dose of *Pulsatilla* every hour during the day, and a dose of *Calcarea carb.* every night. If the patient is addicted to the use of alcoholic or fermented drinks, *Nux vom*, will be of service. *China* may follow the above remedies in debilitated subjects.

GONORRHŒA (CLAP)—GLEET.

This is inflammation of the urethra or the external urinary passage, and is generally caused by an impure connection; although a disease of a similar character may arise from having connection with a healthy woman, during menstruation; and leucorrhœa in the female, in some cases, causes inflammation of the urethra of the male. In the contagious form of the disease, the symptoms commence at uncertain intervals, from the exposure, varying from two or three days to as many weeks; but, in perhaps the majority of cases, at the end of about one week. The first symptom is a tickling or itching sensation at the orifice of the urethra, which is soon attended by a frequent inclination to make water. In a short time the orifice of the urethra becomes red and swollen, and the passage of urine painful. As the disease progresses, a whitish or yellowish white discharge makes its appearance, which sometimes becomes greenish and even bloody, and is often very copious; there is severe scalding and burning during the passage of urine, which is passed with difficulty, and in a small stream. The inflammation travels up the urethra, and sometimes reaches the bladder; the passage is swollen and feels indurated, and the patient is frequently troubled, especially at night, with painful erections, the penis being bent over, and prevented from becoming entirely erect, owing to the inflamed passage. There is generally more or less headache, fever, and restlessness, attending the disease. The acute symptoms, under proper treatment, generally begin to abate in a few days; in some cases they may last a week or ten days, before there is much improvement, and even much longer, if proper care is not used as to diet, exercise, &c. As the disease declines, the discharge, pain, and scalding sensation, diminish; and often at the end of from three to six weeks, the disease is entirely cured; but in some cases, in scrofulous constitutions, or when it has not been properly treated, the discharge may become chronic when it is called gleet. The testicles sometimes become swollen and inflamed during the continuance of this affection, and strictures not unfrequently result from the inflammatory action in and around the passage.

Females do not usually suffer from this disease as severely as males, although in some cases when the inflammation extends to the vagina and uterus as it sometimes does, it may be very severe.

Treatment.—The patient should always abstain from sexual indulgences until the disease is entirely cured, and should restrain his thoughts, and use no animal food, alcoholic or fermented drinks, coffee, green tea, spices or other stimulating condiments, and the stiller he keeps the more certain, safe, and speedy, will be the cure, for exercise generally aggravates the symptoms and prolongs the duration of the disease.

At the commencement of the symptoms, especially if there is any fever, headache, or restlessness, give *Aconite* once in two hours during the afternoon and evening, and *Cannabis* once in two hours during the forenoon. Continue these remedies for three or four days, and longer if there is any improvement, but if the severity of the fever, scalding, and pain, are not lessened, during the morning and forenoon, omit *Cannabis* and give *Cantharis*, but, during the afternoon and evening, give *Aconite*. Continue these remedies when the patient is awake until the fever and restlessness are in a great measure relieved; then, if the difficulty of passing urine and scalding do not abate, omit *Aconite* and give *Cannabis* alternately with *Cantharis* at intervals of two or three hours. *Cantharis* is the best remedy for painful erections or chordee.

After the acute symptoms have been removed by the above remedies, if the discharge lingers and threatens to become chronic, give a dose of *Mercurius viv.* every night, and *Sulphur* in the morning. These remedies are also useful for gleet or chronic inflammation and discharge from the urethra; and if after two or three weeks they fail to afford relief, give *Silicea* every night for a week, and as much longer as there is any improvement; after which return to *Mercurius viv.* and *Sulphur* again. In obstinate cases of either gonorrhœa or gleet, if other remedies fail, weak injections of *Sulphate of zinc* or *Nitrate of silver*, say from one half a grain or grain of the former, or from one fourth to one half a grain of the latter, to an ounce of rain water, once a day, will often relieve, and will not be likely to do harm. Try the *Zinc* first. *Nitrate of silver* injections will permanently stain the patients linen if they come in contact with it. In using injections the finger should be pressed firmly on the passage back of the sore part so as to prevent the fluid passing into the bladder, excepting when the inflammation extends to the bladder.

In the treatment of gonorrhœa avoid large doses of *Balsam copaiba* and *Cubebs*, for these remedies, although they may sometimes afford some relief, are neither reliable nor safe, and may cause swelling of the testicle and stricture.

Strong injections of *Nitrate of silver* are sometimes used, but they are neither reliable nor safe, although they not unfrequently cure the disease when carefully used at its very commencement; in other cases they aggravate the symptoms seriously; and it is best not to use them.

At the commencement of an attack of gonorrhœa wrap the penis in a cotton or linen cloth wrung from cold water, and surround the wet cloth with several thicknesses of dry flannel; wet the cloth once in six hours. If at the end of three or four days the symptoms are not improving, use warm, instead of cold water, and change often; once every hour or less.

INFLAMMATION OF THE GLANS PENIS.

(BALANITIS.)

This affection may be caused by an impure connection, and when this is the case, gonorrhœa generally exists at the same time. It may be caused by an accumulation of the natural secretion beneath the foreskin, when due attention is not paid to cleanliness It may be caused by poisonous plants, and mechanical injuries. When the opening to the prepuce is small, especially with children, it sometimes gets drawn back over the glans, when it cannot be readily returned, and causes constriction, swelling, inflammation, and even mortification of the glans may ensue if the parts are not relieved. This is called PARAPHIMOSIS. When the glans cannot be uncovered it is called PHIMOSIS.

Treatment.—If the disease results from a want of cleanliness, wash the parts two or three times a day with tepid or cool water; if the foreskin cannot be drawn back inject warm water up under it several times a day. If the disease has been caused by constriction of the foreskin back of the glans or paraphimosis, oil the parts well with sweet oil or cream, and take the glans between the thumb and fingers, and gently compress them for several minutes, or until they become so far reduced that you can draw the foreskin over them with the fingers of the other hand. If the disease has been caused by poison ivy or other poisonous plants, wash the parts and give *Bryonia* once in two hours. If it has been caused by mechanical injuries give *Arnica* internally, and put ten drops of the tincture into a cup of water, and wet cloths in the solution and apply to the parts. If the disease exists in connection with gonorrhœa, the remedies proper for that disease will be proper remedies, together with water applied locally. In all other cases apply cloths wet with warm water, and give *Aconite* alternately with *Mercurius viv.* at intervals of two hours. If the disease follows an impure connection, and there are ulcers or sores on or back of the glans on the foreskin, or even on the penis, consult the section on syphilis or the venereal disease.

SWELLING AND INFLAMMATION OF THE TESTICLE (ORCHITIS).

This disease is sometimes caused by gonorrhœa, and when it occurs during the continuance of that disease, the discharge from the urethra usually ceases until the swelling abates and then returns. This affection may be caused by the introduction of a catheter into the urethra, also by mechanical injuries. It not unfrequently occurs after or during the latter stages of an attack of mumps. The testicle becomes swollen, hard, and very painful, and tender on pressure. There are often more or less fever, pain in the loins, colic, nausea, and depression of spirits. In some cases the disease abates suddenly, in other instances it lasts several days. An abscess very rarely forms, although such instances have occurred.

Treatment.—When the disease has been caused by mechanical injuries, give *Arnica* internally and apply it externally. If *Arnica* fails to relieve, give *Pulsatilla* internally once in two hours.

If the disease has been caused by gonorrhœa, give *Pulsatilla* alternately with *Mercurius viv.* at intervals of four hours. If it has been caused by metastasis of the mumps, give *Pulsatilla* and *Mercurius viv.* as above: if they fail, give *Nux vomica* once in two hours. Apply cloths wrung from hot water, or a warm poultice over the parts. For chronic enlargement and induration of the testicle, give a dose of *Sulphur* every night for a month, then give *Lycopodium.*

DROPSY OF THE SCROTUM (HYDROCELE).

This generally occurs only on one side, and the swelling is pear-shaped, more or less elastic, and free from pain. It sometimes occurs in children, even with newly-born infants. In the latter case bathe the parts three or four times a day in a weak solution of *Arnica*, half a teaspoonful to a teacupful of water, and give *Arnica* three times a day. If it does not relieve give the remedies named hereafter. In a majority of cases *Pulsatilla* and *Silicea* are the most important remedies. Give the former at night and the latter in the morning, and continue them for several weeks. *Sulphur* every night may follow the above remedies if it is needed.

Dose, see page 7.

VENEREAL DISEASE (SYPHILIS).

This disease is generally caused by impure connection; although if either of the parents are affected with the disease the child may inherit it; and if a child has a syphilitic disease of the face, it may communicate it to the nurse; or if the nurse has a syphilitic disease about the nipples, breast or face, the child may contract it by contact. The symptoms of this disease are divided into primary, secondary, and tertiary symptoms. The primary symptoms usually make their appearance in from two to ten days after exposure, and consist of one or more sores, or ulcers, called chancres; which appear in the male, usually on some part of the penis, most frequently on either the glans or prepuce, but occasionally on the scrotum, or penis; and in some instances accompanied with, or followed by a bubo, or swelling in the groin. This swelling may be caused by an absorption of the syphilitic virus from the sore on the penis, in which case it is quite sure to maturate, and when it discharges, the sore which results is similar in character to the original ulcer, and does not readily heal or change. Or the swelling in the groin may be simply sympathetic with the irritation on the penis, and may disappear without maturating; or if an abscess forms it may be a simple abscess, and the resulting cavity and opening may heal readily. When the ulcer, or chancre, is on the fold of the mucous membrane of the foreskin or prepuce, beneath the penis which connects the latter to the passage, near the end of the penis, a bubo or swelling in the groin is much more likely to result than when it is at any other point. In the female, chancres may appear on the external parts, on the surface of the vagina, womb, or around the urethra or water passage. Chancres assume various forms; sometimes they are superficial, but in other instances the ulcer inclines to spread and grow deeper, with elevated edges. In the form which is most likely to be followed by secondary symptoms, the edges are elevated, and together with the base of the sore feel hard or indurated. The surface of the ulcer is usually covered with a tough adherent lardy-appearing matter. If there is no induration or hardness about the base of the sore, there is comparatively little danger of its being followed by secondary symptoms. In unhealthy constitutions and persons of bad habits, or when the system is suffering under the causes which produce scurvy, or malignant fevers, the ulcer is apt to spread rapidly by sloughing, and present a dark appearance. The abuse of mercury sometimes causes a healthy sore to assume this character. In other cases the ulcer is attended with violent inflammation, and spreads rapidly, especially if irritating applications are made to the part, or mercury is freely used.

Secondary Symptoms.—These consist of various eruptions, moist warty excrescences, and ulcers on the skin, superficial ulcerations on the tongue, lips, throat, and larynx, or upper portion of the windpipe, inflammation and ulceration about the roots of the finger-nails, and inflammation of the iris, or curtain which forms the pupil of the eye. Pains like those of rheumatism are not uncommon. Such symptoms appear sooner or later after the healing of the primary sore, or even in some instances while it is healing. Syphilitic eruptions on the skin are of various kinds, and are generally chronic; "of a bronze or copper color; frequently scaly, and prone to excoriate; sometimes assuming the form of tubercles of a livid or brown color, surrounded by a coppery areola or circle, and having a tendency to degenerate into foul offensive ulcers." Occasionally they are little more than brown or dirty yellow stains. In rare instances eruptions may assume a bronze or copper color when not caused by syphilis, and on the other hand, in some cases, this color of the eruption may not be very manifest, or even perceptible, when it is caused by syphilis.

Tertiary Symptoms.—These consist in deep-seated affections of the skin, as tubercles, and affections of the glands and bones; enlargement of bones or portions of bones or exostosis; inflammation of the periosteum or external membrane which covers the bones, constituting what are called nodes and caries, or ulceration and death of the bones, especially those of the nose, palate, and shins. These symptoms rarely appear within a year from the healing of the primary sore or chancre, and it may be several years before they show themselves.

It is not always easy to distinguish a chancre from a simple ulcer of the genital organs, or a syphilitic eruption from an ordinary eruption, and the most intelligent and experienced physicians sometimes have been mistaken. A late writer says: "It is only when the symptoms arise in a certain order, that we can positively declare syphilis to be present. If an individual has chancre, which is followed by bubo, or ulcerated throat, and this is accompanied by, or precedes eruptions on the skin, then we may feel pretty confident. Again, when deep-seated pains in the bones follow the previous symptoms, we may consider them to be syphilitic."

Primary and secondary syphilis are contagious, but require contact, and generally an abraded or raw surface, in order that the disease may be communicated. During the continuance of either primary or secondary symptoms, the disease is also liable to be transmitted to offspring. Tertiary syphilis is neither contagious nor transmitable; although it is said that the children of parents suffering from this form of disease, are very apt to be scrofulous, consumptive, or predisposed to cancerous diseases.

Treatment.—Dr. Bennett, a recent allopathic writer, says: "It is now well known that the poison of mercury produces a cachectic disease and secondary sores in the body, which have been to a great extent mistaken for those of syphilis. It consequently has happened that mercury given to cure primary sores has produced a constitutional disorder closely resembling that of syphilis; more mercury has then been administered, increasing the mischief, and so the disease has been perpetuated. The real fact, however, is that the syphilitic poison is no exception to the general rule, which informs us that all contagious diseases of the blood run a certain course, and that we have not yet discovered a specific remedy for one of them. The great proof of this is that the intensity of the disease in modern times has declined exactly in proportion as its treatment by mercury has diminished, and the disorder been left to follow its natural course." In regard to the treatment of the disease by allopathic physicians without mercury, he says: "In various reports now published more than eighty thousand cases have been submitted to experiment, by means of which it has been perfectly established that syphilis is cured in a shorter time, and with less probability of inducing secondary syphilis, by the simple than by the mercurial treatment. These facts are now generally admitted, and malignant syphilis is gradually disappearing. Twenty years ago the most frightful secondary and tertiary cases were met with, and the usual treatment was profuse salivation. At present such cases are rare."

It will be seen from the testimony of this writer that mercury is strictly homœopathic to this disease, and I have made the above quotations to show the danger which results from using homœopathic remedies in crude or allopathic doses; and to prevent, if possible, homœopathic patients from ever resorting to the old empirical treatment, which has made such havoc with the constitutions of thousands. Especially shun quacks who fill the columns of our newspapers with their boastful advertisements If you cannot obtain the services of a homœopathic physician be satisfied to follow the directions contained in this section. A homœopathic physician should always be consulted immediately when practicable.

The homœopathist gives remedies for the sake of exciting a healthy reaction in the organism, and not for the sake of causing the poisonous effects of the drug. In proper homœopathic doses when indicated by the symptoms, this remedy may be given with perfect impunity any length of time, which may be requisite to radically cure this disease, and leave no unpleasant symptoms behind as the result of its administration.

Mercurius viv. is generally the most important remedy at the commencement of the disease, and even later if the patient has not taken mercury in large doses. Give a dose before every meal and at bedtime for four or five days, then night and morning only. Generally after taking the remedy for from one to two weeks, red granulations can be perceived at the bottom of the ulcer; these increase and its lardy appearance gradually disappears. Should proud flesh start up and the ulcer not heal readily, omit *Mercurius viv.* for a few days, and give *Nitric acid* night and morning until the ulcer is healed, then give a dose of *Mercurius viv.* every night for a month; when if there is no appearance of sore throat or eruptions on the skin, the remedy may be discontinued.

Mercurius cor.: If, after giving *Mercurius viv.* for two weeks, there is no change in the ulcer, and the bottom of it still presents the lard-like appearance, give this remedy once in six hours until red granulations make their appearance, then give it only twice a day. If at the end of a week there is no change give *Sulphur* alternately with the *Mercurius cor.* for a few days at intervals of six hours. As soon as an improvement follows omit the *Sulphur* and give the *Mercurius cor.* twice a day. If the chancre has been treated by large doses of mercury, or has been neglected for six or eight weeks until it has become chronic, the lard-like appearance may have disappeared, but the edges remain raised and the bottom hard, in such a case given *Mercurius cor.* night and morning until there is a change for the better; or if no improvement follows at the end of a week give *Sulphur* alternately with it for a few days as directed above. As soon as there is a favorable change in the appearance of the sore, omit the *Sulphur* and give the *Mercurius* night and morning.

If the ulcer presents a dark appearance and spreads rapidly by sloughing, give *Lachesis* alternately with *Mercurius viv.* four hours apart; and if these remedies do not check the progress of the disease, omit the *Mercurius* and give *Arsenicum* alternately with *Lachesis* at intervals of three hours until the sloughing has ceased; then omit these remedies and give *Mercurius cor.*

Buboes require the same remedies as chancre, either *Mercurius viv.* or *Mercurius cor.* is the chief remedy; in obstinate cases *Nitric acid* or *Sulphur* may be required, but follow the directions above for chancre.

Local Applications for Chancre.—The ulcer should be kept clean by the means of water, and lint wet in cold water may be applied to the ulcer, and if it becomes irritable and painful apply warm water.

The diet, in all cases, except when there is a disposition in the ulcer to spread rapidly by sloughing, should be light; if the patient is of a full habit, or stout and healthy, very light; no stimulants, stimulating condiments, or animal food, should be allowed, and the patient should eat moderately, and never fully appease his hunger.

Treatment of Secondary Syphilis.—If ulcerations appear in the throat, or eruptions on the skin, *Mercurius viv.* is still the chief remedy, provided the patient has not taken either *Calomel* or *Mercury* in large doses. Give a dose of the remedy night and morning for one week, then give *Mercurius viv.* at night, and *Sulphur* in the morning, for a week; afterward give a dose of *Mercurius viv.* every night. If, at the end of another week, there is no change for the better, give *Mercurius cor.* night and morning. In obstinate cases, *Lachesis*, night and morning, may follow the mercurial preparations, and afterward *Nitric acid.* The latter remedies are especially useful in cases where allopathic doses of mercury have been taken.

For tertiary syphilis, pains in the bones, swellings, nodes, and caries, or ulceration of the bones, give *Mercurius* every night for one week; *Lachesis* for the next week; if, at the end of four weeks, there is no change, give *Nitric acid.* It is often necessary to continue remedies several months. If other remedies fail, obtain at a druggist's, ten grains of the *Iodide of potassium,* dissolve it in thirty spoonfuls of water, cork it up tight, and give a spoonful three times a day, until gone; if benefit is derived, obtain more. Warm bathing is generally useful, if not carried to the extent of causing debility.

SEMINAL EMISSIONS.

This disease is generally caused by self-pollution, indulging in lascivious thoughts, or by sexual excesses; an excitable state of the seminal vesicles result from such habits, and they expel their contents during sleep, the discharge being generally accompanied by lascivious dreams; the patient, the next day, feeling weak and depressed. If the discharge does not occur more frequently than once in one or two weeks, it is of no great consequence, still it is well to take remedies for it; but if it occurs once or twice a night, or once in two or three nights, it is very important to take measures to lessen or cure this irritability. But above all things, shun quacks and their nostrums. These wretched impostors, in their advertisements in our papers, magnify the evils which result from this affection, for the sake of deceiving the young and swindling them.

Treatment.—This difficulty will generally be very readily relieved in a few weeks or months, by following the directions named. Let the patient keep his thoughts from lascivious subjects, shun all stimulants, stimulating condiments, tobacco, coffee, and tea. Let his diet be light and nourishi g; let him seek the society of virtuous females; dispel all fears as to the result of this affection; let him remember that perhaps more than three fourths of all unmarried men are troubled with these discharges occasionally.

Give a dose of *Pulsatilla* every night for one week, then a dose of *Nux vom.* every night for the next week, and so continue changing every week. Once a week, in the morning, give a dose of *Sulphur*. If there is much debility give a dose of *China* every morning when you do not give *Sulphur*. *Cantharis* and *Calcarea carb.* may be required in obstinate cases. Give one dose of one of them a day, as long as there is any improvement. If there is any slimy discharge while awake, it is in most cases from the prostate gland. *Pulsatilla* at night, and *Sulphur* in the morning, will generally relieve it. If they do not, give *Cantharis* or *Cannabis*, night and morning. A tepid hip-bath in the evening, is sometimes useful.

Every young man, whether troubled with this disease or not, should read the author's work on "Marriage," which is at present bound in the same volume with the "Avoidable Causes of Disease;" and every parent who cares for the moral and physical welfare of his children, will do well to read it; for it has been carefully written expressly to give to husbands and wives the information they need, and also to protect the young from vice and licentiousness. It is a book which parents can safely place in the hands of their sons and daughters, to give them the needed information which delicacy too frequently deters parents from giving orally. It is published by Mason Brothers, New York, and can be had through any bookseller.

CHAPTER VII.

DISEASES OF THE NERVOUS SYSTEM.

BRAIN FEVER,

OR INFLAMMATION OF THE BRAIN AND ITS MEMBRANES, AND HYDROCEPHALUS.

It is generally difficult, if not impossible, to distinguish with certainty between inflammation of the membranes which envelop the brain, and inflammation of the substance of the brain itself; fortunately, this is not important, as similar remedies are required in both affections, and the symptoms will be a safe guide in their selection.

The causes of this disease are various. A predisposition to it is often inherited; males are more subject to it than females; children, from birth to two years of age, are very liable to it; over mental exertion and intemperance, predispose to this disease. The same is true of the cruel practice of confining young children in the school-room six hours a day. An attack may be immediately excited by mechanical injuries, exposure of the head to intense heat, the irritation of teething, disease of the bones of the ear, extending to the brain, alcoholic drinks, violent mental excitement, depressing mental emotions, such as fear or chagrin, retrocession of various cutaneous affections, such as measles and scarlet fever, and a translation of gout or rheumatism; and in children, overtaxing the brain at school, is a fruitful cause of this disease. A form of the disease sometimes occurs between the ages of two and twelve years, which depends on a scrofulous disease of the membranes of the brain, or a deposit of fine tubercles.

Symptoms.—Chills, followed by fever, commence with, precede, or soon follow an attack of violent pains in the head. There are redness of the face and eyes, sensitiveness to light and noise, especially light, a contracted state of the pupils, great restlessness and want of sleep, delirium, either mild or violent, and spasmodic twitchings or convulsive movements. The skin is hot but sometimes moist, the pulse frequent and hard, sometimes irregular, the tongue covered with whitish fur; vomiting is a frequent and often a prominent symptom, and when obstinate vomiting occurs in the case of children, without symptoms of inflammation of the stomach, such as tenderness over and pain in the organ, we have reason to fear the existence of disease of the brain, especially if the nausea and vomiting are aggravated by the patient sitting up. The bowels are generally constipated, but not always.

Pain in the head is one of the most constant symptoms, and it is seldom entirely absent; even when there is a tendency to stupor, it is manifested by moans, cries, contraction of the brows, and putting the hands to the head; and, in case of children, by rolling the head from side to side, or pressing it against the mother's breast. The pain may occupy the whole head, or only the forehead, sides, or back of the head. It may shoot through from side to side, or seem to come from deep in the brain. It is frequently paroxysmal, often seems like the darting pains of neuralgia, and in children it often causes quick short screams. Sometimes the disease commences with convulsions, and they may be repeated so as to constitute a prominent feature of the case; the patient being conscious or unconscious between them. In some cases stupor is a prominent symptom from the commencement. In all cases if the disease continues on uninfluenced by treatment, or the natural efforts of the organism to throw it off, sooner or later, according to the severity of the symptoms, the delirium gradually yields to drowsiness or stupor, at first not so perfect but that the patient can be aroused, but at length profound coma or insensibility ensues. The pupils become dilated, the sight and hearing are destroyed, the surface of the body becomes insensible, and liquids will often lie in the mouth without being swallowed. Convulsions, generally less severe than at first, not unfrequently occur. Rigidity of the muscles, and contraction of one or more of the limbs, are apt to take the place of the convulsions. Sometimes there are picking of the bedclothes, and at imaginary objects in the air, and twitching of the tendons or cords, before the insensibility is complete. Sighing respiration ensues, and the pulse becomes slow and intermittent. The urine may be retained or dribble away involuntarily. If the disease continues on unchecked, great exhaustion ensues. In the place of the spasmodic contractions, or mingled with them, there is partial paralysis; the pulse becomes frequent and scarcely perceptible, the skin is bathed in a cold clammy sweat, the countenance sunken and deathlike, and the patient generally expires either in a state of profound stupor or in convulsions.

Such is the usual course of this disease; but sometimes, in the case of children, as the disease approaches the stage of stupor, there is a treacherous amelioration; the stupor and delirium diminish, and the child recognizes its friends, and even takes an interest in surrounding objects, and all the symptoms seem improved; but after lasting a day or two, either complete insensibility follows, or convulsions, with screaming, tossing, rolling the head, paralysis, and at last death. The duration of the disease is very uncertain. In violent cases death may follow within one or two days, but more frequently between the fourth and seventh days, and when thus early, it is generally from convulsions; but in a majority of fatal cases death occurs somewhere between the end of one and four weeks, and the disease is said seldom to pass the seventh week.

We sometimes have a partial inflammation of the brain or its membranes. This form of the disease generally commences with headache, occasional dizziness, faintness, dimness of sight, loss of appetite, neuralgic pains, prickling and feeling of numbness in different parts of the body, and irritability of temper. There is usually but little fever; the pulse is generally feeble, and often irregular; the face pale, and the surface cool. Nausea and vomiting, on assuming the erect position, are common. Frequently there are squinting, stammering and difficulty of swallowing; and rigidity or continued spasm of an arm or leg or both, on one side, is apt to occur; the attempt to bend the contracted limb generally causes pain. Finally the patient dies in convulsions; or paralysis and stupor ensue, and death follows. The symptoms are sometimes intermittent. After death from this form of the disease, there is sometimes found softening of a portion of the brain; in other cases induration, and occasionally an abscess. This disease may continue for weeks, months, and it is said even for years, before terminating in death.

In the case of children, between the ages of two and ten, or twelve years, we have to fear that the disease is of a scrofulous origin, and depends on the deposition of minute tubercles in the membranes of the brain, when it occurs in those who are subject to scrofulous swellings of the glands of the neck, or who inherit from their parents a strong tendency to consumption or scrofula; and we have especial grounds for such fears, if the disease approaches very gradually and insidiously. Great peevishness and irritability of temper often precede for weeks and months, the full development of the disease in such cases. Sometimes early in the disease, obstinate vomiting and constipation, with slight fever, are the chief symptoms, until perhaps paralysis or convulsions ensue.

From the fact that water is frequently found, after death, within the membranes of the brain, especially in the case of children, both this and the ordinary f rm of inflammation, or that first described, are often denominated dropsy of the brain, or acute hydrocephalus, if the patient dies.

Treatment of Inflammation of the Brain.—Give *Aconite* every hour in all cases when there are chills and fever, hot skin, full pulse, with pain in the head. If the disease has been caused by a fall, blow, or any form of mechanical injury, give *Arnica* alternately with *Aconite*, at intervals of one hour, but if, at the end of twenty-four hours it fails to relieve, give *Belladonna* instead of it, alternately with *Aconite*.

Dose, see page 7.

Belladonna: This is generally by far the most important remedy, after *Aconite;* or if, at the end of twelve hours, *Aconite* fails to relieve the fever, give *Belladonna* alternately with it, especially in all cases where there are severe shooting, darting, or burning pains in the head, with great sensibility to light or noise; red eyes, delirium, twitching, or convulsions. Give these remedies one hour apart, and do not hastily discontinue them. If there is an improvement, lengthen the intervals between the doses to two, and afterward three hours; but if the symptoms seem aggravated after giving the remedies, lengthen the intervals between the doses to six hours.

Bryonia: If the above remedies fail to check the progress of the disease within two or three days, *Bryonia* will generally be required. It should be given earlier if the patient begins to grow drowsy or sleepy, or the delirium becomes less violent with picking at the bedclothes, and cool extremities; also if there is rigidity or contraction of one of the limbs; but if no such symptoms occur until the end of three or four days, then if the fever is less active, and the pains in the head less sharp, or the delirium less violent, omit the *Belladonna* and give *Bryonia* once in four hours; if the head and body are still hot, give *Aconite* once or twice between the doses of *Bryonia;* consult *Helleborus.*

Helleborus: In the case of children if *Bryonia* fails within twelve or twenty-four hours to relieve the symptoms, give this remedy alternately with it at intervals of two hours. If symptoms of drowsiness or stupor appear, dilatation of the pupils, or loss of sight or hearing, sighing respiration, slow or irregular pulse, or symptoms of paralysis make their appearance, our main dependence must be upon the two remedies last named. If, after giving them twenty-four hours, there is no change, omit the *Bryonia* for twenty-four hours, and give *Belladonna* alternately with *Helleborus;* at the end of that period, if the patient seems to be improving, continue the *Belladonna,* otherwise omit this remedy, and give a dose of *Sulphur* at night, and *Helleborus* once in two hours. These are the most important remedies we have to prevent dropsy of the brain, or hydrocephalus; and if effusion has commenced, they are the remedies to check its progress, and promote its absorption. Although when symptoms of effusion exist patients will often die, still if you persevere with the remedies you will sometimes be successful in your treatment when you least expect it. If the disease in children is attended with a scrofulous or a consumptive habit, and you have to fear a tuberculous disease of the membranes of the brain, follow the above directions.

Hyoscyamus: If, in the case of either adults or children, *Belladonna* fails to relieve the delirium, convulsions, or sleeplessness, omit it for a few hours, and give this remedy in its stead; or if *Belladonna* seems to aggravate the symptoms or makes no impression on them, omit it for six or eight hours, and longer if the patient manifestly improves, and give *Hyoscyamus;* if the improvement ceases, return to *Belladonna.*

Stramonium: A few doses of this remedy will sometimes be useful for delirium, frightful visions, and screams, when *Belladonna* fails to relieve such symptoms.

Cuprum: When symptoms of this disease occur during the progress of scarlet fever, or other febrile eruptive diseases, and *Belladonna* does not relieve them, give a dose of *Cuprum* every hour for six or eight hours, and if the patient improves continue it, but if there is no improvement, give *Apis mel.* once in two hours.

In the treatment of the partial and slow inflammation which has been described, and which is often without much fever or heat, other remedies may be required, in addition to those already named. *Belladonna*, *Bryonia*, and *Hyoscyamus*, will often be required in this form of the disease, as well as in the more violent, and the indications for their use which have already been given, are sufficient to guide in their selection. It will be better, generally, to give but one remedy at a time, unless it may be a dose of *Sulphur* once a day; and do not repeat the remedies more frequently than once in three or four hours.

Nux vom: Give this remedy once in six hours when there is drowsiness, severe drawing pain in the head, fullness or pressure, with dizziness, vomiting, pain in the arms, numbness or paralysis of the extremities, or rigidity of the muscles of one extremity.

Pulsatilla may be given once in six hours when there are violent pain in the temples or forehead, which are aggravated by warm air and sitting up, and relieved by cold air and pressure. This remedy is especially useful also in the case of females, even in somewhat acute cases if the disease is connected with a suppression of the menses.

Lachesis: Give this remedy when there is great despondency, with weakness of memory, and of the mental faculties, pressing, darting, or beating pains, dizziness, with nausea and vomiting.

If there are bilious symptoms, such as yellow skin or eyes, give *Mercurius;* and especially if instead of costiveness there are mucous passages from the bowels.

General Directions.—In all acute cases attended with a high fever, hot skin and full pulse, the diet should be light; nothing more than gruel, rice, arrow-root, and at most, toast, cracker, and milk-and-water. If convulsions occur during the early stage when the skin is hot and the fever high, showering the head with a small stream of cold water from a pitcher, holding the head over a tub, and putting the lower extremities into warm water, will often relieve the symptoms. Continue the showering for from five to fifteen minutes, or until the extremities and head become cool, unless the convulsions cease sooner; then omit it until there is heat of the head and extremities, when it may be repeated, even if the convulsions do not return. It may require to be applied several times in the course of the first twenty-four or forty-eight hours; or what is better after the convulsions have ceased, and in cases where there are no convulsions, wring a large towel from cold water, and envelop the entire head with it, excepting the face, as high as the eyebrows, and put over the whole four or five thicknesses of dry flannel, and pin snug so as to exclude the cold air; wet the towel once in six or eight hours. This application often affords very great relief from the pain, restlessness, and heat. If it fails to benefit the patient, sponging the head with warm water generally has a beneficial effect. Sometimes cloths wrung from warm water will do well, and some physicians use them from the commencement, but I have generally preferred the applications named above.

If the bowels are constipated, free injections of warm water once in twenty-four or forty-eight hours will do no harm.

INFLAMMATION OF THE SPINAL CORD AND ITS MEMBRANES (MYELITIS AND CEREBRO-SPINAL MENINGITIS.)

This disease may be either acute or chronic. It may be caused by mechanical injuries, exposure, alcoholic drinks, and other causes of inflammation. The disease may commence suddenly, or be preceded by dull and uneasy feelings in the back and extremities. It may be confined to one part of the spine or extend almost its whole length.

Symptoms.—Severe pain which is increased by pressure and motion, often with a feeling of constriction around the body from the seat of pain; either neuralgic pains, or prickling or tingling, or a sensation of numbness in the parts supplied with nerves from the diseased portion of the spine, frequently occur. If the disease is in the upper portion of the spine, these sensations will be experienced in the upper extremities and the upper part of the chest; if in the middle of the spine, around the chest and abdomen; if in the lower portion of the spine, in the pelvis, and down the lower extremities. The muscles along the spine are often contracted, causing the head to be drawn, and the spine to be bent backward; cramps in the extremities and convulsive movements are not uncommon. Chills and fever usually precede, accompany, or soon follow, the local symptoms. Sooner or later, if the disease is not checked by treatment, symptoms of paralysis make their appearance; there is difficulty of moving one or more of the extremities, the urine may be retained or dribble away, and there may be obstinate constipation from the same cause. If the disease is chronic, the symptoms are similar, but come on more gradually, and without much fever. Inflammation of the spinal cord may be mistaken for rheumatism; but in the latter disease pressure along the sides of the spine causes more suffering than when it is made on the bones of the spine themselves; whereas, in the disease under consideration, the reverse is true. In rheumatism the pain on motion seems to be caused by the contraction of the muscles, instead of being caused by bending the spine. If the spine becomes contracted and bent backward by rigidity of the muscles, or if symptoms of paralysis occur later in the disease, we may be quite certain that the case is one of inflammation of the cord. General convulsions rarely occur in this disease when it does not extend to the brain.

We may have inflammation of the brain and spinal cord occurring at the same time. This form of disease sometimes prevails as an epidemic, when it is apt to be very fatal; patients in some cases dying within forty-eight hours, in other instances within one or two weeks. In this disease we have head symptoms such as pain, often a throbbing pain, generally in the temples or back of the head, intolerance of light and noise, delirium, stupor, perhaps convulsions or drawing back of the head, with great restlessness, incessant movement of the limbs, in some cases fever, thirst, and perhaps vomiting. In some instances there is little or no fever, in other cases the fever assumes a typhoid form, with feeble pulse, cool extremities, and sordes on the teeth, with perhaps black or dark spots in and beneath the skin.

Treatment of Inflammation of the Spinal Cord.—In all cases when the disease is attended with a high inflammatory fever, with a hot skin, give *Aconite* every hour. In fact the treatment is very similar to that required for inflammation of the brain. *Belladonna* will often be required after *Aconite*, or if the fever persists after giving the latter remedy for twelve hours give them alternately.

Dose, see page 7.

Belladonna: After the patient has taken a few doses of *Aconite*, if the fever is not relieved alternate this remedy with it at intervals of one hour; especially when the disease is confined to the upper part of the spine; and if the inflammation extends to the brain this will be a still further indication for the use of *Belladonna;* also when there are neuralgic, prickling, or tingling pains in the direction of the nerves which have their origin from the diseased portion of the spine. *Aconite* may be omitted as soon as the patient is comparatively free from fever, and *Belladonna* may be given alone.

Bryonia is not less important than *Belladonna* when the lower portion of the spine is the seat of the disease, and it may follow the latter remedy when the disease is at any point, provided there is great soreness on motion, with stiffness and contraction of the muscles, which is not relieved by other remedies. Give a dose once in two hours.

Dulcamara: Give this remedy after a few doses of *Aconite*, when the disease has been caused by exposure to wet damp weather, especially when there are drawing pains in the muscles of the spine, lameness with a paralytic feeling, or twitching in the arms and hands. If the patient is not relieved by this remedy select another.

If the disease has been caused by mechanical injuries, give *Arnica* once in two hours, and if it does not relieve the symptoms, give it alternately with *Rhus tox.* at intervals of two hours; or if there is much fever give *Aconite* instead of *Rhus* until it is somewhat relieved. When there are burning pains in the back especially opposite the heart and a little higher up, with difficulty of breathing and palpitation, give *Arsenicum* every hour, and if it does not relieve the symptoms give *Pulsatilla.*

After the acute symptoms are somewhat relieved by some of the above remedies, *Nux vomica* is often required, especially when the disease is in the lower portion of the spine, and there is a bruised sensation, with darting pains increased by contact; numbness or paralysis in the lower extremities, and if there is retention of urine and constipation. This remedy is often useful in chronic cases. Give a dose once in two hours during the day, and a dose of *Sulphur* at night.

In obstinate or chronic cases, in addition to the above remedies, *Lachesis* and *Sulphur* will be required. In a form of the disease which involved both the brain and spinal marrow, which prevailed as an epidemic during the continuance of the Mexican war, through Michigan and some of the other Western states, and was characterized by congestion and prostration of the vital energies, rather than by active inflammatory action, the most important remedies were: *Pulsatilla* when there were violent throbbing pains in the temples and deep in the brain; *Stramonium*, when there were throbbing pains in the back of the head and neck and great restlessness; *Opium* in case complete insensibility ensued and *Stramonium* did not relieve it. *Aconite* and *Belladonna* were of no use as a general rule, and *Bryonia* and *Nux vomica* rarely afforded any relief.

General Directions.—Wet a towel in cold water, and lay over the spine, and cover it with four or five thicknesses of dry flannel, and confine the whole to its place by a bandage or dry towel around the body, Let the diet be light, nothing more than gruel or rice-water, crust-coffee, &c., until the acute symptoms are relieved.

SPINAL IRRITATION.

This is often mistaken for inflammation of the spine, but it is a non-inflammatory affection, and may be distinguished by the absence of fever, by extreme tenderness on slight pressure, and the want of pain under other circumstances, the ability to move without causing much suffering, and the shifting character of the complaint. Females are much more subject to this affection than males, and children are rarely affected. There is simply a nervous sensibility of the ligaments and muscular attachments of the spine. Whatever impairs the general health of an individual, be it indoor confinement, want of general exercise, excesses, profuse discharges, or chronic disease, favors the development of this affection. Sewing, knitting, painting, or sitting a long time in one position, or any occupation which fatigues one set of muscles and part of the spine, to the neglect of the rest, may cause this affection. The irritation of the spine extends to the nerves which pass out between the vertebræ, and we have a great variety of symptoms in the direction of the nerves which pass from the diseased portion of the spine; among which are neuralgic or rheumatic pains, in different parts of the body, or the parts supplied by such nerves; also burning, itching, tingling, prickling, and numbness; palpitation of the heart, faintness, nausea, vomiting, spasms of the stomach, colic, and bearing down pains. This disease, if it is not the cause of hysteria, is often connected with it, and both not unfrequently depend upon irritation, or ulceration of the uterus, as a predisposing cause.

Treatment.—As this is generally a disease of debility, we have first to put away the immediate cause of the affection, and then, by adopting vigorous measures to improve the general health, overcome the predisposition to it. The patient must give up sewing, knitting, writing, or any occupation which has caused this trouble; also avoid sitting, except in a strictly erect position, so that the weight of the head and shoulders may be sustained by the bones of the spine, and not by the ligaments and muscles. Travelling, horseback-riding, walking in the open air, contentment of mind, or, as far as the strength will admit, active useful employment, which shall invigorate the general system, is indispensable. The patient had better spend most of her time in reclining or lying down, so as to relax the spine when she is not taking active exercise.

If the patient is already confined to the bed, or nearly so, and not able to sit up, ride or take exercise, she must be exercised in the horizontal position, until she gains strength, and the tenderness of the spine is relieved so that she can take active exercise. Let an attendant bend and extend her fingers repeatedly, then her wrists, then her shoulders, in every possible direction; then take hold of the hand and turn the hand, or rotate it inward and outward several times; then serve the other arm in the same way, allowing the patient to rest an hour if she becomes fatigued; then bend and extend the toes, then the feet, then the leg, and afterward the thigh; then rotate the toes around in a circle, turn the feet from side to side; separate the feet eighteen or twenty inches, and turn the toes of the two feet together until they touch, then turn them out as far as possible, so as to rotate the whole leg; repeat this several times. Then place one hand on each side of the body, and a few inches below the arms, and vibrate it from side to side; afterward turn the head in every possible direction so as to exercise the muscles of the neck, and finally, gently percuss, or strike with the open hand over the chest, abdomen, and back—but very lightly, if at all, over the tender part. Go over the entire body as above directed at least once in twenty-four hours; and if the patient becomes fatigued, resting an hour or two occasionally. Continue the above exercises a little longer every day, and as soon as the patient feels able, let her resist—slightly at first—the various motions which her assistant gives her. Continue the above exercises, and she will soon be able to ride out, and at last walk out and take exercise herself. Remove all blinds and curtains from her windows without fail, during the day, and have her room if possible on the south side of the house; the sun need not shine in her face, but it must in her room, and the more freely, the sooner she will recover. Fresh air i also important. Give her a good nourishing diet, brown bread, beefsteak, &c.; but no tea, coffee, or stimulants. And as soon as she is able, let her read, or read to her, from the beginning to the end, the author's work on the "Avoidable Causes of Disease;" and she will find the directions there, which will keep her well if she will follow them.

Medicines will be useful to palliate the symptoms when the patient suffers severely; but, so far as curing the disease is concerned, they are far less important than the measures named above.

If the disease occurs during nursing, or after the loss of blood or other fluids, give a dose of *China* night and morning. If the menses are profuse and frequent, *China* may prove beneficial; but if it fails to relieve, give *Platina* night and morning, and if necessary, afterward, *Calcarea carb.* If the menses are suppressed, give *Pulsatilla*, followed by *Sepia.* For palpitation of the heart give *Nux vom. Belladonna*, or *Pulsatilla.* For numbness, prickling, or neuralgic pains, give *Belladonna, Nux vom*, or *Pulsatilla;* also give these remedies for spasms of the stomach and colic pains. For nausea and vomiting, give *Ipecac* or *Nux vomica*, and if they fail, give very weak *Coffee* after eating, once or twice a day.

CONGESTION OF THE BRAIN FROM DEBILITY.

The symptoms are similar to those of the first stage of inflammation in many respects. The patient complains of a rush of blood to the head, and sometimes there is in different parts of the body a sensation of numbness, prickling or twitching, and slight convulsions or stupor may occur; but the patient is pale, the flesh thin and flabby, the pulse small, weak, and slow, and the least exertion or excitement causes palpitation of the heart. The pain in the head is generally in the back of the head, or over the top of the head, lengthwise; there is great languor and debility. This disease may be caused by the loss of blood from blood-letting, abortion, bleeding piles, or by long-continued nursing, over-exertion, indigestion, diarrhœa, unnutricious diet, damp, confined, and dark air, want of exercise, or any other cause of debility.

Treatment.—The cause should be shunned as far as possible, and the diet should be nutritious, and contain more or less animal food, especially beef, mutton, and milk.

China: Give this remedy night and morning, when there is severe headache with pressure from within, out; aggravation of the headache from pressure or touch, or a contractive pain in the scalp. *China* is especially useful when the disease has been caused by the loss of blood, diarrhœa, nursing, &c.

Pulsatilla once in four hours will often afford temporary relief, when there is pain in the head which is relieved by cool air, lying down, and by pressure; *Belladonna*, when the pain is in the forehead, *Nux vom.* when it is in the top and back of the head.

CONGESTION OF THE BRAIN AND APOPLEXY.

Apoplexy is caused by pressure on the brain, by some cause within the skull, producing a sudden loss, to a greater or less extent, of sensation, voluntary motion, and consciousness, without a suspension of respiration and circulation. The symptoms may be caused by simple congestion of the blood-vessels of the brain; and when this is the case, if the patient recovers, no paralysis, or other traces of the disease, is necessarily left behind; or the symptoms may be caused by hemorrhage within the skull. The blood may be effused beneath or within the membranes or within the substance of the brain. Paralysis, more or less complete, is very apt to follow this form of the disease. Lastly, the symptoms may be caused by a sudden effusion of water or serum. We cannot often, at the time of the attack determine, with any degree of certainty, which of these conditions exists; but if the patient soon recovers without paralysis or impairment of the mental faculties, we may conclude that the case was one of simple congestion.

The attack of apoplexy is often preceded by symptoms of congestion of the brain, such as a feeling of weight and fullness in the head, dizziness or a whirling sensation, headache, drowsiness, confusion and loss of memory, apprehensions of impending evil, dimness or derangement of sight, temporary deafness and noises in the ears, bleeding from the nose, numbness or prickling in some part of the body, faltering speech, unsteady gait, and vomiting. One or more of the above symptoms may precede the attack for weeks or months, or only for a few moments. When attacked, the patient, if in the erect position, usually falls, and is deprived either completely or to a greater or less extent, of consciousness, sensation, and the power of moving.

In severe cases, there is neither sensation, sight, nor hearing, and if a limb is raised, it falls as if destitute of life. The countenance is expressionless, and often flushed, and sometimes the arteries of the neck throb violently. The pulse is usually full and slow, but sometimes intermittent. The respiration is slow and snoring, with puffing ont of the cheeks or lips. The pupils of the eyes are generally immovable, and insensible to light, and may be either dilated or contracted. There is difficulty in swallowing, the bowels are usually constipated, and the urine is either retained or passes involuntarily. There is sometimes a spasmodic contraction of the muscles of one side. This state of insensibility may last but for a few moments before consciousness returns, or it may continue for hours or days, sometimes to the sixth or seventh day, when, if the disease does not terminate fatally, the patient slowly recovers. He may recover entirely, but more frequently, after severe attacks, there remains more or less paralysis of either sensation or motion, or both, on one side of the body, or of some one organ or part. If an effusion of blood occurs on one side of the brain, paralysis results on the opposite side of the body. A predisposition to this affection is sometimes inherited; high living, the use of fermented and alcoholic drinks, and disease of the heart, favor its development. This disease may be mistaken for drunkenness, or the stupor caused by opium, or other narcotics; but if you cannot detect alcohol in the breath, and can derive from attendants, or from other sources, no evidence that the patient has taken any substance which is capable of causing stupor, you have a right to infer that the case is one of apoplexy; and if one side of the face or mouth seems settled down lower than the other, this is very good evidence; but this symptom is not always present in apoplexy.

Treatment.—The premonitory symptoms denote congestion of the brain, and it is all-important when such symptoms appear, without fever, to attend promptly to them, so as to prevent an attack of apoplexy if possible. The patient should live on vegetable food, eat moderately, and avoid stimulants. When such symptoms occur in an individual of full habit, give a dose of *Aconite* every hour, especially when there seems to be a determination of blood to the head, with redness and fullness of the face, sensation of fullness in the head, and dizziness, especially when stooping. If the patient improves, lengthen the intervals between the doses. If *Aconite* alone fails to relieve such symptoms, alternate it with *Belladonna*, at intervals of one hour.

Dose, see page 7.

Belladonna should be given either alone, or alternately with *Aconite*, when there is fullness and pressure in the head, with redness of the eyes and face, derangement of sight or hearing, sleepiness, prickling or numbness in various parts, difficulty of speaking, or other paralytic symptoms.

Nux Vomica: This remedy is perhaps as frequently required as any other, especially when there is neither heat nor redness of the face, and the patient is addicted to the use of coffee, fermented or alcoholic drinks, and if there is an aggravation of the symptoms in the morning, and in the open air; also when there are great heaviness of the head, and sleepiness; painful sensitiveness of the brain, when walking, dimness of sight, dizziness during or after a meal, with a sensation as if the head were turning, with danger of falling; buzzing in the ears, fainting, or temporary loss of consciousness, numbness, prickling, with difficulty of moving parts of the body. Give a dose every hour, until the severe symptoms are removed, then two or three times a day, to prevent their returning.

Give *Arnica* when there is dull pressure in the brain, buzzing in the ears, dimness of sight, and dizziness after or while eating.

Give *Lachesis* when there are pale face and absence of mind.

Give *Pulsatilla* when there are pains in one side of the head, which are relieved by pressure, dizziness on lifting the eyes, or when sitting or stooping, buzzing in the ears, and dimness of sight.

Give *Opium* to old people, when there is stupor, sleepiness, dizziness, heaviness in the head, pressure in the forehead, throbbing in the temples, dry mouth, nausea, or vomiting. If the symptoms of congestion of the brain have been caused by grief, give *Ignatia*.

When you have selected your remedy, give it every hour until the severe symptoms are removed; then give it before every meal, and a dose of *Sulphur* every night.

Treatment of the Apoplectic Attack.—Place the patient in a recumbent position, with the head and shoulders elevated by pillows; remove everything that is tight from around the neck, unbutton his shirt collar, admit fresh air, and make warm applications to his feet in all cases. If the patient's face is red, his head hot, and the pulse full, apply cold water to the head, but if his face is pale and the pulse is feeble, do not apply it.

Belladonna: Give this remedy at the commencement of the disease when the face is red or bloated, the pupils of the eyes dilated, or the mouth is drawn to one side with paralysis of the right side; also if convulsive symptoms occur. Give a dose every hour. *Nux vomica* is often required after this remedy, or alternately with it.

Nux vomica: Give this remedy when there is snoring respiration, hanging down of the lower jaw, or when the attack was preceded by headache, dizziness, buzzing in the ears, nausea or vomiting. Give a dose every hour until there is some improvement, then lengthen the intervals to three or four hours. Give *Opium* when the attack is severe, the pulse slow and irregular, snoring respiration, red bloated face, hot head covered with perspiration, dilated or contracted pupils, or convulsive movements.

Give *Pulsatilla*, especially in the case of females, when there is violent palpitation of the heart, small pulse, and bluish red face with loss of consciousness.

Give *Arnica* when the pulse is full and strong, and there are involuntary discharges from the bowels, and of urine, and there is paralysis of the limbs on the left side.

If the bowels remain costive, give a free injection of warm water. If the urine is retained it must be drawn off at the end of twelve hours, and afterward at least once in twenty-four hours. Any physician can perform this operation.

PALSY (PARALYSIS).

This disease frequently results from an attack of apoplexy, or rather from the diseased condition which causes the apoplectic symptoms. In some cases, we have an attack of paralysis without its being either preceded or accompanied by an apoplectic attack, owing to the pressure on, or change in the brain, being so slight, or coming on so gradually, as not to cause insensibility or stupor. In other cases, there may be slight symptoms of apoplexy at the commencement of the paralytic symptoms. Paralysis may also result from inflammation of the brain or spinal cord, and from the pressure of bone in cases of fracture of the skull or spine.

Local palsy may result from injury or disease of individual nerves. We may have palsy of one half of the body laterally, the other half remaining sound ; this is called hemiplegia. The palsy may be confined to the lower extremities, or the lower half of the body; this is called paraplegia. When a single part is paralyzed it is called local palsy. Both sensation and motion may be impaired or lost, or sensation may be impaired or lost, and the power of moving the part remain; or the ability to move may be impaired or lost and sensation may remain. Palsy may come on suddenly or gradually. In aged persons we sometimes have what is called paralysis agitans or shaking palsy. Lead palsy sometimes occurs from the poisonous influence of lead.

Treatment.—When this disease results from apoplexy, the remedies named under the head of that disease are useful; especially *Belladonna*, *Nux vomica*, and *Arnica*. Give a dose of *Sulphur* every night at bedtime, and if the paralysis is on the right side, give a dose of *Belladonna* before every meal, and if it fails to relieve, give *Nux vomica* in the same manner. If the paralysis is on the left side, give *Lachesis* before every meal, and if it fails, give *Arnica*, and afterwards, if necessary, *Nux vomica*. When the lower half of the body is paralyzed, give *Nux vomica*. Give *Arnica* when the disease results from rheumatism, and if it does not relieve, give *Sulphur* at night and *Bryonia* in the morning. If the fingers are paralyzed, give *Calcarea carb*. night and morning, and at the end of two weeks give *Silicea*. *Rhus tox.* is often useful when there is paralysis of the extremities, especially the lower extremities. If paralysis causes difficulty of swallowing, give *Lachesis*, *Belladonna*, or *Silicea*. If it causes loss of voice give *Belladonna*, *Hyoscyamus*, or *Lachesis*. For paralysis of the eyelids give *Belladonna* or *Sepia*. Electricity is a very uncertain remedy, and never should be used except under the direction of a skilful physician.

If the paralysis has been of some standing, and all pain, dizziness, or irritation in the head, has been removed, regular exercise of the part paralyzed becomes not less important than medicine. Let an assistant two or three times a day for a few moments bend and extend the paralyzed limb or part in every direction, if the muscles are contracted, gradually stretch them out; also with the open hand slap repeatedly the palsied part or limb over its entire surface. After thus exercising the part for a few days, the patient by an effort of his will, may try to assist in moving the weak part or limb, but he should never attempt to move it except when the assistant is moving it, until he feels that he has gained sufficient control over the part to be able to move it readily without assistance. As soon as the patient is able to move the part without assistance, let him exercise it regularly himself two or three times a day, but never to the extent of fatigue, or until there is increased feeling of weakness. His assistant may continue to rub and slap the part; and, as strength returns, he may offer a little resistance to the movements of the patient, and this may be cautiously increased until the part becomes strong.

HEADACHE (CEPHALALGIA).

Headache is a general attendant on all febrile affections, also on congestion and inflammation of the brain, and other inflammatory affections. In this section, headaches, which are independent of all such diseases, will be considered. Often headache is external to the brain, being seated in the scalp or cranium. Such is the case with many rheumatic, gouty, and neuralgic headaches;

also with the pains which result from various inflammatory affections of the external coverings of the skull; and this is true of syphilitic affections of the periosteum or covering of the bones, and of the bones themselves. Headaches are of every variety as to severity, location, extent, and duration. The pain may be on both sides of the head, or on one side; it may be over the eyes, in the forehead, temples, on the sides, on the top, or in the back of the head. It may be confined to a small spot, as if a nail were driven in, or it may extend over the entire head. It may last but for a single instant, or for hours, days, and weeks. Sometimes it is periodical or intermittent. The pain may be shooting, darting, aching, throbbing, tearing or burning; it may be superficial or deep-seated; there may be simply pain, or it may be mingled with dizziness, fullness, lightness, a sensation of emptiness, heat or coldness, noises in the ears, and perversions of vision. Temporary dimness of sight, or even blindness, sometimes precedes the attack of pain. Occasionally headache depends on disease of the heart, and it may be sympathetic with derangements of the stomach, constituting sick headache, or with derangements of the liver, constituting bilious headache; ulceration and chronic inflammation of the uterus, frequently cause headache in the back of the head, extending up to the crown, perhaps with a numb sensation. Nervous headache is common. Coffee causes a headache, which commences in the morning, grows worse until noon, and then gradually abates. Tea, tobacco, and decayed teeth, frequently cause this affection.

Treatment.—If the patient is subject to rheumatism or gout, and the pain seems to be external to the skull, if the scalp is sore to the touch, and the pain is dull and tearing, or shooting, give *Bryonia* once in two hours, especially when the pains are aggravated by walking, stooping, or contact, and if such pains are confined to one side of the head. If *Bryonia* fails to relieve, give *Rhus tox.*, especially if the pains are burning or beating, and if there is wavering of the brain when stepping, and creeping in the head, or if the pains are excited by walking in the open air.

Dose of these remedies, see page 7.

Belladonna will perhaps relieve more cases of headache than any other remedy, especially when the pain is aggravated by light, also when noise increases it. Shooting, darting pain, or aching and throbbing over the eyes, especially over the right eye and through the forehead, worse on motion, or on moving the eyes, red face and eyes, perversions of vision and of hearing, and temporary dimness of sight before the attack, are all indications for this remedy. Give a dose once an hour until the pain is relieved, unless it aggravates the symptoms; in that case discontinue the remedy and give *Hyoscyamus.*

Pulsatilla: Next to *Belladonna*, this remedy will perhaps relieve more cases of headache than any other, especially with females; also with males, if the following symptoms occur. Aching, beating, tearing, or shooting pains, especially when the pains are aggravated by heat, hot air, hot applications, and also by sitting up; and when the symptoms are relieved by cold air, pressure, and lying down. If there is a sour stomach, or acid vomiting, or pale face, with little or no thirst, *Pulsatilla* will be still further indicated. Give a dose every hour.

Nux Vomica: Give this remedy when there is constipation, with a tendency of blood to the head, especially with individuals of sedentary habits, or those addicted to the use of alcoholic and fermented drinks, or coffee. Also if there is sensitiveness of the brain, with contusive pains, headache every morning, on walking, after eating, or in the open air, while stooping, or during motion, or pain as if a nail were driven into the brain, or pain in the top or back of the head. Bilious or sick headache is often relieved by this remedy. Give a dose once in two hours.

Aconite may be given when there are violent, stupifying, compressive, contractive, drawing, or burning pains, through the brain, with red face and eyes, and especially if the pain is worse on the left side, over the left eye, and is aggravated by talking, raising one's self, drinking, and moving, and relieved in the open air. Give a dose every hour.

For sick headache, select, from the remedies already named, either *Pulsatilla, Nux vom.* or *Belladonna*, according to the symptoms, and give a dose every hour during the attack, and give the same remedy every night, to prevent a return; also give a dose of

Sulphur every morning, especially if the pain during the attack was most severe on the left side of the head, but if it was worse on the right side, give *Sepia;* if it was alike on both sides, give *Sulphur* for one week, and *Sepia* the next, and so continue.

If the headache is intermittent, give *China* once in four hours during the intermission, especially when the pains are aggravated by contact, and whenever the hair of the head is very sensitive. If *China* fails to relieve intermittent headache, or those in which the patient has a return of the pain regularly every day, or every other day, give *Arsenicum* once in four hours, when the patient is free from pain; *Nux vom.* or *Belladonna* may be given during the pain.

When the headache has been caused by grief, give *Ignatia;* when by anger, give *Chamomilla* or *Nux vom.*

Give *Calcarea carb.* for chronic headache, especially when it occurs either through the upper or the front portion of the head, and when the pains are stupifying, throbbing, or boring, aggravated by mental efforts; also if there is a sensation of coldness in the head, or if there is falling off of the hair.

In addition to the use of remedies for headache in nervous and chronic cases, let the patient, or what is better, an assistant, rub briskly with the ends of the fingers of both hands, from the root of the nose over the top of the head, to the neck, back and forth, for a minute or two; then rub from the centre of the back of the head, sidewise, in the direction of the lower part of the ears; also gently slap or percuss the head with ends of the fingers, or palm of the hand, for a few moments.

DELIRIUM TREMENS.

This is a disease which follows the suspension of the habitual use of alcoholic or fermented drinks. It occurs more frequently with steady drinkers than with those who only occasionally get drunk; and persons of sedentary habits, or inactive life, are much more liable to have the disease than those who take active exercise. If habitual drinkers receive a mechanical injury, or are attacked with an acute disease, they are very liable to have delirium tremens; and this is one reason why injuries and acute diseases are so much more fatal with rum-drinkers than with others. This disease is said to sometimes follow the sudden omission of opium, or tobacco, where individuals have been long addicted to the use of these poisons.

Trembling of the tongue when the patient attempts to protrude it, and twitching of the tendons or cords in his wrists, are among the first symptoms of this disease; and when such symptoms occur without fever, with an individual who is in the habit of using stimulants, we always have reason to suspect the commencement of delirium tremens. Anxiety and agitation soon follow, the pulse is soft, feeble, and generally frequent; the mind weak, and sooner or later the perceptive faculties begin to take cognizance of matters and things which do not exist, in the natural world at least. The patient seems frightened, and begins to see the most grotesque, frightful or disgusting objects, such as serpents, rats, mice, toads, and other loathsome reptiles and vermin, crawling over his bed or person, or running about his room; he hunts them among his bedclothes. The sufferer is always afraid; robbers, officers, or creditors, he imagines, after him; he hears them conspiring against him; he sees knives, swords, and firearms, pointed at him, and strives to escape from his tormentors, and may injure himself or others, in striving to protect himself or escape; although patients in this disease rarely make a malicious attempt to injure others, for they have enough to do to attend to the affairs of their own spiritual household. This disease under proper treatment is attended with very little danger, except when it is complicated with mechanical injuries, or other severe diseases. Patients may die from exhaustion resulting from over-exertion, and this should be guarded against. Without treatment the patient either gadually becomes exhausted from over-mental and physical exertion, and the want of sleep, and dies, or, after from three to seven days, he falls into a quiet slumber from which he awakens after sleeping from a few hours to twelve, eighteen, twenty-four, and, in some instances, it is said, thirty-six hours, feeling weak and feeble, and looking pale, but free in a great measure from his tormentors.

Treatment.—He who shuns the use of alcoholic and fermented drinks, opium and tobacco, as every one should do, has not to fear this disease ; but no man who uses them can count himself safe. The only sure preventive measure, then, is total abstinence.

We have seen that this disease is caused by leaving off suddenly the use of stimulants. The appetite for the accustomed stimulant fails, and it is omitted, when symptoms of delirium tremens make their appearance. To prevent the full development of the disease, or cure it after it is developed, in most cases we have but to give the patient moderate, but regular doses of brandy, and then withdraw it as the disease abates. There is no danger of cultivating an appetite for it, by giving it during the disease, as the patient has no desire for it, although he will generally take anything which is offered him. A tablespoonful of brandy in water, sweetened, once in two hours, will, in many cases, be sufficient, but if the patient has been a hard drinker he may require two tablespoonfuls once in two hours, or even more frequently in some rare cases; and the brandy should be continued until the patient falls into a quiet sleep. When he awakens it need not be repeated unless symptoms of the disease return, and it should *never* be continued longer than is absolutely necessary to relieve the visions and sleeplessness To relieve the debility never give stimulants, but beef tea, chicken broth, mutton, and beef; and *China* night and morning.

Nux vomica: This remedy will sometimes relieve the disease if given early. It is indicated when there are trembling of the tongue and limbs, frightful visions with desire to escape, and also when there is nausea and vomiting at any stage of the disease. Give a dose once in two hours. Give *Belladonna* when there are frightful visions, also visions of mice and rats, and when the face is red and bloated. Give *Arsenicum* when there are great weakness, cold extremities, with fear of thieves and desire to hide. Give *Opium* when there are symptoms of convulsions or approaching stupor. Give a dose of either of the above remedies every hour.

LOCKJAW (TETANUS).

This, although not very frequent, is one of the most formidable and dangerous diseases when it does occur. It sometimes follows wounds, even slight wounds, and occasionally attacks newborn infants, especially colored children in hot climates. It may occur without any assignable cause, perhaps depending on atmospheric changes or states. In this disease the muscles are in a state of constant spasmodic contraction, with periods of partial relaxation; the body may remain straight, it may be bent backward so as to rest on the head and heels; or, less frequently, it may be bent forward or even sidewise. As the disease progresses, in addition to the permanent rigidity named above, paroxysms or spasms make their appearance, at first light, but at length they may become terribly severe, throwing the body about in different directions. This affection generally commences either with stiffness in the muscles of the jaws and throat, or of those on the back of the neck, which more or less rapidly extends to other muscles. Swallowing becomes difficult, respiration more or less hurried and anxious, the pulse is often quite regular until late in the disease, except during active spasms, the skin is moist. The mental faculties remain unimpaired throughout the disease, or until very near its close, when there may be light wandering. Tetanus is more common with men than with women. Patients most frequently die between the end of the first and fifth days; if they live until the ninth day they generally recover.

Treatment.—When the disease is caused by a wound or mechanical injury, if the patient has previously taken *Arnica*, give a dose of *Belladonna* every hour; but if he has not taken *Arnica*, give a dose of *Arnica* one hour, and *Belladonna* the next. *Belladonna* is often useful when the disease occurs with young children, and when it arises from unknown causes, or atmospheric changes, especially if *Hyoscyamus* fails to relieve such cases. If *Belladonna* does not lessen the severity of the symptoms at the end of twelve hours, give *Nux vom.* every hour. If, at the end of twenty-four hours, this remedy does not lessen the severity of the symptoms, give *Hyoscyamus* for twelve hours at least. *Ignatia* or *Lachesis* may follow the latter remedy if necessary. Do not discontinue any remedy until the patient has taken it at least twelve hours, and if there is the slightest improvement continue the remedy without fail, or even if the patient ceases to get worse under its use, continue it.

If the disease has not been caused by a wound, and commences with stiffness of the jaws, give *Hyoscyamus* every hour. If this fails at the end of twelve hours, follow it with *Belladonna.* If the last remedy fails, give *Nux vom.* *Ignatia* and *Lachesis* are also remedies which may be required in lingering cases.

HYDROPHOBIA (RABIES).

This disease is usually caused by the bite of a dog, cat, or some other animal, suffering from this affection, although it may be caused by the saliva from an animal suffering from the disease coming in contact with a raw or abraded surface of the skin, and possibly with the mucous membrane of the lips or mouth. In the human species it is estimated as the result of observation, that only one in ten or fifteen of those who are actually bitten by rabid animals, contract the disease. If the bite is through garments, the saliva is generally wiped from the teeth, so that none enters the wound; but if on an exposed surface like the hand or face, there is far more danger. The disease rarely if ever appears within the period of eighteen days after the reception of the wound; and in cases where it follows at all, it is rarely delayed beyond three or four months, although in rare instances it is said to have appeared at the end of twelve or eighteen months after the bite, and even at a later period.

Symptoms.—Often the first warning of an approaching attack, is pain, or an uneasy sensation near or in the seat of the wound, perhaps nothing more than burning, coldness, tingling, aching, or stiffness. If, in such cases the wound is unhealed, it assumes an unhealthy appearance, and discharges a thin watery fluid, instead of healthy matter; if the wound is healed, the scar is apt to become swollen, reddish, or livid, and sometimes breaks out into an open sore. About the same time the patient becomes restless, irritable, and dejected, light disturbs him, he is restless during sleep, and sooner or later he begins to feel some difficulty of swallowing, with stiffness about the throat; at length swallowing becomes almost impossible; even the attempt to swallow causes great suffering and spasms. There occurs oppression of the chest, with sighs and sobs; there is trembling of the whole frame, mental anxiety, terror, or despair. The attempt to swallow liquids, or even the sight of water, or hearing it running, or anything which brings to his mind this fluid, causes convulsive spasms about the throat, and great agitation and oppression. Sharp pains, like an electric shock, are often experienced through the regions of the stomach, neck, and back. There is a profuse secretion of saliva or spittle, which the patient spits rapidly and indifferently around him. He is generally conscious, although sometimes, at intervals, delirious, in other cases suspicious, and sometimes furious until exhausted. There may be great thirst which cannot be gratified; the pulse is excited at first, but as the disease progresses, it becomes frequent, feeble, and perhaps wanting. The skin, at first warm, becomes cold, and covered with a profuse offensive perspiration. If the patient dies, death may occur quietly or in convulsions; generally between the second and fifth day, or not until the end of a week or ten days.

Treatment.—This disease is so frightful in its character, and fatal in its tendency, that in case a person has been bitten by an animal suffering from it, every possible means should be used to prevent an attack. Experience has shown that if the skin and wound are washed, and the entire wound is removed by a knife so as to remove every part which has been in contact with the animal's teeth, when this is practicable, it is very sure to prevent the disease. The sooner the operation is performed the better; immediately if possible; but it has been urgently recommended even after the commencement of premonitory symptoms, especially when there is swelling, discoloration of the scar, or an unhealthy appearance of the ulcer if the wound has not healed. After the operation, or when the latter is not practicable owing to the extent, depth or location of the wound, the following recommendation of Dr. Hering may be followed. Apply radiating heat, by the means of a hot iron, or a live coal, held as near the surface of the wound as the patient can well bear without causing too great pain, or burning the part, and continue it for half an hour or hour, or until chills set in. This may be repeated two or three times a day until the wound is healed. Also give a dose of *Belladonna* once in three days, and continue it for three or four weeks, then alternate this remedy with *Lachesis* at intervals of three days, for three or four months.

If symptoms of the disease already exist, give *Belladonna* every hour, especially if there is difficulty of swallowing, spasms in the throat, and later in the disease, if the patient is furious, or frightened and disposed to strike, spit and bite. Give a dose every hour. If at the end of twelve hours there is no improvement, omit *Belladonna* and give *Lachesis* every hour for twelve doses; if the patient improves under its use continue it; but if there is no improvement, return to *Belladonna*. If neither of the above remedies check the onward progress of the disease, give *Hyoscyamus* every hour for six hours; then if there is no improvement give *Belladonna* for six hours; afterward *Hyoscyamus* again. *Cantharis* is sometimes useful. Dose of either of the above remedies: six globules, or one drop of the tincture on a little sugar dry on the tongue.

EPILEPSY (FALLING SICKNESS).

Very little is known in regard to the causes of this disease. It is supposed that a predisposition to it is sometimes transmitted from parents to their children, although it often occurs where there is no evidence of a hereditary taint. It is more common with the young than with the old. It sometimes results from an attack of inflammation of the brain; it may be caused by a fracture of the skull, and depression of a portion of it; also by fright, and the present method of forcing or cramming children in our schools, the suppression of eruptions on the skin, the sudden healing up of old ulcers, worms, and irritation of the stomach and bowels from other causes, self-pollution, and sexual excesses. When the disease is fully developed it is characterized by attacks of convulsions with loss of sensibility and consciousness, and usually followed by stupor; but the paroxysms are without fever.

Sometimes this disease commences with very slight paroxysms of giddiness, confusion of mind, inability to stand, although without loss of consciousness; but, as the paroxsyms continue, they become gradually more severe, until the patient becomes unconscious during them, and finally convulsed. In other instances the first paroxsyms manifest distinctly the character of the disease. Sometimes the paroxsyms are preceded by certain premonitory symptoms, such as unusual states of temper or feeling, failure of memory, confusion of thought, dizziness, drowsiness, fullness, or emptiness in the head, dimness or perversions of sight, ringing in the ears, unpleasant odors which are not real, &c. In rare instances a sensation of coldness, heat, pain, itching or tingling commences in one of the extremities, or some other part of the body, and proceeds toward the brain. When the sensation reaches either the stomach or head the paroxysm commences. After the continuance of the above premonitory symptoms for a longer or shorter period, or without any of them, the patient falls down in convulsions, sometimes uttering a fearful cry at the moment of the attack. There is generally more or less rigidity of the body, and one side is frequently more convulsed than the other; the head is twisted round and the face is drawn to one side, and the limbs are violently convulsed by sudden contractions and relaxations of the muscles. The eyes and face twitch and are often greatly distorted, the face is generally swollen, and of a reddish or purple hue, respiration is difficult, there is frothing at the mouth, and the pulse is small, frequent, and often irregular. The paroxysm may last from a few moments to several hours, and even with occasional periods of relaxation, for twenty-four hours or more, the patient being either convulsed or in a state of stupor all the time. A state of stupor follows the paroxysm, but gradually passes off and the patient awakens, perhaps a little confused at first, and soon returns to his usual state. In some instances headache, paralytic symptoms, or temporary insanity follows the paroxysm. At first the paroxysms may only occur at intervals of months or even years, but they are apt to become more frequent as the disease continues. Sometimes they are very frequent at their commencement. When the disease is fully developed they may occur, only at intervals of weeks or months, or they may return daily, or even several times a day. Patients sometimes, but very rarely, die during the paroxysms. The mental faculties may become impaired from the long continuance of the disease, and even idiocy sometimes results.

Treatment.—This is, in most cases, a very obstinate disease, and sometimes baffles the skill of the most eminent physicians, yet it is often cured by a persevering use of homœopathic remedies, and it is generally ameliorated by treatment.

Belladonna: Give this remedy three times a day, one half an hour before eating, at the commencement of the disease, or even at any stage, if there are severe convulsions, with distortion and twitching of the eyes and face, if the paroxysms are excited by mental emotions, and there are great irritability of temper and sleeplessness between the paroxysms. At the same time, give a dose of *Sulphur* every night. If any change either in the frequency or severity of the paroxysms follows, either for better or worse, give the remedies less frequently, or give but one dose a day; *Belladonna* three nights, and *Sulphur* one, and so continue as long as there is any improvement.

Dose of either of the remedies, see page 7.

Ignatia before meals, and *Calcarea carb.* at bedtime, may follow *Belladonna* and *Sulphur*, and be given in the same manner, especially in the case of children. If the paroxysms occur at night, these remedies may be given before *Belladonna* and *Sulphur*.

Nux Vomica: Give a dose of this remedy before every meal, and *Silicea* on retiring at night, in case the remedies already named fail to relieve or cure the patient. If any change follows, lengthen the intervals as directed for *Belladonna* and *Sulphur*. *Lachesis* and *Hepar sulph.* may follow the above remedies, if necessary. *Hyoscyamus* and *Sepia* are remedies which have sometimes been found useful.

Do not change your remedies too frequently, and never change them so long as there is any improvement, either in the frequency or in the severity of the paroxysms. You will generally have to give a remedy several weeks before you can be fully satisfied as to the effect. If you can cure the disease by administering remedies from six months to two years, you may regard yourself as very fortunate. Look well to the diet of the patient. Read the author's work on the "Avoidable Causes of Disease," and you will find a vast fund of instruction, not less important to epileptics than medicine. If you fail to cure the patient, call on a homœopathic physician, for he may be able to cure, by the use of higher or lower dilutions, or other remedies which you do not have.

CONVULSIONS OR SPASMS, IN CHILDREN AND OTHERS.

It not frequently happens, especially with children, and occasionally with adults, that, from transient causes, such as sudden fright, anger, or other mental emotions, exposure to great heat, mechanical injuries, the irritation from teething, also from indigestible substances in the stomach and bowels, convulsions are caused, which are without fever, and more or less resemble those of epilepsy. There may be starting and twitching, and other nervous symptoms before the attack, or they may come on suddenly. They may last but for a few moments, or for hours, with occasional relaxation, but generally from ten to twenty minutes. They may extend over the whole body, or be confined to one half of it, to one limb, or to the face. The face may be pale or purplish, and often apparently swollen. The patient generally sleeps at the termination of the paroxysm. There may occur but a single attack, or several, at irregular intervals. There is very little danger attending such convulsions, as patients rarely die in them. If the attack is preceded or accompanied by fever, hot skin, headache, or delirium, consult the section on inflammation of the brain, and follow the directions there given. If the paroxysms occur repeatedly, are without fever, and come on suddenly, and you cannot trace them to swollen state of the gums, improper diet, strong mental emotions, worms, or any other cause, consult the section on epilepsy, and follow the directions you there find, in the intervals between the attacks If the patient is a female between the ages of ten or twelve and forty-five, especially if there is a disposition to sob, cry, or laugh, at the commencement, or at the termination of the paroxysm, consult the section on hysteria and hysterical convulsions. But in other cases, follow the directions below.

Treatment.—During the attack, make warm applications to the lower part of the body, and lower extremities, or put the lower half or two thirds of the body into warm water. If the head is hot, and the face red, you may shower the head for a few moments with cold water, especially if the disease has been caused by the irritation of teething. If the attack has been caused by eating green fruit, or other indigestible food, as soon as the patient can swallow, let him drink freely of warm water—all he can swallow —then tickle the throat with a feather, so as to cause vomiting; even if vomiting does not ensue, the warm water may benefit the patient. In all cases where the bowels are costive, or you have the least reason to suppose the attack is caused by irritation of the stomach and bowels, or by worms, give a free injection of warm water, and repeat it in one hour, if the bowels do not move feeely.

Belladonna: Give this remedy every half hour or hour, when the disease has been caused by teething, chagrin, or insults; also when you cannot ascertain the cause. In the case of children, give a dose two or three times a day, and a dose of *Calcarea carb.* at bedtime, to prevent a return of the symptoms, after the paroxysm is over.

Dose: Dissolve twelve globules, or one drop of the above, or any of the following remedies, in half a glass of water, and during the convulsions, put a few drops of the solution into the mouth, but as soon as the paroxysm is over, give a teaspoonful for a dose. If the medicine is in powder, give as much as will lie on the end of a penknife blade.

Chamomilla: Give this remedy if the disease has been caused by irritation of the bowels, colic, diarrhœa, anger, disappointment, or by teething, if *Belladonna* fails to relieve in the latter instance. Give a dose every half hour or hour, until a disposition to spasms has been relieved, and then give a dose three times during the day, and if the disease has been caused by irritation of the bowels, give a dose of *Mercurius viv.* at bedtime, to prevent a return of the paroxysms.

Opium: If the convulsions are the result of fright, give *Opium*, and if it fails to relieve give *Ignatia*.

Ignatia: If the attack has been caused by grief or fright, give this remedy every half hour or hour, also in other cases where *Belladonna* or *Chamomilla* fails to relieve the symptoms. *Stramonium* when there is trembling and nervous excitement or convulsions without loss of consciousness.

If the attack has been caused by indigestible food, give *Nux vom.*, but if the bowels are loose give *Pulsatilla* or *Chamomilla*. If the spasms seem to be caused by worms, give *Cina*, and consult the section on worms.

ST. VITUS' DANCE (CHOREA).

This disease generally occurs between the ages of five and twenty, although there is no period of life absolutely exempt. Females are more subject to it than males. Whatever tends to impair the general health and increase nervous irritability predisposes to this disease. It may be caused by strong mental emotions or over-excitement, deranged stomach and bowels, self-pollution, spinal irritation, suppression of the menses, &c.

Symptoms.—This disease is characterized by involuntary movements, sometimes of the whole or almost the whole body, often worse on one side than on the other, and occasionally confined to one limb or part. The patient does not lose her consciousness, and has the power to commence moving, but cannot control her movements, or at least until after several efforts. These irregular movements may be so incessant as to interfere with sleep; and are generally increased by mental emotions, especially by the consciousness that others are observing her. The face often becomes distorted into all sorts of fantastical shapes, and walking is frequently difficult, and in bad cases, walking, or even standing or sitting, may be impossible. Stammering is but a variety of this affection.

This disease may only continue for a few days, or it may last for months and years, when improperly treated, or without treatment.

Treatment.—Sun-light, out-door air, exercise, brown bread, loose dresses and absence from heated school-rooms and confinement; and relief from close study, are the essential conditions necessary for a cure, without which remedies will be of little avail.

Give *Belladonna* once in six hours, if the face is implicated, if the patient stammers, or has headache, and also, if, with the above symptoms, the disease extends to the extremities. If this remedy fails to relieve, give *Cuprum* at night and *Belladonna* before every meal. Give *Hyoscyamus* before every meal, if there are stammering, involuntary action of the under jaw, neck, head, and of the extremities, and give *Cuprum* at bedtime. *Stramonium* may follow the above remedies once in three or four hours, if it is required.

If the extremities are more affected than the face, or, in other cases, if the above remedies fail, give *Arsenicum* three or four times a day, and if it does not relieve the symptoms within a few days, give it at night only, and if the patient is a male, give *Nux vom.* before every meal; if relief does not follow, give *Pulsatilla.* If the patient is a female, give *Pulsatilla* before every meal; if it fails to relieve, give *Nux vom.* *Ignatia* before meals and *Sulphur* at night will be useful in obstinate cases.

HYSTERICS (HYSTERIA).

This affection generally occurs in females between the ages of twelve and forty-five, and it is more frequent at the menstrual periods than at other times. The present cruel method of bringing up young ladies, favors the development of the disease, by rendering the whole system delicate and nervous. They are deprived to a great extent of the all-important necessaries of life—sunlight, pure air, active labor, and exercise. Hot rooms, unnatural confinement in schools, crowding the intellect to the neglect of the body, solitary vice, and novel-reading, are among the many causes of this disease; also disappointments in love, domestic troubles, strong mental emotions, and an irregular or vicious life. It is often connected with if not caused by spinal irritation, also by diseases and derangements of the womb.

Symptoms.—The symptoms all manifest a state of unnatural excitement of the nervous system, and they are apt to occur in paroxysms. The patient may be troubled more or less constantly with aches, pains, palpitation of the heart, nausea, irregular action of the bowels and kidneys, prickling, and numb sensations; also choking, a disposition to sob, laugh, or sigh, great sensitiveness on pressure, and soreness of parts, and all from this affection. The soreness and tenderness on pressure over the spine, bowels, breasts, and many other parts, often simulate inflammation, but may be known from the latter disease by the absence of fever, and by the tenderness being as great, and often greater on slight pressure, than it is on heavy pressure; and then moving the parts often causes but little if any pain. After having been troubled for a longer or shorter time by some of the above hysterical symptoms, or without them, an individual predisposed to this disease is liable to be attacked with a sensation as if a ball were ascending from the left side of the abdomen, stomach, or chest, up to the throat: or more frequently there is simply a sensation of uneasiness or oppression at the stomach, or in the chest, when the patient falls, if standing, throws her limbs about convulsively, beats her stomach or breast, pulls her hair, perhaps attempts to bite, and twists the body into all sorts of shape. Sometimes there is simply rigidity with perhaps the body bent backward as in tetanus. The patient not unfrequently cries out, but is generally partially, and in some instances entirely unconscious. The face is rarely distorted to any great extent. The paroxysm may continue but for a few moments, or it may last for hours, or even days, with intervals of sleep or stupor. When it passes off the patient sometimes breaks out in a fit of laughing or sobbing; in other instances quiet sleep follows, and she awakes comparatively well. In another form of the disease, instead of convulsions the patient becomes stupid and insensible, and cannot be aroused; the breathing becomes feeble, the pulse small and the extremities cold. This state may continue from a few hours to two or three days, and sometimes the paroxysms are followed by temporary paralysis of some part of the body. Hysterical paroxysms with those who are subject to them, may occur at intervals of from a few days to a month, or several months This disease is attended with very little danger to life.

Treatment.—Medicine is good, for it may and will palliate the symptoms, but it alone can never cure. If a husband, father, or brother, would avoid spending his living on doctors or nostrums, or if a lady would avoid a life of suffering and wretched uselessness, let him or her obtain the author's work on the "Avoidable Causes of Disease," and read it carefully through from beginning to end, and then profit by the information therein contained; and this disease can be cured, but first the whole life and habits must be revolutionized.

If a paroxysm of hysterical convulsions occurs at about the time of the menstrual flow, give a dose of *Coffea* every hour, and if, after two doses, the symptoms are not relieved, give *Pulsatilla* every hour; also in all cases, if there is a disposition to sigh, sob, or laugh. This remedy, *Pulsatilla*, is also useful for hysterical stupor, and the same is true of *Belladonna* and *Nux vom.*

Dose, see page 7.

If the paroxysm has been caused by grief, disappointment, contradiction, or even fright, give *Ignatia* every hour; and if three or four doses do not relieve, give *Pulsatilla*. *Nux vom.* will sometimes be useful when either fright or anger has caused the paroxysm. If jealousy is the cause, give *Hyoscyamus* every hour.

At the commencement of a hysterical paroxysm, dash a handful or two of cold water into the patient's face, on to her neck and breast; admit fresh air, and unfasten everything that is tight about the breast and waist. These measures will often prevent the paroxysm, and sometimes even relieve it after it has commenced. To overcome a tendency to this disease, *Calcarea carb.*, *Sulphur*, and *Sepia*, are among the remedies, in addition to those named above. If the menses are profuse and frequent, give *Calcarea carb.* every third night; and if they are attended with severe pain, give *Nux vom.* on the two nights when you do not give *Calcarea.* If these remedies, at the end of two months, do not relieve, give *Platina* night and morning. When the menses are scanty or suppressed, give *Pulsatilla* and *Sulphur* alternately, two nights apart, and if, at the end of two months, there is no change, omit them, and give *Sepia* once in three nights. Also consult the sections on spinal irritation, dyspepsia, and uterine diseases.

CATALEPSY.

In this disease, there is a more or less perfect loss of consciousness, with rigidity of all the muscles of the body, or only of a part, or a single limb. The body or limbs are not usually so stiff but that they can be bent without much difficulty, but the peculiarity is, that they retain the position in which they are placed, however awkward it may be. If an arm is raised, it retains its position. The paroxysm may last but a few minutes, or it may continue for hours or days. This is a very rare disease, and resembles, in many respects, hysteria, and arises from the same causes.

Treatment.—Give *Chamomilla* every hour, and if it fails, give *Belladonna*. *Platina* may be given night and morning, to prevent a return of the paroxysm.

SLEEPLESSNESS.

Hearty or late suppers frequently cause disturbed sleep, and sometimes sleeplessness. The use of coffee and tea, late rising in the morning, strong mental emotions, reading, writing, and mental application, during the evening, are among the chief causes of this derangement.

Treatment.—If sleeplessness or disturbed sleep, arises either from eating too much at supper, or from late suppers, let the patient avoid the former, and abandon forever the latter, and take *Pulsatilla* about one hour before retiring. Give *Aconite* when sleeplessness is caused by mental anxiety, or by alarming events, fear, fright, or chagrin, especially if there is fullness of the head.

Give *Belladonna* one hour before retiring, when the patient feels sleepy, but no sleep follows; also when he cannot restrain his thoughts; and when frightful visions occur during sleep.

Nux vomica is the proper remedy when the sleeplessness is caused by thinking, reading, or writing late at night, and when all sorts of ideas crowd upon the patient's mind; it is especially useful in the case of coffee-drinkers, and of those who use alcoholic and fermented drinks.

Ignatia, when the sleeplessness is caused by grief, sadness, care, mental anxiety, and depressing emotions. *Opium* will be required for the sleeplessness of aged people; also give it to others if *Aconite* does not relieve this symptom, when it is caused by fear or fright.

Give *Hyoscyamus* when sleeplessness occurs during the progress of fevers, and other diseases, or while recovering from them. If it fails, select some other remedy.

For sleeplessness of young children, give *Aconite*, especially if there is any fever or restlessness, and if the symptoms are not relieved in an hour, give *Coffea;* repeat these remedies if necessary. *Belladonna* may be given if the child cries without apparent cause; and if there is sudden starting or twitching which is not relieved by it, give *Chamomilla.* Give *Chamomilla* when the child is troubled with colic, or earache, and if it fails give *Belladonna.* Repeat the dose of either every hour until relief follows.

DROWSINESS OR SLEEPINESS

When this occurs between the regular hours of sleep, if it occurs soon after eating, it may be caused either by over-eating, especially of animal food, or by debility of the digestive organs. It may also be caused by derangements of the liver, and by a tendency to congestion of the brain.

Treatment: If the sleepiness occurs soon after eating, eat less, and take a dose of *Nux vom.* before each meal, and if you do not get relief consult the section on dyspepsia. If the skin and eyes are yellow, or if there is more or less uneasiness in the right side, just beneath the right lower ribs, give *Nux vom.* at night and *Bryonia* in the morning. In all other cases, especially when there is a tendency to profound sleep, consult the section on congestion of the brain and apoplexy. In case of nervous females, consult also the section on hysterics.

NIGHTMARE (INCUBUS).

This is an affection which comes on during sleep, and is characterized especially by a sense of weight on the chest, with an inability to move or speak; sometimes accompanied with a dream of being held down by some horrid monster, or of trying to escape from some great danger. It may be caused by late or hearty suppers, cold feet, the habitual use of tobacco, and by whatever interferes with sound sleep.

Treatment.—Let the patient eat light suppers, go to bed early, use no tobacco, tea, coffee, or stimulating drinks. Give a dose of *Nux vomica* one hour before the patient retires, when the disease results from over-eating, the use of coffee or stimulating drinks. *Pulsatilla* may be given if *Nux vomica* fails to relieve, especially in the case of females. Give *Aconite* if there are feverish heat and palpitation of the heart; *Opium*, if other remedies fail, and the paroxysms are very severe; if the breathing is snoring, the surface cold, and if there are twitchings of the extremities. Give *Sulphur* mornings.

MENTAL EMOTIONS.

As strong mental emotions often cause disease, it is not always best to wait until manifest symptoms occur, before resorting to the use of the proper remedy, for the early administration of the remedy may aid in restoring harmony to the mental faculties, and thereby prevent suffering. If unpleasant symptoms already exist, consult the section on the form of disease which is manifested. Give, among the different remedies mentioned below, under the different heads, the first one named, and repeat the dose every hour, when the emotions are very violent, until four or five doses have been taken, when, if no relief follows, give the next remedy. As soon as relief begins to be experienced, lengthen the intervals between the doses to four, six, or eight hours.

For fear or fright, give *Opium*, *Aconite*, *Ignatia*, or *Pulsatilla*.

For excessive joy, give *Coffea* or *Pulsatilla*.

For grief, give *Ignatia* or *Lachesis.*

For disappointment in love, give *Hyoscyamus* or *Ignatia.*

For jealousy, give *Hyoscyamus, Nux vom.*, or *Lachesis.*

For mortification, resulting from insults, disappointed ambition, &c., give *Belladonna, Ignatia, Pulsatilla,* or *Platina.*

For violent anger, give *Aconite, Nux vom., Chamomilla* or *Bryonia.*

For chagrin and the effects of contradiction, give *Aconite, Chamomilla, Ignatia,* or *Bryonia.*

For religious excitement, give *Belladonna, Lachesis, Hyoscyamus,* or *Sulphur.*

INSANITY OR MENTAL DERANGEMENT.

It would require too much space to enter into a full description of the various forms of insanity, nor do I propose to do more than to allude to this subject and point out some of the most important remedies to be tried at the commencement of the disease, by those who have not access to a homœopathic physician, before sending the patient to an insane asylum. It is to be hoped that the day is not far distant, when some of our noble charitable institutions, devoted to the treatment of this disease, will be under homœopathic treatment. Never, until then, shall we be able to know the full measure of success which may be attained in the treatment of mental diseases.

Delirium is common during febrile and inflammatory diseases, and will be found frequently noticed in other sections, in connection with such diseases, but what little is said here has reference to continued or intermittent derangement of the intellectual and moral faculties. A predisposition to insanity is sometimes inherited, and it is often acquired. The intermarrying of blood relations, overtaxing the brain and intellectual faculties in our schools, and neglect of the body, are perhaps the most fruitful causes of a predisposition to this disease in our country. Solitary vice is a very frequent cause; and the same is true of strong mental emotions.

We have, first, cases of mental alienation, which consist in a mere perversion of the mental and moral faculties; and second, of those which consist in the impairment or loss of the same faculties. Under the first head may be recorded what is called mania, in which the intellect is perverted on all subjects. Second, what is called monomania, or partial insanity, in which the perversion is restricted to one subject. Third, moral insanity, which consists in a perversion of the natural feelings, of the affections, inclinations, temper, habits, moral disposition, or natural impulses, without any remarkable disorder of the intellect, and particularly without any insane illusions. Under the second head, we have first, what is called dementia, in which the intellect has been impaired or destroyed; second, idiocy, where the deficiency is congenital, or the patient was born with it.

Treatment.—Let every parent who has the least ground to fear that his child may inherit a tendency to insanity, also every individual who fears this disease, obtain the author's work on the "Avoidable Causes of Disease, Insanity, and Deformity," and read the chapters on children, education, amusements, marriage; and especially on the mental causes of disease and insanity.

If this affection has been caused by mental emotions, consult the section on mental emotions, which precedes this, and follow the directions there given for the treatment of the different emotions.

If the disease has been caused by excessive study or mental application, give *Lachesis* night and morning, afterward, if necessary, *Nux vomica, Platina,* and *Sulphur;* do not change as long as there is any improvement.

If caused by suppression of the menses, give *Pulsatilla* night and morning; *Platina* and *Belladonna* may be of use in such cases after *Pulsatilla.*

If caused by solitary vice, give *Nux vomica* at night and *Sulphur* in the morning. Follow these remedies, if necessary, by *Pulsatilla* at night and *Calcarea carb.* in the morning.

If there is a disposition to commit suicide, give *Arsenicum* in the morning and *Nux vomica* at night; afterward if the symptoms are not relieved, give *Pulsatilla* or *Belladonna.* If the patient desires to commit acts of violence to others, give *Belladonna* or *Hyoscyamus.*

For imbecility or idiocy, give *Belladonna* one night and *Sulphur* the next. If at the end of a month there is any improvement, give them at intervals of three days. Follow the above remedies, if necessary, with *Hyoscyamus* and *Lachesis* in the same manner.

MELANCHOLY OR HYPOCHONDRIASIS.

This is often but the first stage of insanity or monomania, although it may depend on dyspepsia; and when that seems to be the case, consult the section on that disease. For religious melancholy, give *Sulphur* every night and *Pulsatilla* every morning until there is some improvement, then give them two or three days apart. *Belladonna* and *Lachesis* may be required. When it results from disappointment, give *Belladonna*, *Ignatia*, or *Pulsatilla*. Consult the section on insanity, and the one on mental emotions.

CRAMPS IN THE LEGS.

If this affection occurs at night, give *Nux vomica* night and morning until the paroxysms cease, then give it at night and *Sulphur* in the morning to prevent a return. If the above remedies do not cure, give *Veratrum*, in the place of *Nux vomica*, and afterward give *Secale cor.* if it is needed. If this symptom occurs while sitting, or after violent exercise, give *Rhus tox.* If on stretching out the limbs, give *Calcarea carb.* *Colocynth* is sometimes useful.

CHAPTER VIII.

DISEASES OF THE EYE, EAR, AND NOSE.

NEAR-SIGHTEDNESS (MYOPIA).

THIS affection is generally congenital, or the individual is born with it. It is usually caused by the cornea, or front transparent part of the eye being too convex; sometimes it arises from too great convexity of the lens, or both may be in fault.

Treatment.—Close one eye, and look straight forward with the open eye, then press gently with the fingers over the centre of the ball of the closed eye, for a minute or two, afterward serve the the other eye in the same manner. Repeat this two or three times a day, until the near-sightedness is relieved by gradually reducing the convexity of the eye. Another measure of relief is derived from wearing concave glasses, or spectacles. Glasses should not be worn constantly, but only when especially required. Give a dose of *Sulphur* once a week, as this remedy, in some cases, is useful; afterward give *Pulsatilla* once a week. Continue each for some months.

LONG-SIGHTEDNESS (PRESBYOPIA).

This is often one of the earliest indications of advancing years, and is caused either by a flattening of the cornea or front part of the eye, and perhaps of the lens, or by a change in the density of the various structures of the eye. Distant objects are distinctly seen, while those near cannot be distinguished.

Treatment.—Place the ends of the thumb and two or three fingers at different points around the ball of the eye, as far back in the socket as possible, and gently press upon the eyeball for a minute or two at a time, two or three times a day, carefully avoiding all pressure on the transparent portion of the eye. Convex glasses relieve while they are worn.

PARALYSIS OF THE OPTIC NERVE—BLINDNESS (AMAUROSIS).

This disease may be caused by overtaxing the eyes, in looking at minute objects, or by looking at a very strong light, as at the sun; and even the absence of light, or living in dark rooms, may cause this affection. Symptoms of this disease are very common with females who live in dark parlors, sew, and take little exercise, but in such cases they are generally accompanied by a general impairment of health, and the eyes suffer with the rest of the body. This affection sometimes comes on suddenly, when it arises from some violent cause, such as a strong light, great exertion, excessive heat, or disease of the brain, but generally it is preceded by various derangements of sight, such as sparks, dark or various colored spots, or a blur, mist, or floating specks, before the eyes. There is sometimes, but not always, pain through the eyes and temples.

Treatment.—Shun the direct rays of the sun, and of artificial lights, also strong reflected rays from brilliant objects; avoid dark rooms and veils, and remember that the undimmed light of day is a natural stimulant to the eyes; therefore, live in open air and light as much of the time as possible, and take active and regular exercise, especially if you have been living a sedentary or indoor life. If debilitated from any cause, a good nourishing diet is requisite, and a dose of *China* may be taken every night. *Gelsemium semp.* when there is wavering before the eyes, and confusion of sight, with uneasiness through the temples

Belladonna: Give this remedy night and morning, if there are sparks or bright objects before the eyes, or if there is pain or heat in the eyes or temples. *Sepia*, especially in the case of females, often follows *Belladonna* to advantage, and may be given every night. *Phosphorus, Calcarea carb.*, and also *Sulphur*, are important remedies, especially in obstinate cases. If there is any dizziness, or fullness in the head, do not fail to consult the sections on congestion of the brain and apoplexy, and follow the directions found there.

CATARACT.

This is an opacity of the crystalline lens, or of the capsule or sack, which surrounds it, and can generally be distinguished by a change in color within the pupil or sight of the eye. Children are sometimes born with this affection. In some instances it results from an injury, and in other cases the origin of the disease can be traced to no definite cause.

Treatment.—If the disease has been caused by an injury, give *Arnica* night and morning; follow it if necessary by *Pulsatilla* at the end of a few weeks. In other cases give *Pulsatilla* every night for a week, then give *Phosphorus* every night for a week, and so continue, alternating every week. If remedies fail, and both eyes are becoming blind, a surgical operation will be necessary, but if one eye is sound, be satisfied with that, without an operation.

Squinting, when not of long standing, can sometimes be cured by *Belladonna*, given every night and morning, followed if necessary by *Hyoscyamus*, and afterward by *Stramonium*. Old cases can be relieved by an operation which is neither dangerous to vision, severe, nor very painful.

STYE ON THE EYELID.

This disease consists of inflammation of the meibomian glands, situated on the edge of the eyelid; an abscess soon forms, if the inflammation is not checked.

Treatment.—*Pulsatilla* is the chief remedy, and it is much more certain to cure if used at the thirtieth dilution, than when used stronger, although any dilution will often check the progress of the disease. Give six globules or one drop of the tincture internally once in six hours; and dissolve the same quantity in a tablespoonful of water, and wash the swelling frequently with the solution. To prevent a return of the disease, give *Pulsatilla* and *Sepia* alternately three days apart.

CATARRHAL INFLAMMATION OF THE EYES.

(CONJUNCTIVITIS.)

This consists of inflammation of the conjunctiva, or of the external coat of the eye, which also lines the under surface of the lids. It may be caused by cold, foreign or irritating substances, and a strong light. Newborn children are very subject to this disease. With them it is generally caused by a too strong light, cold air, or contact with the leucorrhœal or gonorrhœal discharge during the passage of the head through the vagina, when the mother is suffering from either of the latter diseases. One of the worst forms of this disease is caused by the accidental contact of the eyes, with the discharge, in cases of gonorrhœa or clap. Catarrhal inflammation sometimes prevails as an epidemic, and is often contagious, or the discharge from a diseased eye, if brought in contact with a healthy one, will cause a similar disease; therefore every one should avoid washing in the same dish or wiping on the same towel, with those suffering from this disease.

Symptoms.—There is every degree in the severity of the symptoms, from a trifling disease of little moment, to a most formidable affection, rapidly endangering sight. Itching, burning, smarting, intolerance of light, redness, swelling, and a more or less profuse discharge of tears and mucus, are among the prominent local symptoms. If the disease is severe, there are fever, headache, and loss of appetite; and if the inflammation is not checked, ulceration and disorganization of the cornea, with impairment and even loss of sight, may result. If the disease is slow in its progress, or continues long, the under surface of the lids are apt to become rough or granulated, and this may prolong the duration of the disease indefinitely.

Treatment.—If the disease is slight, with or without fever, give a dose of *Aconite* in the morning, and a dose of *Belladonna* at night. In all cases avoid reading, sewing, and a strong light. If the symptoms are more severe; if there is great redness, heat, intolerance of light, pain, or fever, give a dose of *Aconite* once in two hours during the day, and a dose of *Belladonna* as frequently during the evening and night, when the patient is awake. Six globules of the remedy you are giving internally, may be dissolved in two tablespoonfuls of water, warm or cold, as is most grateful to the patient, and the eyes may be frequently washed in the solution; and a soft cloth may be wet in it and placed over them, and confined by a dry handkerchief, every night. Persevere with the above remedies, if necessary, several days. And at the end of three or four days, and even sooner, if the fever and heat have abated, and the discharge is mattery, omit the *Aconite* and give *Mercurius viv.* during the evening and night, and *Belladonna* during the day—each once in two or three hours when the patient is awake. Continue the above remedies as long as there is any improvement. If the disease threatens to become chronic, give *Sulphur* night and morning. In chronic cases *Sulphur*, *Mercurius viv.*, and *Calcarea carb.*, are the chief remedies.

If the disease occurs with newborn infants, the above is your treatment, also when it occurs with adults; but if it has been caused by the discharge in cases of gonorrhœa or clap, give *Pulsatilla* instead of *Belladonna*, after the first few days, but otherwise the same treatment.

The diet should be light; in severe cases no animal food, stimulants, or stimulating condiments, should be allowed. Generally warm applications do better than cold. Sometimes cloths wet in cold water, and dry flannel placed over them, changing only once in three or four hours, will do well.

SCROFULOUS INFLAMMATION OF THE EYES.

This affection is very common with children. There is great intolerance of light, profuse flow of tears, sometimes an eruption on the skin around the eyes; and often pimples, pustules, and even ulcers make their appearance around, and on the transparent portion of the ball. The edges of the lids are frequently inflamed, red, and swollen.

Treatment.—Outdoor air and sunlight, with active exercise, are indispensable; and good nourishing diet is important, especially bread made from unbolted or coarse flour. You need not expect to cure this disease, while you allow the patient to live on superfine flour bread, and high-seasoned food; allow neither coffee nor tea.

Give *China* morning and noon, and *Belladonna* before teatime, and on retiring. Continue these remedies at least one week, and as much longer as there is any improvement. If there is an eruption about the eyes or face, and the above remedies fail to relieve, give a dose of *Mercurius cor.* at night, and *Rhus tox.* in the morning. If the patient is a child of a full habit, or disposed to bleed at the nose, give a dose of *Calcarea carb.* every night, and if, at the end of a week, there is no improvement, give *Sulphur;* afterward give *Hepar sulph.* night and morning for several weeks. *Arsenicum* every night may be required in very obstinate cases. If water is applied externally, it should generally be warm.

RHEUMATIC INFLAMMATION OF THE EYES.

This affection generally occurs in those who are subject to rheumatism elsewhere, although it may attack the eyes first; and it involves either the dense structure or coat of the eye beneath the conjunctiva, what is called the sclerotic coat, or it attacks the iris, the curtain which surrounds the pupil or sight, or it may involve both. There is generally more pain and less discharge than in catarrhal inflammation, and there is less redness and itching.

The treatment is similar to that required in acute rheumatism in other parts of the body. *Aconite*, *Bryonia*, *Rhus tox.*, and *Belladonna*, are the chief remedies. *Mercurius viv.* will often be useful. At the commencement of the attack, give *Aconite* every hour for twelve or twenty-four hours; then if the pains are sharp, and there is much intolerance of light, give *Belladonna* alternately with *Aconite*, one or two hours apart. If the pain is dull, heavy, and tearing, and increased by every motion of the eyes, give *Bryonia* once in six hours, and *Aconite* every hour between. After *Bryonia*, *Rhus tox.* may be required, or *Mercurius viv.*, especially the latter, if there is much perspiration, or, if the iris is involved, and other remedies do not relieve. Give a dose once in six hours. If the patient is subject to the gout, *Pulsatilla* or *Nux vom.* may be required. Consult also the section on rheumatism.

INFLAMMATION OF THE IRIS, OR OF THE CURTAIN WHICH SURROUNDS THE PUPIL OR SIGHT (IRITIS).

This affection is generally caused by rheumatism, the abuse of mercury, or by syphilitic (venereal) poison, although it sometimes arises from exposure or a strong light. There are, in severe cases, heat and fever, and a red circle of enlarged vessels may be seen surrounding the cornea or transparent portion of the eye. The iris often changes color when compared with the other eye, is less brilliant, and of a dusky hue, and its edges become irregular, as the disease progresses, from the presence of lymph, which is poured out. By the contraction of this lymph, the pupil is sometimes destroyed and vision lost.

Treatment.—If the disease has been caused by rheumatism, consult the sections on rheumatic inflammation of the eyes and rheumatism. If caused by an abuse of mercury, give *Nitric acid* alternately with *Belladonna*, two hours apart, afterward give *Sulphur*, if necessary. If the disease has been caused by syphilis (the venereal disease), *Mercurius* is the chief remedy, provided its use has not recently been abused by the taking of large doses. Give a dose of *Mercurius viv.* once in two hours. If, at the end of two or three days, there is no improvement, give *Mercurius cor.* once in four hours, and give a dose of *Belladonna* between the doses of this remedy.

In all cases of iritis, without regard to the cause, if the pupil becomes much contracted and irregular with shreds of lymph projecting from the edges of the iris, put two or three drops of the tincture of *Belladonna* into a tablespoonful of water, and wash the eyelids, and around the eye, once in four or five hours. If you have not the tincture you can get a little of the extract of *Belladonna* at any druggist's, and a piece as large as a small pea dissolved and used in the same manner will answer. *Belladonna* causes dilatation of the pupil, and it will sometimes prevent its obliteration in cases of iritis; but it will not often be required.

FOREIGN SUBSTANCES IN THE EYES.

If the substance is beneath the lower lid, with the fingers draw the lid down, and ask the patient to look up, then with the head of a pin covered with a soft silk or cambric handkerchief, remove the foreign body. If the offending substance is beneath the upper lid, which is generally the case, take a knitting or tape needle, or the small end of a metal pencil in one hand, place the end across the upper lid about half an inch from its edge, take hold of the eyelashes with the fingers of the other hand, and gently raise the edge of the lid while you press the pencil or needle downward, so as to turn the lid inside out over the pencil, when you will be able to see the foreign substance on the under surface of the lid, and an assistant can readily remove it, as directed in case of the lower lid. With mechanics small particles of steel are often driven into the ball or cornea; they can be removed with the sharp point of a needle or knife, but it requires great care not to injure the eye, and when practicable you had much better apply to a physician, than to attempt it yourself.

DISEASES OF THE EAR.

EARACHE (OTALGIA).

This may be purely a neuralgic affection ; it may be caused by decaying teeth, or it may arise from inflammation of the ear. In either case the pain is most intense, often making the patient almost frantic. Children frequently suffer from this affection, and before they can make known their sufferings by words, the seat and character of the disease may be suspected when the child screams violently, frequently brings its hands to the side of the head, moves its head uneasily, and does not draw up its legs and bend forward as in colic. A child will cry from severe colic, but generally not as violently and continuously as from the earache. If the pain is caused by inflammation, there is usually tenderness on pressing immediately in front of the ear, there may be swelling and redness in the passage; and if the disease is not checked, an abscess forms in a few days, upon the breaking of which the pain abates. The discharge in some cases, especially if not properly treated, may continue for years. If the internal ear is involved in the inflammation, the bones and other structures are sometimes so far involved in the disease and destroyed, as to seriously impair the hearing. Measles and scarlet fever frequently cause this affection or it occurs in connection with these diseases. The inflammation may become chronic, with more or less ulceration, keeping up a constant mattery discharge for years. In rare cases the inflammation and ulceration cause death of the entire thickness of bone and reach the brain and its membranes, and matter or pus is found on the inside of the skull, which presses on the brain, and we have symptoms of inflammation and congestion of the brain, followed usually by death at no distant period. As there is a liability that chronic inflammation of the ear may take this turn, it is always desirable to cure such an inflammation as soon as practicable, by a careful and persevering homœopathic treatment.

Treatment of Earache.—In all cases there is no objection to applying dry warm cloths over the ear, or the same wet in warm water.

Chamomilla: This remedy is especially useful in the case of children, and also in that of adults, if the pains are shooting or darting from within outward. In the case of children, if you have any doubt whether the cause of the crying of the child is earache or colic, give this remedy. Give a dose every hour, unless the pains are aggravated after the doses; in that case, omit the remedy. If relief follows the use of this or either of the other remedies, lengthen the intervals between the doses to three or four hours. *Pulsatilla* is often required after *Chamomilla.*

Pulsatilla: This is the chief remedy when there is inflammation, swelling, heat, or tenderness, on pressure. Give a dose once in two hours. If, at the end of twelve hours, there is no improvement, omit this remedy for six hours and give a dose of *Belladonna* every hour; if the patient improves under this remedy, continue it, but lengthen the intervals between the doses; but if there is no improvement, return to *Pulsatilla.* In severe cases of inflammation, it may be necessary to continue the two remedies, changing occasionally, for two or three days before the disease will be cured. If the above remedies fail, *Nux vom.* will often relieve the symptoms, but if that does not check the progress of the disease, or afford some relief, give *Mercurius viv.* once in two hours. If the pains become throbbing, and there is a roaring sound, give *Hepar sulph.*

Nux vom.: This remedy is sometimes useful in inflammatory earache, especially after *Pulsatilla;* but in neuralgic earache, it is often useful at the commencement, or after *Chamomilla.* Give a dose once in two hours. If the pains are in paroxysms, worse mornings and evenings in bed, and are very violent, tearing and stitching, extorting cries, give this remedy.

If the patient is very sensitive and nervous, and there are no signs of inflammatory action, if *Chamomilla* does not relieve, give *Arnica,* especially if there is great sensitiveness to noise. Give *China,* if the pains seem to be external, and are aggravated by contact, and if there is ringing in the ears. If the pain in the ear is caused by decaying teeth, which may be suspected when the pain commences in the teeth, or when the latter are sore to the touch, *Belladonna* or *Chamomilla* will often relieve it. *Phosphorus* should be given if the teeth are decayed and broken nearly to the gums, and the sockets are inflamed. Have worthless teeth and roots extracted.

RUNNING FROM THE EARS (OTORRHŒA).

This affection frequently follows an abscess or inflammation, when treatment has been neglected or discontinued too soon. The discharge in chronic cases is often offensive, and of a white, yellowish, or greenish color.

Treatment.—In an acute or recent attack of inflammation, if notwithstanding the treatment, a discharge of matter follows, never wait to see whether it will stop spontaneously or not, but give *Pulsatilla* one night, and *Sulphur* the next; at the end of a week, lengthen the intervals between the doses of the above remedies, to forty-eight hours, and continue these remedies for several weeks. In all cases of long standing, which have been neglected, or inefficiently treated by allopathic measures, you may commence with the above remedies. In chronic cases, you will need to continue a remedy several weeks, gradually lengthening the intervals as the symptoms improve.

If the discharge follows scarlet fever, small-pox, or measles, give *Mercurius viv.* alternately with *Belladonna*, the former at night and the latter in the morning. If in the course of two or three weeks, the discharge does not cease, give *Pulsatilla* and *Sulphur* as directed above.

Calcarea Carb.: In obstinate cases, give a dose of this remedy once a week, and continue it as long as there is any improvement. *Silicea* may follow it, especially if the discharge is offensive. *Carbo veg.* is also useful in such cases.

DEAFNESS—DEFECTIVE HEARING (DYSECŒA).

Deafness may arise from an excessive secretion and accumulation of earwax. In such cases it usually comes on gradually, and is often attended by buzzing and other noises. By a careful examination, you can see that the passage is filled with hardened wax. When this is the case, drop two or three drops of sweet oil into the ear, and after a few hours, syringe out the ear carefully, but thoroughly, with warm water, so as to wash out the wax; let the head, while using the syringe, be leaning over in the direction of the obstructed ear. Repeat the above once a day, until the wax is entirely removed. Also give *Pulsatilla* alternately with *Sulphur*, one week apart, to prevent a return of the obstruction.

If the deafness results from inflammation, or is connected with a discharge from the ears, the treatment which has been recommended for earache, and running from the ears, is the proper treatment.

NERVOUS DEAFNESS is another form of this affection. It may come on gradually or rapidly, from a sudden paralysis of the auditory nerve. Together with hardness of hearing, there are often buzzing, roaring, singing, and various noises in the ears. Sometimes there is great dryness in the ears. If there are buzzing in the ears, pressure and fullness in the head, with deafness, consult the sections on congestion of the brain and apoplexy, and follow the directions therein given.

Treatment of Nervous Deafness.—If there are dryness of the ears, with deafness, as if the ears were closed, and singing, buzzing, or ringing in the ears, give a dose of *Calcarea carb.* every night, until there is some change, then gradually lengthen the intervals between the doses. This is one of the most important remedies for nervous deafness, especially in young persons. If the patient is a female, once a month omit the *Calcarea carb.* for a week or ten days, and give *Pulsatilla* every night in its stead.

If the deafness has followed the disappearance of an eruption about the head, face, or ears, give *Sulphur* every night, and after a few weeks give *Hepar sulph.* If the patient is a male, lives high, or if his habits are sedentary, and he has buzzing in the ears, or whistling, give *Sulphur* in the morning and *Nux vom.* at night.

BUZZING OR OTHER NOISES IN THE EARS.

This affection is often connected with congestion of the brain, and in all cases when there is a sensation of fullness, pressure or pain in the head, consult the section on that disease. It may be caused by a cold, if so, *Nux vom.*, *Mercurius*, *Aconite*, or other remedis appropriate for cold in the head, are proper. Noises in the ears are common in cases of great debility from the loss of blood, or other fluids of the body ; when this is the case, *China* may be given before every meal. *Pulsatilla* will be necessary if *China* fails to cure.

Noises in the ears are often the premonitory symptoms of deafness. In such cases, *Pulsatilla*, *Calcarea carb.*, *Belladonna*, and *Nux vom.*, are among the proper remedies. Consult the sections on deafness and earache.

DISEASES OF THE NOSE.

Under the head of coryza, or cold in the head, commencing on page 124, acute inflammation of the mucous membrane of the nostrils, has been considered. For a description of the symptoms and proper treatment of chronic inflammation of the nostrils, or catarrh and ozæna, see page 126. For the symptoms caused by foreign bodies in the nostrils, and the way to remove them, see page 127.

BLEEDING FROM THE NOSE (EPISTAXIS).

This is a very common affection with young persons, and frequently occurs during adult life. Generally the quantity of blood discharged is moderate, and it is only occasionally that it becomes so great as to injure the general health or endanger life. With some individuals there is a strong tendency to alarming hemorrhages from the nose, gums, or other organs ; and in such cases, if prompt measures are not adopted to arrest the flow of blood, death may result. Bleeding from the nose is a common symptom in various febrile affections; sometimes as a critical discharge inaugurating a favorable change, but in other cases it becomes a dangerous symptom. It may result from mechanical injuries ; also from a watery state of the blood, or from a loss of vitality in this fluid, and the vessels which contain it, as in scurvy, typhus fever, &c.

Treatment.—*Arnica* may be given when it results from mechanical injuries, or from lifting, or straining, or when, in other cases, there is itching in the nostril. Give a dose every fifteen minutes; and if it fails to check the flow of blood at the end of one hour, give *Rhus tox.*

Dose of this or other remedies, see page 7.

Aconite should be given if the patient is of a full habit, with red face, or if there is a sensation of fullness in the head, and when this symptom has been caused by heat. If *Aconite* alone fails to check the bleeding at the end of an hour, alternate it with *Belladonna* at intervals of half an hour.

China.—Give this remedy every half hour when the patient is weak and exhausted, and if it does not soon check the discharge, follow it with *Secale cor.*

Pulsatilla is especially efficacious in the case of females, when this symptom occurs before the first menses, or if they are scanty or delayed. Give a dose every hour.

If bleeding from the nose occurs during typhoid or typhus fever, follow the directions given in the section on that fever, so far as remedies are concerned, but remember the mechanical measures described below.

To overcome a tendency to this affection, if the patient is young and of a full habit, give *Aconite* one night, and *Calcarea carb.* the next, for one week, then lengthen the intervals between the remedies to three days. If the patient is weak and exhausted, give *China* and *Secale cor.*, in the same manner. If the vitality of the blood is impaired, and dark spots appear in and beneath the skin, give *Arnica* in the morning and *Carbo veg.*, at night.

General Measures.—Keep the patient either in a sitting or standing position, or at least the head elevated, excepting in cases where there is fainting, when it should be lowered, until this symptom is relieved. Cold water or ice may be applied to the nose, lower part of the forehead, and back of the neck. If the attack is severe, the feet may be put into warm water. Elevating the arm of the same side from which the blood comes will sometimes check the flow. The same is true of pressing with the finger on the side of the nose, letting the pressure extend up an inch or so.

Mechanical Measures.—In serious cases, where remedies and

the measures already named fail to prevent a dangerous loss of blood, the nose must be plugged, and this must be properly done or it will be useless. To simply fill up the external orifice will do little or no good, for the blood will flow down the throat. A clot of blood often forms in the nostril and answers as a plug if the patient will only let it alone and avoid blowing or clearing his nose. Tear eight or ten pieces of old cambric or soft cotton or linen cloth, about one and a half inches square; take a needle with a stout double thread and fasten it securely to the centre of one of the pieces, and then simply string all the rest of the pieces upon this double thread by passing the needle through each toward one corner; having done this, take another needle with a single thread, and fasten it to the first piece of cloth, or the same to which the other thread is fastened, then catch up a stitch in the centre of the next piece and tie it securely so that it will not slip, but leaving a slack thread of about three inches between the two pieces of cloth, then fasten all the rest of the pieces to the single thread in the same way about three inches apart. Having done this, with a knitting or tape needle carry the piece of cloth to which both threads are fastened into the nostril nearly as far back as the further end of the soft palate, and hold it there firmly by the double thread while you carry in the other pieces one by one, allowing them to slide on the double thread and pack the entire nostril full, crowding some of the pieces up well toward the ridge of the nose. Having filled the nostril, lay a little roll of cloth across the opening (but so large that it cannot enter) between the double thread, and tie the thread snugly around it, so as to confine the whole to its place, and prevent any part from passing back into the throat. In this way you can with the greatest certainty stop the flow of blood. To be certain that you have succeeded you can look into the patient's mouth and see that the blood is not running down the throat, or ask him to hawk and ascertain if he raises blood. You may allow the plug to remain in for twenty-four hours before removing it; and then put in another if the bleeding returns. In one instance I was obliged to plug both nostrils to stop the hemorrhage. Of course the patient had to breathe through his mouth.

SWELLING AND INFLAMMATION OF THE NOSE.

Swelling and inflammation may result from mechanical injuries, scrofula, syphilis, whiskey drinking, or erysipelas. Small abscesses not unfrequently form in the wings of the nostrils.

Treatment.—If the disease results from a mechanical injury, give *Arnica* and apply it externally—a few drops in a tablespoonful of water may be used for a wash.

Belladonna may be given once in two hours when there is redness, swelling, or symptoms of an abscess. It is also useful when erysipelas attacks this organ. If in either case this remedy does not relieve, apply warm water to the nose. Give *Rhus tox.* once in two hours.

Dose of either of the remedies, see page 7.

If the disease has arisen from whiskey drinking, let the patient stop drinking and take *Nux vom.* at night and *Sulphur* in the morning.

SYPHILITIC INFLAMMATION will require *Mercurius viv.* or *Mercurius cor.*, followed by *Nitric acid.* Consult the section on syphilis.

SCROFULOUS INFLAMMATION OF THE NOSE will be benefited by *Sulphur*, *Colcarea carb.*, *Phosphorus*, or *Mercurius viv.* Consult the section on scrofula.

For warts on the nose, give *Calcarea carb.*

CANCER OF THE NOSE.—Give for this affliction, *Arsenicum* night and morning, and continue it at least a month, and as much longer as there is any improvement. Afterward give *Silicea*, *Sulphur*, or *Carbo veg.*

For POLYPUS OF THE NOSE, give *Calcarea carb.* night and morning; afterward give *Sepia* every night.

CHAPTER IX.

DISEASES OF FEMALES.

TARDY APPEARANCE OF THE FIRST MENSES.

Menstruation is a natural process, and with a healthy female there should be little or no suffering. There is a great variety in regard to the age at which the menses make their first appearance. Climate makes a great difference; in hot climates they may appear as early as the tenth year, and even earlier; in very cold climates, they may be delayed until the twentieth year, or later; whereas, in temperate climates, usually between the thirteenth and the sixteenth years, although they not unfrequently appear a year or two earlier, or are delayed three or four years later. If they appear early in life, they are apt to cease early; and if they commence late, they continue late. They usually cease, in temperate climates, at about the age of forty-five years. The duration of the menstrual flow is generally four or five days, but it may last but for a day, or it may continue for nine or ten days, and the patient remain healthy; it should return once in twenty-eight days, although it may vary a few days without serious harm. I have alluded to the variations which occur in regard to the menses, as to age, duration, &c., to impress upon the reader the important fact that a deviation from the usual habit, does not necessarily denote a diseased state, and require treatment. Much injury is often done by uncalled-for anxiety and unnecessary medication.

So long as the health is good and the spirits are buoyant, no anxiety need be felt owing to the delay of the menses, even though the young lady may be eighteen or twenty years of age; but if she becomes nervous, pale, or has a flushed face, with symptoms of congestion of the brain or chest, with palpitation of the heart, it will be best to give proper attention to her case. Sunlight, outdoor air, and active exercise, are by far the most important measures, for they will invigorate the entire body, and generally soon relieve the existing symptoms, and bring on the menses; without them, remedies may fail, or only partially relieve the case.

Pulsatilla: This is one of the most important remedies, and may be given alternately with *Sulphur*, forty-eight hours apart. If the patient is of a full habit, *Calcarea carb.* may take the place of *Sulphur* at the end of one month.

Give *Bryonia* every morning in obstinate cases.

Sepia: If, notwithstanding the above remedies, especially *Pulsatilla* and *Calcarea carb.*, there ensue great debility, pale and bloodless face and lips, emaciation, unnatural craving for chalk, slate, &c., give *Sepia* every third night.

Lycopodium is sometimes useful, and may be given every night, when relief is not obtained from the above remedies.

SUPPRESSION OF THE MENSES.

(AMENORRHŒA.)

This may result from exposure, getting the feet wet, fright, or other strong mental emotions; and it frequently occurs, during the progress of diseases of the lungs, liver, bowels, and uterus; and in such cases is either symptomatic, or the result of debility; and we can only expect relief when the disease is cured, and health and strength begin to return. In all such cases, the principal attention should be paid to curing the existing disease, which has caused the suppression, and not to the removal of this symptom.

Treatment of Suppression of the Menses.—If it is the result of exposure, or getting the feet wet, give a dose of *Pulsatilla* every night. If there are headache and fullness in the head, give in addition to this remedy a dose of *Belladonna* in the morning; and continue these remedies until the next period arrives; or if the menses have been some time suppressed, continue them for a month, if relief is not sooner afforded. If they fail, give *Sepia* alternately with *Pulsatilla* two days apart.

If the suppression has been caused by fright, or other violent mental emotions, give *Aconite* once in six hours; also when it arises from other causes, if there is fullness in the head, or a flushed face, with palpitation of the heart. As soon as these unpleasant symptoms are relieved, give but one dose a day. *Lycopodium* may follow *Aconite* if the latter fails to bring on a return of the menses. Give a dose every night for one week, then only twice a week. This remedy is also proper when the face is pale, the spirits depressed, and the patient suffers from the whites or leucorrhœa.

If the patient is of a full habit, and other remedies, especially *Aconite*, *Belladonna*, or *Pulsatilla*, fail, give a dose of *Calcarea carb.*, every night.

If there is great debility, give a dose of *China* every night.

In obstinate cases, give *Bryonia* every morning. If there are frequent chills, or a disposition to cough. Give *Sulphur*, if there are aching pains in the back of the head, disposition to take cold readily, leucorrhœa, exhaustion after talking, and if the mind is irritable and dejected.

SCANTY MENSTRUATION, BUT NOT ENTIRE SUPPRESSION.—The remedies named for suppression are the most important remedies for this affection.

Pulsatilla, if there is headache, which is aggravated by warmth, and relieved in the cold air, palpitation of the heart, leucorrhœa (whites), diarrhœa, sadness and weeping.

Calcarea carb. may be given every night if the patient is of a full habit, with rush of blood to the head, buzzing in the ears, languor and heaviness in the whole body.

Give *China* when there is great debility. *Sepia*, *Lycopodium*, or *Sulphur*, may be required in obstinate cases.

THE MENSES ARE SOMETIMES TARDY IN MAKING THEIR APPEARANCE. Instead of occurring once in twenty-eight days, they may return only once in five, six, or more weeks. When this is the case, and the patient seems otherwise well, give a dose of *Sulphur* once a week, until within four or five days of the time when the menses should occur, then give *Pulsatilla* night and morning until they commence. During the next two or three months, pursue the same course. If relief does not follow, give *Sepia* and *Bryonia* in the same manner as directed for *Sulphur* and *Pulsatilla.*

In all cases when the menses are retarded, deficient or suppressed, during the progress of disease of the lungs or of other organs, you must consult the section on such disease as well as the directions given above.

PROFUSE MENSTRUATION.

The menses may be regular as to time, or delayed when they are profuse, but generally they are too frequent occurring, once in two or three weeks. The secretion may be natural, or it may contain clots of blood ; it may continue an unusual length of time, or no longer than natural. There is sometimes severe pain in the back, and through the womb, and in the left side, with soreness.

Treatment.—The patient should use her drinks cold, avoid tea, coffee, stimulants, shun feather-beds, and live on plain food; if there is much pain, soreness, and fullness, mostly vegetable food; if there is great debility with little pain or soreness, animal food, beef or mutton, should be used at least once a day.

When the menses are too frequent with more or less pain and soreness, give a dose of *Calcarea carb.* every third night in the intervals between the menstrual periods. During the flow if the discharge is bright red give *Ipecac* once in two hours. If there is much pain or flowing and *Ipecac* does not relieve it, give *Belladonna* every hour. Continue this treatment for two months, and longer if the patient is steadily improving; but if no relief follows, or if the patient has ceased to improve, give *Platina* every night between the periods, and if there is much pain or flowing, give *Nux vomica* once in two hours during the period. *Chamomilla* is sometimes useful after *Nux vomica* when there are severe pains with the discharge of dark clots. Give *Sabina* once in four hours if other remedies fail to relieve the flowing.

If there is great weakness with but little pain, give a dose of *China* every night. This remedy will also be found useful in obstinate cases where there are spasmodic pains through the womb, especially if the discharge has been very profuse or causes faintness. *China* may be given both during the interval and the period, but if it has been given during the interval and has not prevented severe flowing at the period, give *Secale cor.* every hour until it ceases. If notwithstanding the use of *China* for one or two months, the menses still remain profuse without pain and with great debility, give *Sepia* once in two days during the interval, and *Secale cor.* every hour during the flowing. *Pulsatilla* will sometimes be found useful; if the above remedies fail, it may be given instead of *Secale* once in three hours. If the patient does not improve under this treatment a dose of *Sulphur* may be given one night in a week instead of either *China* or *Sepia.*

If the flowing is very profuse let the patient keep the horizontal position, with the hips elevated, and apply cloths from cold water to the lower part of the abdomen and between the thighs.

PAINFUL MENSTRUATION OR MENSTRUAL COLIC.

This may occur when the menses are natural, scanty or profuse, and when as to time the patient is regular or irregular.

Treatment.—If the menses are profuse, last too long, or return too frequently with severe spasmodic pains, and pressure in the region of the womb, give a dose of *Platina* every night between the periods, and night and morning during the flow. Continue this remedy at least one month, and as much longer as there is any improvement. *Nux vomica* may follow *Platina* and be given in the same manner. If the menses as to time of appearance are either regular or delayed, natural as to quantity, or scanty give *Pulsatilla* and *Sulphur* alternately two days apart on retiring at night. During the pain give a dose of *Pulsatilla* once in two or three hours. *Belladonna* or *Chamomilla*, will sometimes relieve the pain if *Pulsatilla* fails. If at the end of two months the patient is not relieved, omit the above remedies and give a dose of *Sepia* once in three days, at night, and give at the commencement of the pain a dose of *Nux vomica*, and repeat it at the end of two hours if necessary.

If the flow is scanty, and the pain severe, apply cloths wrung from warm water, over the lower part of the abdomen, and between the thighs.

CESSATION OF THE MENSES, OR CHANGE OF LIFE.

This generally occurs, in this climate, when females arrive at about forty-five years of age, or at some other period between the fortieth and fifthieth years. With healthy females, there is usually little or no serious disturbance of the system ; the change approaching gradually, the menses becoming less profuse, and perhaps less frequent, until they cease. But in other instances, there is a tendency to hemorrhage ; even profuse flowing is not uncommon. And when there is no hemorrhage, especially if the courses stop suddenly, there is frequently dizziness, headache, nervousness, flashes of heat, disturbances in the urinary secretion and discharges, debility, pains in the back and lower part of the abdomen, with heat ; sometimes there is violent itching of the external parts.

Treatment.—This period of life, under homœopathic treatment, is attended with very little danger, as the various disturbances which result, are generally soon relieved by our remedies.

Pulsatilla is perhaps more frequently required than any other remedy, especially when, with a cessation of the menses, there are dizziness, headache, nervousness, urinary derangement, pain, heat, and itching. Give a dose night and morning, until the symptoms are relieved. This remedy, when there is profuse flowing, is sometimes useful, if either *Belladonna* or *Lachesis*, which should generally be tried first, does not relieve the symptoms.

If *Pulsatilla* fails to relieve the various symptoms named, give *Lachesis* night and morning. *Sepia*, and finally, *Sulphur*, may follow *Lachesis*, if required by any remaining symptoms.

WHITES (LEUCORRHŒA)—UTERINE ULCERATION.

The chief causes of these affections, which are so prevalent, are : too much indoor confinement, the want of *sunlight*, air, and active exercise, during childhood; and too lengthy confinement in school and neglect of active exercise during early youth; also tight dressing, and the use of tea, coffee, and stimulating food. These influences all weaken the system, prevent robust and perfect development, and predispose to these affections, so that even unmarried females become subject to them. The above bad habits, by causing delicacy and deformity, render multitudes of our young ladies incapable of enjoying the pleasures, or bearing the necessary burdens of married life, without causing these diseases, and also falling of the womb. Let the mother who cares for the health of herself or daughters, read carefully the author's works on the "Avoidable Causes of Disease and Deformity," and on "Marriage," and have her daughters read them.

Symptoms.—At first the discharge may be slight, and transparent, but gradually it becomes whitish, sometimes yellowish, and in bad cases, green, bloody, or dirty brown, and it may be acrid, so as to excoriate the external parts. When it becomes excessive, the general health begins to fail, the appetite is poor, the pulse becomes weak, and there are great debility, lowness of spirits, and pains in the back. If excoriation or ulceration on the neck of the womb ensues, there are often pains, soreness, and a sensation of rawness, with perhaps heat and smarting in that region. Pain in the right side of the abdomen, and pain in the back of the head, and in the back part of the top of the head, with a numb sensation, are common symptoms which attend uterine congestion and ulceration. Leucorrhœa may exist without ulceration, or even much if any inflammation, but the latter affections rarely occur, without causing more or less discharge. Leucorrhœa or a whitish discharge, is not uncommon in young girls, and even in children.

Treatment.—Sunlight, outdoor air, and exercise, are all-important in the treatment of these affections; in fact, if these are neglected, remedies of any kind can only palliate the symptoms. All blinds and curtains should be removed from the windows during the day, and the patient should, if possible, occupy a south room. She should sit in the sunlight and open air, ride and walk out, if able; she must have exercise in order to have pure blood, good digestion, and gain strength, and thus be in a favorable condition for the cause of the symptoms, be it debility, congestion, inflammation, or ulceration, to be relieved. But here is the difficulty: if the disease is at all severe, the patient cannot walk, ride, or perhaps even sit, without causing severe suffering, and aggravating the symptoms and disease. How is she to obtain the needed exercise? First, if she is not able to exercise herself, she is to be exercised. Second, she is to take exercise, or be exercised, while in a position in which exercise will not increase the congestion or sufferings in the region of the womb, generally at first while lying down, perhaps with the hips elevated; afterward, while sitting up, and still later, while standing. Commence with the extremities, stretching, bending, and extending them, rotating them in every possible direction; if the patient is able, let her resist. Thus exercise her for half an hour (allowing her to rest occasionally), once a day, after a little, twice a day. As soon as she is able, let her exercise herself. Such exercise will not only increase the digestive powers, purify the blood, and give strength, but it will also call off the blood from the congested parts to the extremities, and thus relieve the congestion. Follow the above directions, and give the appropriate homœopathic remedies, and a cure will generally follow. There are many specific exercises appropriate in this disease, but it would be difficult to describe them here, and the knowledge and skill of a physician should direct their application in individual cases, when practicable. If you do not obtain relief from the measures and remedies described, consult a physician, one if possible, who not only understands how to select the right homœopathic remedy, but also one who has the skill to select and direct you in regard to such exercises and general measures as you may need, to effect a cure by the aid of the remedies.

Pulsatilla: This is one of the most important remedies in a majority of cases, especially if the discharge is white and thick, or watery and irritating, with pain, heat, and burning. Give a dose every night for one week, then alternate it with *Sulphur*, twenty-four hours apart, gradually lengthening the intervals to three or four days.

Sepia: Give this remedy every night, gradually lengthening the intervals, to two or three nights, if the discharge is yellowish, or green and corrosive, and is attended with smarting or itching, and pains in the abdomen. *Lycopodium* may follow *Sepia* in such cases, after a few weeks, and may be given in the same manner.

Calcarea carb.: If the discharge is worse before the menses, or if it is bloody and thin, and if there are pain, soreness, smarting and itching, give a dose of this remedy every night for one week, afterward twice a week. *Sulphur* and *Lycopodium* may be required after *Calcarea*, and may be given in the same manner. In cases of great debility from a profuse discharge, a dose of *China* in the morning will be useful.

For leucorrhœa, or a whitish discharge, in the case of young girls or children, *Cannabis sat.* is the chief remedy. Give a dose night and morning for three weeks, then give a dose of *Calcarea carb.* once a week. Washing the external organs once or twice a day with tepid water is useful in such cases.

In all cases of leucorrhœa the patient should avoid high-seasoned food, tea, coffee, and stimulants, eat brown bread and plain meats, vegetables and fruits.

FALLING OF THE WOMB (PROLAPSUS UTERI).

For the causes which predispose to this disease consult the above section on leucorrhœa. Over-exertion, and getting up too soon after child-birth, and especially the use of cathartic remedies during confinement, are often the immediate cause of this difficulty. The womb sometimes settles down so as to be seen externally, and in some instances so as to project one or two inches. There is a bearing down pain, and a dragging sensation in the lower part of the abdomen, and pressure toward the external parts. There are faintness at the pit of the stomach, sometimes numbness of the lower extremities, nervousness, and a frequent inclination to pass urine. There is sometimes pain in the left side beneath the short ribs. The above symptoms are aggravated by lifting, over-exertion, and a long walk. It is important to state that these symptoms very frequently exist with very great severity when there is but little if any prolapsus.

Treatment.—Patients who are predisposed to this disease should retain the horizontal position an unusual length of time, without sitting or even raising up after child-birth, and especially avoid cathartic remedies during this period. They should avoid tight-dressing, lifting, over-exertion, and long walks, at all times. The wearing of pessaries and supporters is only a palliative measure, and often does great harm by weakening, relaxing and irritating the parts, and weakening the abdominal and other muscles. They should rarely be worn, and never if they can be avoided, for they do not cure. It is much better to cure this affection by a persevering use of homœopathic remedies, and proper exercise, and I am happy to say that this can generally be accomplished; only in extreme cases, and then only for a temporary period, is it necessary to resort to such mechanical support.

I have space here only to allude to a few of the movements which are useful for the cure of prolapsus or falling of the womb. Let the patient lie on her back, and let one assistant take hold of her hands and another hold of her feet, and gradually stretch her; if she is not too weak she may resist. Then the same may be done when she is lying on her face, the assistant gradually raising her feet as she draws. This tends to raise the ribs, enlarge the abdominal cavity, and causes a flow of blood to the extremities. Also exercise the extremities as directed under the head of leucorrhœa. Let the patient lie on her face and rest the entire weight of her body on her elbows and toes, and gradually raise her hips and lower them several times. If the patient is very weak, an assistant may support part of her weight and assist her. This simple exercise, practised for a short time two or three times a day, is worth more for the relief, and radical cure of falling of the womb than all the supporters and pessaries ever invented. Let the patient lie on her back with her hips elevated and her knees drawn up, then let an assistant repeatedly draw her knees apart, the patient resisting; then let the patient bring them together, the assistant resisting. All the above exercises are taken in the horizontal position and do not increase the prolapsus, but tend to restore the womb to its natural position, and to strengthen tne muscles and parts which should retain it in its true position. Persevere then with such exercises, until cured. Homœopathic remedies will also greatly aid in restoring the patient to sound health, and in relieving the unpleasant symptoms which attend this displacement of the womb. In fact the remedies alone will cure many cases, where the displacement is not too great. Falling of the womb is frequently caused by congestion and enlargement of that organ, and homœopathic remedies cure by relieving the congestion.

Nux vomica: If prolapsus, or symptoms of this affection follow confinement, give a dose of this remedy every night, and let the patient keep the horizontal position until she is entirely relieved. In other cases you may commence the treatment with this remedy, giving a dose every night. If the patient's menses are profuse or frequent, give also a dose of *Calcarea carb.* every third morning, but if the menses are natural or scanty, give a dose of *Sepia* every third morning instead of that remedy.

If, at the end of a month, the patient is not relieved, omit *Nux vomica* and give *Belladonna* every night, and give either *Calcarea carb.* or *Sepia* once a week in the morning. At the end of another month, *Nux vomica* can be given again if necessary, but it will be better to consult a homœopathic physician if the patient is not cured.

INFLAMMATION OF THE WOMB (METRITIS).

This disease may occur at any age, although it is very rare before puberty; it not unfrequently attacks newly-married females; it occasionally occurs during pregnancy, but is far more frequent during confinement than at any other period; and when it attacks lying-in females it constitutes one form of childbed fever. It may be caused by mechanical injuries, exposure, the extension of inflammation from other organs, &c. The disease may be acute or chronic.

Symptoms.—If the attack is acute and severe there are chills followed by fever, a sensation of uneasiness, and heat in the region of the womb with more or less pain, which may be sharp and in paroxysms, or dull, and may extend to the back and groin. The irritation may extend to the bladder and cause irritation in the urinary passages, or to the bowels and cause diarrhœa. There is generally tenderness on pressure, and nausea and vomiting are not uncommon.

Treatment.—*Aconite* is the most important remedy at the commencement of the disease when the skin is hot, and there are burning and pain in the region of the womb; give a dose every hour.

Dose, see page 7.

Belladonna, at the end of twelve hours, should take the place of *Aconite*, or, if the skin is hot and dry, it should be given alternately with it at intervals of one hour. These remedies one or both should be continued until the acute symptoms are relieved. It is necessary sometimes to continue them several days.

Chamomilla may be given when passion or disappointment has caused the disease. Give *Mercurius viv.* when there are shooting pressive pains with little heat but free perspiration. Give *Nux vomica* after the acute symptoms have been somewhat relieved by other remedies, where there remains a burning, aching sensation in the region of the womb, with pain in the back, and aggravation of the symptoms in the morning. Give a dose once in six hours.

Consult the section on childbed or puerperal fever.

INFLAMMATION OF THE OVARIES.

There is pain, more or less acute, in the lower part of the abdomen, on one or both sides in front of the hips. There is generally tenderness on pressure and sometimes swelling. If the disease is acute there are perhaps chills, fever, and loss of appetite. This disease, when overlooked or neglected, is very apt to become chronic.

Treatment.—If the symptoms are acute, give *Aconite* once in two hours, and if it fails to relieve within twenty-four hours, give

Belladonna, once in four hours; and if, at the end of two or three days, the symptoms are not relieved, give it alternately with *Lachesis*, at intervals of two hours. In chronic cases, or cases which threaten to become chronic, give *Platina* every night, if *Belladonna* and *Lachesis* do not cure the disease; afterward give *Sepia* every night.

INFLAMMATION OF THE LABIA

It is not uncommon for the lips of the vagina or passage to the womb to become inflamed, red, swollen, and hot; and if the inflammation is not subdued, an abscess is apt to form. This affection may be caused by the rupture of the hymen, difficult labor, exposure, or it may occur without apparent cause.

Treatment.—If the disease has been caused by mechanical injuries, give *Arnica* once in three hours. In other cases, give *Belladonna* once in two hours. If at the end of twelve hours, there is no improvement, alternate it with *Rhus tox.*, at intervals of two hours. Wash the parts three or four times a day, with a weak solution of *Arnica;* half a teaspoonful of the tincture, to a teacupful of water, is about the right strength. If the above remedies fail to relieve, give *Mercurius viv.* once in four hours.

PREGNANCY.

Although females should enjoy good health while in this condition, still, in the present artificial state of society, it is not unfrequently attended with distressing symptoms, severe diseases and dangerous accidents. To point out all the causes of such difficulties would require a volume, and such a volume the author has written, and every female who would shun suffering and disease, should read the "Avoidable Causes of Disease."

The pregnant female should take regular exercise in the open air and sunlight, riding and walking. Active indoor exercise and labor are useful. The patient should shun over-exertion, hard lifting, and too long walks. She should, above all, carefully avoid tight-dressing, even about the waist and chest, for it may not only injure her, but destroy her child, or cause it to be deformed. She should cultivate cheerfulness and contentment, avoid strong mental emotions and outbursts of passion, and have no fears as to the result; for under homœopathic treatment, during pregnancy and confinement, when compared with the allopathic treatment, there is very little danger Nowhere is the wonderful superiority of homœopathy more manifest, than in the success which attends the treatment of females during pregnancy, labor, and confinement, when compared with the best results of any other system of practice.

DIZZINESS AND HEADACHE.

A sense of fullness in the head, chest, and, in fact, of the whole body, with dizziness or headache, is not uncommon. When such symptoms occur, give a dose of *Aconite* in the morning, and a dose of *Belladonna* at night. If these remedies do not give relief soon, consult the sections on headache, and congestion of the brain, on pages 309, 303, and 304.

MORNING SICKNESS.

Heartburn, sour stomach, nausea, and vomiting, are common symptoms, generally commencing about six weeks after conception, and continuing, when not relieved by treatment, for eight or ten weeks; sometimes in fact not abating until after delivery. These symptoms are generally more troublesome in the morning than at any other time of day.

Treatment.—For heartburn or sour stomach, give a dose of *Pulsatilla* every night. If *Pulsatilla* fails to relieve the symptoms, give a dose of *Nux vom.* every night, and a dose of *Pulsatilla* every morning.

For nausea and vomiting, give a dose of *Nux vom.* every night, and a dose of *Ipecac* at any time when there is any nausea, but not more frequently than once in four hours.

If the above remedies fail, give *Natrum mur.* night and morning.

Arsenicum will be required in obstinate cases, when there is great heat and burning in the stomach.

Opium, when the nausea is aggravated on sitting up. *Sepia*, in obstinate cases. The remedies last named may be given two or three times a day.

CONSTIPATION.

This is not an uncommon symptom during pregnancy. The patient should take regular exercise, eat coarse bread and fruits, and attend to the bowels at a regular hour every day. Give a dose of *Nux vom.* every night and a dose of *Sulphur* in the morning. If these remedies do not relieve, give *Natrum mur.* night and morning; if this fails, give *Lycopodium* at night, and *Bryonia* in the morning. *Opium* three times a day is sometimes useful. Consult the section on constipation, page 238.

DIARRHŒA.

This affection is less frequent during pregnancy than constipation, but it is much more injurious when it does occur. The chief remedies are *Phosphorus*, *Sepia*, *Sulphur*, and *Dulcamara*, although other remedies may be required. For the indications for the use of individual remedies, consult the section on diarrhœa, page 233.

ITCHING OF THE PRIVATE PARTS.

It may be accompanied by a thrushlike eruption. In that case, wash the parts with a weak solution of *Borax*, and give *Mercurius viv.* one night and *Sulphur* the next, and so continue. If the parts are of a dark red color, and there is oozing of a watery fluid, give *Rhus tox.* one night and *Sulphur* the next. If there is dryness of the parts, give *Bryonia* three times a day. *Lycopodium* every night is sometimes useful.

Painful and Involuntary Passage of Urine—Retention.—The chief remedies for these affections, are *Pulsatilla, Nux vom.* and *Sulphur*. Select the proper remedy, according to the indications given on pages 272, 273, and 276.

Toothache.—The chief remedies are *Nux vom.*, *Pulsatilla*, *Belladonna* and *Calcarea carb.* Give a dose of one of them once in two hours until relief is obtained. Consult the section on toothache, page 191, for the particular indications for these remedies.

Pains in the back and side, more frequently in the right side, are not uncommon. Give *Nux vom.*, at night and *Bryonia* in the morning; if these fail, give *Sepia* at night and *Belladonna* in the morning. If the pains are worse while at rest, or lying down, give *Rhus tox.*, night and morning. *Arnica* sometimes will be found useful.

Cramps in the lower extremities, hips, or abdomen, are not uncommon. If in the legs, give *Nux vom.*, every night and *Calcarea carb.*, once in three mornings. If they fail, give *Hyoscyamus* night and morning. Afterward if required, give *Secale cor.* If the cramps extend to the back, and *Hyoscyamus* does not relieve, give *Ignatia* night and morning. For cramps in the abdomen, give *Belladonna, Nux vom., Pulsatilla,* or *Hyoscyamus.*

SWELLING OF THE VEINS OF THE LOWER EXTREMITIES (VARICOSE VEINS).

This is quite common during pregnancy. The veins of the leg, and perhaps of the thigh, become enlarged, swollen and knotty, Give a dose of *Arnica* night and morning, and put one teaspoonful of the tincture of *Arnica* into half a pint of water, and wash the swollen veins. If this does not soon relieve the symptoms, wet a cloth in the solution, lay it over the veins, and apply a laced stocking or a bandage (commencing always at the toes) smoothly over the wet cloth. Make this application in the morning.

If *Arnica* does not relieve the disease, give *Pulsatilla* night and morning, and afterward *Lycopodium, Lachesis,* and finally *Carbo veg.*, may be required in some cases.

MISCARRIAGE—ABORTION—PREMATURE LABOR.

Although this accident may occur at any period of pregnancy, still it is most common about the third or fourth month, and it is less dangerous at that period. It may be caused by mechanical injuries, strong mental emotions, the abuse of drugs, over-exertion, tight-dressing, sexual excesses, &c. It often depends upon a debilitated state of the system, or a constitutional defect, either inherited or acquired. If a patient has once miscarried, there is always great danger that it will happen again at about the same period of pregnancy; and it is sometimes very difficult to break up this habit. Although a miscarriage, when properly treated, is not necessarily attended with very great danger, yet it is far more dangerous than child-birth at the full period, and a frequent recurrence of this accident is sure to impair seriously the health of the female. The shock to the nervous system is far more serious than that which results from natural child-birth, and the liability to hemorrhage and inflammation is greater. It is therefore very important to prevent this accident when possible, on account of the mother, as well as for the preservation of her offspring.

Symptoms.—Sometimes the first symptom of a threatened miscarriage is a discharge of blood, in other instances pain resembling labor pains, or perhaps aching in the back, extending through the womb. Chills not unfrequently attend the above symptoms, and sometimes fainting, especially when there is much flowing. If there are both pains and flowing there is always much greater danger of miscarriage, or premature birth, than when there is but one of these symptoms, even though it be severe.

Treatment.—First: to overcome a predisposition to this accident, if the patient is subject to profuse or frequent menstruation, which is often the case, consult the section on that affection, and follow the directions there given when the patient is not pregnant. If she is troubled with leucorrhœa, or falling of the womb, consult the section on that difficulty. During pregnancy the patient should avoid undue mental excitement, over-exertion, and if she is subject to frequent and profuse menstruation when not pregnant, give her during pregnancy *Calcarea carb.* alternately with *Sabina*, at intervals of two weeks. You should never give the *Colored tincture of Sabina* during pregnancy; the globules of a high dilution are the best. If the patient's menses are usually, when not pregnant, either regular or scanty, give *Sabina* alternately with *Sulphur* two weeks apart.

If symptoms of miscarriage occur, such as pains or flowing, the patient should assume the horizontal position immediately, and rigidly keep it until such symptoms are entirely relieved.

Arnica: Give a dose of this remedy once in two hours, when symptoms of miscarriage have been caused by mechanical injuries or over-exertion. If *Arnica* fails, to relieve give *Belladonna* every hour.

Belladonna: Give this remedy every hour, when there are severe labor-like pains, with or without the discharge of blood. If the flowing is very profuse, give *Ipecac* alternately with *Belladonna*, at intervals of one hour.

If there are flowing and chilliness without pains, give *Ipecac* every hour until there is an improvement, then lengthen the intervals between the doses. If *Ipecac* does not relieve the flowing, give *Sabina* once in two hours.

Chamomilla: If there are severe labor-like or cutting pains without much flowing, and *Belladonna* does not relieve them, give a dose of this remedy every hour.

If other remedies fail, give *Sabina* once in two hours. In obstinate cases of flowing with threatening miscarriage, if the above remedies do not afford relief, give *Platina* once in two hours.

FALSE PAINS.

Some females are very subject to labor-like pains for weeks and even months before confinement. False pains are not attended by flowing, and are generally less regular in their recurrence than natural pains. It is always well to relieve such pains promptly by the use of the proper remedy, and the remedies which are proper for these pains will do no harm if they are given through mistake, when genuine labor pains are present.

Treatment.—*Belladonna* is one of the most important remedies for these pains, and may be given every hour, until they cease.

Give *Coffea* if the pains are violent, and there is great nervous excitability. Give a dose every hour. If *Coffea* does not relieve the pains, give, in such cases, *Aconite*.

Nux Vomica: Give this remedy once an hour, when there is either a constant urging to urinate, or to go to stool. If it does not relieve, give *Pulsatilla*. *Chamomilla* is sometimes useful for false pains, in sensitive individuals.

PUERPERAL CONVULSIONS.

This is a disease which sometimes attacks females during the last months of pregnancy, during labor, or after child-birth. If the attack is during labor, the convulsions generally occur during the pains; sometimes they commence with the very first pains.

There are three forms of these convulsions. *First:* Hysterical convulsions, in which the paroxysms are preceded, accompanied, or followed, by laughing, sobbing, crying, or singing, or other hysterical symptoms; but there is no frothing at the mouth, and the patient is generally not insensible, though she cannot speak. In this form, there is very little if any dauger. *Second:* Epileptic convulsions. In this form of the disease, there is a total loss of consciousness during the convulsions, great twitching of the limbs and muscles, and frothing at the mouth. This is by far the most common form of the disease. *Third:* Apoplectic convulsions. This is the worst form of the disease, but, fortunately, it is very rare. Convulsions, more or less severe, are followed by complete stupor, snoring respiration, and paralysis of muscles; generally there is no frothing at the mouth, and but one paroxysm of convulsions.

Both epileptic and apoplectic convulsions are frequently preceded by violent pains in the head, dizziness, and humming in the ears.

Treatment.—In the hysterical form of the disease, or when there is no frothing at the mouth, and the patient is not entirely unconscious, give *Pulsatilla* every hour, and if it fails to relieve at the end of four hours, give *Nux vom.* *Belladonna* or *Ignatia* may be required, in case *Nux vom.* fails. At the very commencement of each convulsion, dash a handful of cold water in the patient's face; this will often prevent the paroxysm.

In the epileptic form, or when there are frothing at the mouth, twitching of limbs and body, with insensibility, *Hyoscyamus* is perhaps more frequently required than any other remedy, especially when there are great oppression of the chest, and red and staring eyes. Give a dose after each paroxysm, and every hour when the convulsions cease, so as to prevent a return. If this remedy fails to relieve at the end of a few hours, either *Ignatia* or *Chamomilla* will often be required.

If the patient is delicate, very excitable and nervous, *Chamomilla* may precede or follow *Hyoscyamus*, and may be given every half hour or hour.

Ignatia: This remedy may be given if *Hyoscyamus* or *Chamomilla* fails to relieve the symptoms, if the patient is of a mild disposition, and there are unconsciousness, frothing at the mouth, and great oppression at the chest. If the disposition is irritable, *Nux vom.* will often do better than *Ignatia.* Either of these remedies may be given as often as the paroxysms return, and every hour or two after they cease.

Opium: If, notwithstanding the use of the above remedies, the paroxysms continue and become more frequent, and there is a greater degree of stupor between them, the countenance becoming more purple, and the oppression of breathing greater, the pulse small or nearly extinct, give a dose of *Opium* after every paroxysm. It should not be given early in the disease. If you give the globules of this remedy, and you see no effect from two or three doses, give either one drop of the *Tincture of opium*, or a drop of *Laudanum*, after every paroxysm. In the most critical stage, when other remedies fail and death threatens, there is no remedy equ to this, when thus administered.

For the apoplectic form of the disease, or when one or two paroxysms of convulsions are followed by stupor and paralysis, give *Belladonna* alternately with *Nux vom.*, one hour apart. If at the end of six or eight hours there is no improvement, omit the above remedies for six or eight hours and give *Opium* every hour. If you use the *Tincture of opium* in such cases, put one drop in a glassful of water, and give a teaspoonful for a dose. The globules are strong enough for this form of the disease, in fact are to be preferred.

Cloths wet in cold water may be applied to the head, and changed often, in all cases where the head is hot.

As the epileptic form of childbed convulsions is a frightful disease, and fearfully fatal under allopathic treatment, it may not be amiss for the author to state, for the encouragement of those who rely upon the homœopathic treatment, that he has seen, since he has practised homœopathy, thirteen cases, some occurring before, some during, and some after labor, which have been treated with homœopathic remedies, and but one out of the thirteen has died, and that one took an allopathic dose of an anodyne mixture, before he saw her. In that case and in that only, chloroform was tried.

LABOR.

Conception generally takes place within ten days after the cessation of one of the menstrual periods, and labor usually, but not invariably commences within ten days after the termination of nine full months from the last show. Quickening, or the first sensation which the mother experiences of life or motion, generally occurs at the end of four months and a half from conception.

Labor is often preceded for a few hours, by nervous trembling, depression of spirits, looseness of the bowels, frequent inclination to pass urine, and a slight discharge of reddish mucus.

During labor a physician should be called to attend, if one can be found, but a few suggestions to be heeded before his arrival, or in case a physician cannot be found, may not be amiss. First, when, from the regularity and frequent return of the pains, you are satisfied labor has commenced, you will do well to prepare the bed for the patient to lie on during labor and confinement. First, make up your bed as you wish it to be after labor, with the under

16*

sheet only spread on; and a folded blanket, or an oil cloth beneath it, to protect the bed; then on the right side of the bed toward the foot spread folded blankets, coverlets, or an oil cloth with a folded sheet over it, to protect the bed during labor; be careful and always place these over the under sheet, so that they can be drawn out from under the patient when she is through, without changing the sheet; then over the under sheet, place another folded sheet, beneath the patient's hips, as she is carried to her proper place in bed after labor. If the labor pains are very violent, with great suffering, and nervous excitability, give *Coffea* every half hour.

Dose of this or other remedies, see page 7.

For tedious labor, or severe but ineffectual pains, give *Belladonna* every hour. For deficient pains give *Pulsatilla* every hour.

Give the patient no stimulants or herb drinks. She may drink black tea, crust-coffee, or cold water, as she may prefer. If there is much flowing during or after labor give *Sabina* every half hour, and if it does not relieve, give *Secale cor.;* if that remedy is not sufficient give *Platina.* If there is much faintness give *China* every half hour. If the flowing is very profuse apply cloths wrung from cold water over the lower part of the abdomen until it ceases. Wait until respiration is well established with the child before you attempt to tie and cut the cord, and do not be in a hurry about delivering the afterbirth; wait for pains, and if within an hour they do not come on rub the lower part of the abdomen with the cold hand, and when you feel the womb contracting beneath the hand, draw gently on the cord, but never violently.

APPARENT DEATH OF A NEWBORN INFANT.

If the skin is pale or slightly dark, and the pulsations in the cord are very small and frequent, or imperceptible, and the child does not breathe, immediately wrap it up in dry warm flannel, and gently rub it with the warm hand or dry flannel; turn the child on its face, and clear its throat carefully with piece of soft cambric drawn over the end of the finger. Dissolve a globule or two of *Tartar emetic* in a drop of water, and put it on the tongue.

If the child does not commence breathing, wash the lips, and press the sides of the child's nose between the thumb and finger, so that the air cannot escape through it, and place your lips over the lips of the child, and gently blow into its mouth until the lungs are distended, then carefully press the walls of the chest down so as to expel the air, after which blow in the mouth again, and repeat this process of alternately filling the lungs and pressing out the air, repeatedly. If the above measures fail, put the child into a warm bath, and afterward rub it dry, and repeat the inflation of its lungs. But if the face is very purple or dark, the pulsations in the cord very slow and full, if these symptoms do not very soon abate, and the child commence to breathe regularly, cut the cord three or four inches from the navel before tying a string around it, and let a few jets of blood escape, until the pulse becomes more frequent, the face lighter colored, and respiration commences. Do not let the blood flow too rapidly, and stop it the moment there is any improvement. Dissolve two globules of *Opium* in a drop of water and put on the child's tongue, and rub the surface with dry flannel.

Swelling of the scalp and elongation of the head frequently result in tedious or severe labor. Gentle pressure two or three times a day with the hands will bring the head into shape in a few days, and six or eight drops of *Arnica* in a tablespoonful of water, used as a wash, will relieve the swollen scalp.

TREATMENT AFTER DELIVERY.

You have to fear fever and inflammation ; therefore let the patient's diet be light, and carefully avoid stimulants, and animal food for the first week or ten days ; toast, rice, farina, gruel, roasted apples, &c., are sufficient. The patient should avoid sitting up too soon, as it frequently causes falling and inflammation of the womb.

AFTER-PAINS.

Give *Arnica* once an hour, and if it does not soon relieve them, give *Chamomilla* alternately with it at intervals of one hour. *Pul-*

satilla may follow these remedies, if they do not suffice. *Nux vom.*, is often useful in obstinate cases, and if that fails, give *Cuprum* every hour. If there is no flowing of moment, apply warm cloths over the lower part of the abdomen.

Dose of either of the remedies, see page 7.

MILK FEVER.

Until about the third day the secretion of milk is usually not very free; and as the breasts begin to fill on this day, there is often more or less fever, headache, and restlessness. For these symptoms, give *Aconite* once in two hours.

NURSING.

As soon after delivery as the mother is rested, always apply the infant to the breast, and never fail to do this before feeding it; for the child, before it has been fed, always knows how to nurse, but it sometimes loses this instinctive knowledge afterward. Then the breasts always contain a small quantity of milk which should be drawn off, and this is of the exact quality the child needs. The infant should be nursed regularly three or four times a day. There are many advantages which result from nursing the child early and regularly, if proper care is exercised, even though the breasts may contain but little milk, or, to appearance, none. The child thereby retains the faculty of nursing, an early secretion of milk is excited, and it is regularly drawn off, so that the breasts do not become suddenly congested, thereby we avoid, to a great extent, the milk fever, and the danger of inflammation in the breasts. Then the nipples become gradually accustomed to being used, and there is less danger of their becoming sore and inflamed than when the child is not applied until the breasts are full; provided, always, that when the breasts are comparatively empty, before the third day, you never allow the child to nurse but a minute or two at a time, and do not allow it to draw on the breasts when the mother feels that they are empty. If you neglect this precaution, yon are very liable to cause sore nipples, and even inflammation of the breasts.

SORE NIPPLES.

Before confinement it is well to wash the nipples several times a day with cold water, or weak brandy-and-water, and after delivery, do not allow tbe child to remain long at the breast, and never, for a single moment, after the breast is empty. Apply the child to the breast as soon after delivery as the mother is rested, and do not wait for the filling of the breasts, when nursing will be more difficult. If the nipples become excoriated, sore, or painful, wash them in a solution of *Arnica* and water—six or eight drops of *Arnica*, to a tablespoonful of water, is the proper strength. Before nursing, wash the nipples with tepid water, or milk-and-water. Also give *Arnica* internally, once in two hours; and if there is much pain and soreness, give it alternately with *Chamomilla*, at intervals of two hours. If the nipples, notwithstanding the above treatment, become cracked or ulcerated, give *Sulphur* every night, and *Silicea* in the morning; and if, at the end of one week, they are not well, give *Calcarca carb.* night and morning. *Hepar sulph.* may follow the last named remedy if it is required.

AGUE IN THE BREAST; OR, INFLAMMATION AND ABSCESS IN THE BREAST.

Indurations in the breasts are often caused by the wearing of stays and tight dresses while young, and such indurations are very liable to become inflamed when the breasts fill with milk. This disease may also result from exposure, or taking cold. Inflammation of the breasts is a very painful affection, and if not soon checked, is very liable to result in the formation of an abscess. If the breasts become distended, and feel full and painful, give *Apis mel.* once in two hours, and if, at the end of twelve hours, there is no improvement, give *Bryonia* once in two hours; if they become inflamed and red, and the patient is troubled with chills and fever, give *Belladonna* alternately with *Bryonia*, at intervals of one hour, and apply to the breast a plaster composed of one part of yellow beeswax, and two parts of lard, melted together and spread on a cloth; or, what is equally as good, and perhaps better, cover the entire breast with cabbage leaves, first warming and slightly wilting them, by holding them to the fire a minute or two. If, at the end of two days, the inflammation is not subdued, omit the *Bryonia*, and give *Phosphorus* alternately with *Belladonna*, at intervals of two hours. If these remedies fail to check the disease, omit them at the end of forty-eight hours, and give *Hepar sulph.* morning and noon, and *Silicea* before tea, and at bedtime, until the abscess breaks, then give *Sulphur* at night, and *Phosphorus* in the morning. Generally, by prompt treatment, you will be able to prevent the formation of an abscess.

THE LOCHIA,

OR THE DISCHARGE WHICH FOLLOWS CONFINEMENT.

This discharge should gradually grow lighter and cease at the end of one or two weeks. It should not stop suddenly; but if it should be suppressed, owing to damp or chilly weather, or mental emotions, give *Pulsatilla* every hour; if there is violent headache with pain in the back, give *Bryonia* alternately with *Pulsatilla* at intervals of two hours. If these remedies do not relieve the symptoms, give *Platina*.

If the discharge is profuse or long continued, give a dose of *Platina* once in six hours, and if after two or three days it fails to relieve, give *Pulsatilla* once in six hours. If this remedy does not relieve, give *Calcarea carb.* night and morning.

Dose of either of the remedies, see page 7.

MILK LEG (PHLEGMASIA ALBA DOLENS).

In this disease, to which lying-in females are subject, one of the legs becomes swollen without redness, very tender to the touch and painful. There are also chills followed by fever.

If such symptoms appear give *Arnica* alternately with *Belladonna* one hour apart, and put one teaspoonful of the tincture of

Arnica into a pint of water, and wring a towel from the solution thus made, and wrap it around the leg, and over that four or five thickness of dry flannel; wet the towel once in eight hours.

If at the end of twenty-four hours there is no improvement, give internally *Rhus tox.* instead of *Arnica*, alternately with *Belladonna*, at the same intervals. If the symptoms do not soon yield, omit the above remedies for twelve hours, and give a dose of *Sulphur* once in two hours, then return to them again.

If swelling remains after the acute symptoms are removed, give *Arsenicum* once in six hours; afterward *Pulsatilla*, and then *Nux vomica*, continuing each remedy several days.

CHILD-BED FEVER (PUERPERAL FEVER)

The attack generally commences within from twelve hours to three or four days after delivery. There occur chills followed by fever, a flushed face, and frequent pulse, headache, perhaps nausea and vomiting, with pain in the lower part of the abdomen, with tenderness on pressure, which extends and increases; the lochia is generally suppressed, the urine scanty and high-colored. This disease sometimes prevails as an epidemic, and is always formidable. A homœopathic physician should be called when practicable. This fever is not as common, nor as dangerous under the new treatment, as under the old practice. It is frequently caused by cathartics, stimulants, and other drugs.

Treatment.—At the commencement of the attack give *Aconite* every hour for twelve hours, then alternate it with *Belladonna* at intervals of an hour. If at the end of twenty-four hours there is no improvement, but there is increased tenderness of the abdomen, give *Bryonia* once in six hours, and *Aconite* every hour between. Also fold a flannel blanket in one direction so that it will be wide enough to extend from the knees to the shoulders, then lay it lengthwise across the bed; fold a sheet in the same manner, but not quite as wide as the blanket; wring the sheet out of warm water, and wrap it around the body and hips, and wrap the ends of the flannel blanket as the patient lies upon it, over the wet sheet; wet the sheet again as soon as it becomes cool.

A few doses of *Chamomilla* will be useful when there are very severe pains like after-pains, which are not relieved by the remedies already named, give it instead of *Bryonia*.

In desperate cases when the pulse becomes small and the extremities cool, give *Rhus tox.* every hour, and if no improvement follows, alternate it with *Arsenicum*.

Consult the section on peritonitis on page 223. If with fever, and pain and soreness of the bowels, there is diarrhœa, consult the section on enteritis, page 226. Also consult the section on inflammation of the womb, page 359.

STATE OF THE BOWELS DURING CONFINEMENT.

It is desirable that the bowels should not move for from five to eight days after delivery, and they generally will not if they are let alone. This is natural, and gives time for the swollen and sometimes almost lacerated organs to return to their natural size and position, and for the soreness to disappear. Untold injury and suffering often arise from the use of cathartic remedies during confinement or after labor. I have known a single dose of castor oil cause the most intense suffering, which was not even mitigated at the end of six months.

If at the end of eight days the bowels do not move, give a dose of *Bryonia* once in six hours, and if at the end of twenty-four hours more there is no action, give *Nux vom.*, and also give a free injection of tepid water night and morning, until there is a free discharge. Eat brown or coarse bread, baked apples, and potatoes.

IF THERE IS A DIARRHŒA, *Dulcamara*, *Rheum*, *Hyoscyamus*, and *Phosphorus*, are the chief remedies. For particular indications, consult the section on this complaint, page 234.

FOR A KNOWLEDGE OF THE PROPER TREATMENT OF ANY OTHER AFFECTION which may occur during confinement, or while nursing, consult the section on that disease, in the forepart of this work.

CHAPTER X.

DISEASES OF CHILDREN.

For information in regard to the proper management of children from the hour of birth until the completion of their education, and how to prevent disease and deformity, the author earnestly refers the reader to his work on the "Avoidable Causes of Disease." That work should be read carefully by every parent, for it contains in a small compass, an amount of practical information, such as can be found in no other single volume, as to the wants of very young children, frequency of nursing, deficiency of milk, weaning, bringing up children by hand, cows' milk, food proper for children after weaning, exercise, light, air, playgrounds, moral management of children, dress, education—physical, moral, and intellectual, &c.

As, of course, the diseases of children are similar to the same diseases in adults, and the treatment nearly the same, to save unnecessary repetition, and to have the treatment as full as possible, any variation which is required in the treatment of any disease to which both the adult and children are subject, has been noticed, in speaking of such disease under its appropriate head, so that, with a few exceptions, the reader will simply be referred to the appropriate pages, where he will find a description of the diseases and treatment much more full than it would be possible to give it here without repeating much of the volume.

CRYING AND WAKEFULNESS OF INFANTS.

If the child cries suddenly, see that a pin is not pricking it. In other cases, see that the belly-band is not too tight, for when it is it sometimes causes intense suffering. If the child draws itself up as if from colic, give *Chamomilla* every half hour, and consult the section on colic, page 240. Also consult the section on earache, page 340. For wakefulness, give *Coffea* every night, and if it fails, give *Belladonna*, and finally *Hyoscyamus*.

SWELLING OF THE BREASTS.

The breasts in infants are sometimes found swollen and hard, but not from the presence of milk, as is sometimes supposed. Do not rub them, but wash them in a tablespoonful of water into which has been dropped six drops of *Arnica*, then cover them with a piece of cotton or linen cloth, wet with *Sweet oil*, and give a dose of *Belladonna* night and morning.

JAUNDICE.

The skin and eyes sometimes become yellow within a few days after birth. Give a dose of *Mercurius viv.*, night and morning for two days, then give *China* night and morning. If these remedies do not relieve the symptoms consult the section on jaundice, p. 255.

EXCORIATIONS.

The utmost attention to cleanliness is requisite to guard against this difficulty. Wash frequently with cool water, and between folds of the skin where there is redness, or excoriation, place a piece of fine linen wet with cold water, or cold water which contains eight or ten drops of *Arnica*, to the teacupful. If this does not relieve, wash with cold water, wipe dry, and dust with wheat starch. Give internally *Chamomilla* night and morning, and if at the end of four or five days there is no improvement, give *Mercurius viv.* every night and *Sulphur* every morning; follow these at the end of a week, if necessary, by *Calcarea carb.*, every night.

THRUSH—SORE MOUTH—APHTHÆ.

In one form of the disease white curdy points or patches make their appearance on the mucous membrane of the mouth, which can be wiped off without much difficulty. In another variety, white vesicles appear over the tongue and mouth, which form, after a time, superficial ulcerations. The stomach and bowels are frequently deranged, and the disease may be attended with fever. Improper food, often causes this disease, and there is sometimes a constitutional predisposition which favors its development.

Treatment.—Dissolve a piece of *Borax* as large as a pea in a teacupful of water, wash the mouth three times a day with this solution, and give *Mercurius viv.*, night and morning for five days, then give *Sulphur* night and morning. If a watery diarrhœa attends this affection, and the above remedies do not relieve it, give *Arsenicum* once in six hours. If the passages contain undigested food, give *China* morning and noon, and *Arsenicum* before tea and at bedtime.

Red Gum—see diseases of the skin, page 102.
Prickly Heat—see Eczema and Lichen, pages 90 and 94.
Constipation—see page 238.
Diarrhœa—see pages 233 and 237.
Intestinal Worms—see page 250.

CHOLERA INFANTUM.

This affection is common with children under three years of age. Vomiting and purging, more or less severe, are the prominent symptoms at the commencement of the disease. After a few days the vomiting may cease and the diarrhœa continue. In very severe cases the patient may die within twenty-four or forty-eight hours, but milder cases may last for weeks. Rapid emaciation, sunken eyes, and great debility soon result, and sleepiness, stupor, and symptoms of disease of the brain, are apt to ensue in severe cases.

Treatment.—Give *Veratrum* every half hour at the commencement, and if it does not soon relieve the nausea and vomiting, give it alternately with *Ipecac* at intervals of one half an hour. If, notwithstanding the above remedies, there ensue great prostration, cold extremities, and sunken eyes, give *Arsenicum* alternately with *Veratrum* fifteen minutes apart. If symptoms resembling disease of the brain appear, give *Belladonna* and *China* alternately two hours apart. For nourishment give milk, and if this disagrees, give rice water or oatmeal gruel; milk is generally the best.

Consult the sections on cholera morbus, page 216, and diarrhœa, on page 233.

RETENTION OF URINE.

This frequently occurs in newborn infants, and sometimes causes great distress and danger. Give *Aconite* once in two hours, and if three or four doses do not relieve the symptoms, give *Pulsatilla* in the same manner. Put cloths from warm water over the lower part of the abdomen and between the thighs.

Inflammation of the Eyes—see page 336.

Earache and Discharge from the Ear—see pages 340 and 343.

Convulsions—see page 321.

Inflammation and Dropsy of the Brain—see pages 291 and 295.

Croup—see page 135.

Hooping Cough—see page 150.

Vaccination—see page 63.

Scald Head—see pages 89 and 90.

Milk Crust—see page 88.

Erysipelas—see page 80.

Measles—see page 75.

Scarlet Fever—see page 67,

Rupture—see page 246.

Wetting the Bed—see page 276.

INFANTILE REMITTENT FEVER.

Children under ten years of age are subject to this disease. It is characterized by one or more daily paroxysms of fever, with intervening remissions. There is usually headache, drowsiness, loss of appetite, pain in the bowels, and at first constipation. At the end of eight or ten days, if the symptoms are not relieved, they are apt to become more marked; chills, followed by more violent paroxysms of fever, vomiting, increased drowsiness, starting or twitching of the muscles, flushed cheeks, picking at the nose, mouth, and eyes, cough, and grinding of the teeth. The symptoms are often improperly attributed to worms, and this affection is sometimes called worm-fever. As the disease advances, the breath becomes offensive, there is vomiting of undigested food, and there are offensive discharges from the bowels; sometimes worms are discharged, and there is frequently delirium. The disease may be caused by improper food, impure air, and exposure.

Treatment.—At the commencement of this fever, when the bowels are constipated, give *Bryonia* once in two hours. If there is violent pain in the head, or drowsiness, which this remedy fails to relieve, give *Belladonna* alternately with it, at intervals of one hour. If there is nausea or vomiting, give *Ipecac* alternately with *Bryonia,* one or two hours apart.

If, as the disease progresses, there are offensive discharges from the bowels, with pain in and distension of the abdomen, give *Pulsatilla* once in two hours. If there are griping pains, with mucus or slimy passages, with straining, give *Mercurius viv.* once in two hours.

If the disease does not soon abate, under the above treatment, give a dose of *Sulphur* every night, and continue during the day the remedy which seems most appropriate.

Give *Cina* once in two hours, when there are picking at the nose, starting during sleep, diarrhœa, with colic. *Chamomilla* will often relieve such symptoms, if *Cina* fails If the brain becomes seriously disordered, and there is stupor or delirium, give *Bella-*

donna alternately with *Bryonia;* and if these remedies do not relieve, give *Helleborus* alternately with *Bryonia*, two hours apart.

The diet, throughout the disease, should be light—gruels, rice, milk, baked apples, and, at most, toast or cracker. A daily warm-bath, and frequently sponging of the surface of the body, face, and head, with tepid water, will be useful, so long as there is much fever.

Dentition.—This process is sometimes attended with severe suffering from an inflamed state of the gums, which gives rise to pain, headache, and fever; also to diarrhœa. If there is diarrhœa, consult the section on that affection, or if any other manifest symptoms of disease occur, consult the section on such disease. To facilitate the process of teething, and allay the irritation of the gums, give *Calcarea carb.* every night, and *Belladonna* every morning, when the gums seem to be sore and swollen. If there is much heat about the head, *Aconite* may be given morning and noon, instead of *Belladonna.*

SUGGESTIONS TO PARENTS.

Please remember that the essential conditions for the substantial development and health of children, are first, sunlight, out-door air, and play; second, plain wholesome food and drink, free from spices and stimulating condiments. Never allow children or the young either tea or coffee, for these drinks are far more injurious to the growing child than to the adult. If you would have your child healthy, do not allow him to stay in-doors during daylight longer than is necessary for meals, for if you do his blood will become watery and thin, and he will become pale and unable to withstand the diseases of childhood. Do not allow him to sleep in a room where the sun has not shone during the day, if you can help it.

CHAPTER XI.

EXTERNAL INJURIES, APPARENT DEATH, POISONS AND THEIR ANTIDOTES, &c.

EXTERNAL INJURIES.

As such injuries are often sudden and alarming, it is desirable that every one should have some knowledge as to the best treatment.

BURNS AND SCALDS.

For a superficial burn, where the skin is not blistered, hold the part to the fire until the pain ceases.

A linament, composed of equal parts of *Lime-water* and *Sweet oil*, spread on a piece of cotton cloth and applied, is one of the best applications for a burn.

Raw cotton applied to the surface, does very well, also wheat flour, dusted over the surface repeatedly, so as to protect it from air, is a very good application. A teaspoonful of the tincture of *Urtica urens*, may be put into a teacupful of water, and cloths dipped in this solution, may be applied. This is an excellent application. Also a solution containing half a teaspoonful of the tincture of *Rhus tox.* to a half-pint of water, and applied in the same manner, as *Urtica urens*, does well, if you have it.

If there are severe pains and nervous excitement give *Rhus tox.* once an hour. If head symptoms should be developed, give *Belladonna* alternately with *Rhus tox.*, one or two hours apart. If there is great debility from an excessive discharge, give *China*, night and morning. If the ulcer which results from a deep burn, is in a healthy condition, a simple plaster of either mutton tallow, or of beeswax and lard, is a suitable dressing.

FROZEN LIMBS AND PARTS, AND APPARENT DEATH FROM FREEZING.

In case of frost-bitten parts, or apparent death from freezing, we have especially to guard against a sudden transition from cold to heat. Warm applications or a warm atmosphere, applied to a frozen part, is destructive to the part, and a warm room and heat, are death to the patient, in critical cases of freezing.

In all cases let the patient be kept in a cool room, out of draughts of air, and apply to the frozen parts snow, ice-water, or as cold water as you can get, if you can get neither snow nor ice-water. If the whole body is apparently dead from cold, cover it with snow, or put it into cold water, leaving, of course, the nostrils and mouth uncovered in either case; and after the frozen parts are relieved of the frost, as they soon will be, take the patient from the snow or water, and gently rub the frozen parts with snow or cold water, until they begin to look natural; then rub them with the warm hand.

For the severe pains which follow, give *Carbo veg.* every hour, and if at the end of five or six hours they are not relieved, give *Arsenicum.*

SPRAINS AND BRUISES.

Apply to the injured parts cloths wet in a solution containing a teaspoonful of *Arnica* to a teacupful of water, and over the wet cloths apply dry flannel. Also give *Arnica* internally once in three hours. If after a few days the symptoms are not relieved, give *Rhus tox.*, once in two hours.

DISLOCATIONS AND FRACTURES.

A physician or surgeon should always be called in such cases; if a homœopathist cannot be obtained, an allopathic physician or surgeon should be called.

Arnica may be applied to the injured part as directed in cases of bruises and sprains, and the limb should be kept in an easy and as natural position as possible until the surgeon arrives.

CONCUSSION OF THE BRAIN.

This results from a sudden jar, which may stun the individual for a time, or only partially do this. The face is pale, the pulse small, and nausea and vomiting frequently follow.

Give *Arnica* every half hour, and if dizziness, headache, or convulsions follow, give *Belladonna* alternately with it at intervals of one hour. If fever and inflammation follow, give *Arnica* alternately with *Aconite*, and consult the section on inflammation of the brain, page 291.

WOUNDS.

Simple incised wounds, or such as are made with a sharp-cutting instrument, will heal in four or five days without any discharge if the edges are carefully kept in contact by adhesive plaster, bandages, and perhaps stitches; but if the irritating substances, which are so popular with the public, are applied, it will require several weeks for the wound to heal, and there will be a profuse discharge, and a large scar. Then, from a wound which has been made with a sharp instrument, carefully remove all foreign substances and bring the edges together with long strips of adhesive plaster, from one fourth to one half an inch wide; and support these with a bandage around the part, if practicable. If there is much bleeding, that should first be checked.

TO STOP HEMORRHAGE.

If the flow of blood is slight, simply pressing the edges of the wound together, and bathing it in cold water will stop the bleeding in a few moments. If the blood flows very freely, and in jets, it denotes that an artery has been wounded, in that case, if it is of any magnitude it will require ligaturing, or tying; but you can generally stop the flow of blood for the time-being by pressing with a finger directly on the end of the bleeding vessel in the wound, or by pressing over the course of the vessel between the wound and the heart. The pressure will require to be kept up until the artery can be tied.

If the wound is in one of the extremities, you may tie a handkerchief, a cord, or suspender, around the extremity above the knee or elbow, and then place beneath the handkerchief or cord a compress made of cloth, a stone, or stick, half as large as a hen's egg, on the inside of the thigh or arm, over the course of the main artery, and with a stick twist the cord until the bleeding stops; if it does not readily stop change the position of the compress a little either inward or outward until you get it right. But if the flow of blood is very rapid, do not wait a moment, but press directly with your finger, if possible, on the end of the bleeding vessel, until the ligature can be applied, as directed above, around the limb, or the artery can be tied. Never pile on a wound rags or cloths with a view to stop the flow of blood, for they only absorb it. If the patient faints from the loss of blood, lay him on his back with his head low, and give him *China* or a spoonful of brandy-and-water, or a drop or two of *Camphor*, and dash cold water in his face. If a surgeon cannot be had readily, bend the point of a pin and hook it into the end of the artery draw, it down and tie a stout thread around it tightly; then dress the wound, but leave one end of the ligature hanging out.

LACERATED AND CONTUSED WOUNDS.

If the parts are not too badly bruised, but simply torn or cut, you can bring the edges together with stitches and adhesive plaster, as in the case of incised wounds, and they will generally unite readily; but if the parts are much bruised or swollen, apply cloths wet in cold water, or what is better, a solution which contains a teaspoonful of *Calendula* to half a pint of water. If fever and inflammation ensue, give *Aconite* every hour, and if it does not relieve, give *Belladonna* alternately with it one hour apart, and apply warm water or a warm poultice, if the inflammation is violent.

In gunshot and punctured wounds, it is not desirable to heal up the external opening until the bottom is healed, a little lint may be put into the external orifice to prevent the edges from uniting, and the wound may be dressed with cold water or *Calendula* and water, as directed for contused wounds to prevent inflammation ; and if inflammation ensues treat it in the same manner as directed in case of inflamed contused wounds. If in any case the discharge is very profuse, and causes great debility, give *China* night and morning. If the discharge is unhealthy give *Silicea* at night and *Hepar sulph.* in the morning.

POISONED WOUNDS.

STINGS OF INSECTS AND BITES OF SERPENTS.

For the sting of a bee or wasp, apply a slice of an onion, and give *Belladonna* internally, or bathe the parts in a weak solution of *Arnica.*

For the bite of a serpent, suck the part with the mouth, and if you are careful to swallow nothing, and rinse the mouth afterward, no injury will result to any one from doing this. If a cupping glass is applied it will do well, but this usually is not at hand.

If a band or a handkerchief is tied tightly around the limb above the injury immediately, so as to retard the return of blood to the heart, it will be of some service. If at hand hold a coal of fire, or a hot iron, as near the wound as the patient can bear it, until a shivering or stretching sensation is experienced. Give internally *Belladonna* alternately with *Arsenicum* ten or fifteen minutes apart, or give brandy-and-water, in small but repeated doses, or a little salt and water, if you have nothing else handy.

For the proper treatment for a bite of a rabid or mad dog, or other animal, consult the section on hydrophobia, page 316.

APPARENT DEATH FROM DROWNING.

The wet garments should immediately be removed, and dry warm blankets or flannels, applied to the body, and the latter should be placed in a horizontal position, with the head and chest raised, with the mouth and nostrils open. Warmth should be diligently applied to the extremities and body, by the means of hot flannels, bricks, &c., and the surface may be rubbed with the dry warm hand, and warm flannels.

As soon as practicable, artificial respiration should be commenced. The tube of a common pair of bellows may be fitted into one nostril, and the other nostril and the mouth may be closed with the fingers, so as to prevent the escape of air, and at the same time gently draw downward, and press backward the upper part of the windpipe, so as to open that tube, and prevent the air from passing into the stomach; then blow the bellows gently, so as to fill the lungs When this is done, remove them, and let the nose and mouth be free, while you press down the walls of the chest, so as to expel the air; then go through the same process of inflating the lungs, and expelling the air, repeatedly, until natural respiration commences, and is well established, or until the limbs become rigid or stiff, showing that the patient is actually dying. If a pair of bellows is not at hand, the mouth of the operator can be applied over the mouth of the patient, closing the nostrils with the fingers, air can be blown into the lungs, and expelled as directed above, and this can be repeated until a pair of bellows can be obtained, or the patient is restored. A slight current of electricity or galvanism, passed through the chest is sometimes useful.

APPARENT DEATH FROM HANGING OR CHOKING.

The treatment is the same as recommended for apparent death from drowning.

APPARENT DEATH FROM NOXIOUS GASES.

Persons in descending into old wells, or wells near a recent fire, or into casks or large vessels where fermentation is going on, or by sleeping in a tight room, where burning charcoal has been permitted to stand, are not unfrequently suffocated by carbonic acid gas. Other gases may also cause death by their poisonous effects. In all cases of apparent death, or a near approach to it, which result from an exposure to such gases, remove the patient immediately into a current of fresh, cool air, and dash cold water freely over the face, neck, and chest, and wipe the patient dry, and apply warmth by the means of warm flannels and blankets; also resort to artificial respiration, as directed in the case of apparent death from drowning; if relief is not soon afforded, electricity may be tried, and as soon as respiration is established, give a dose of *Opium* every half hour.

APPARENT DEATH FROM LIGHTNING.

The general measures are the same as in apparent death from noxious gases; namely: cool air, dashing with cold water, artificial respiration, and the application of warmth. In addition to the above, give *Nux vom.* every half hour, dry on the tongue, or in a single drop of water.

APPARENT DEATH FROM A FALL.

Place a drop of *Arnica* on the tongue, and resort to artificial respiration and warmth, as directed in cases of drowning.

OVERHEATING—SUN-STROKE.

Give *Aconite* every fifteen minutes, and if it does not soon relieve, give *Belladonna* alternately with it one half hour apart. *Bryonia* may follow the above remedies at the end of a few hours, if necessary, and *Carbo veg.*, if at the end of a day or two any unpleasant symptoms, such as headache and pressure over the eyes remain.

POISONS AND THEIR ANTIDOTES.

As it is no uncommon thing for poisonous substances to be taken through mistake or for the sake of committing suicide, or for them to be given to others with a criminal intent, and as the life of the patient often depends on the most prompt measures, it is important that proper instructions in regard to treating such cases, should be accessible to all.

If a poison has been taken into the stomach, the first thing to be done is to remove it as soon as possible by exciting vomiting, or by the use of the stomach pump. Then some remedy may be given which will neutralize or destroy the action of the poison.

Vomiting can generally be excited by drinking a large quantity of tepid water, and then tickling the throat with the finger, or a feather. If this fails, a teaspoonful of powdered *Mustard* in a glass of warm water may be given, or an emetic dose of *Ipecac*, or even of *Sulphate of zinc*, or of *Sulphate of copper*, or *Blue vitrol*, may be given. Generally the tepid water and tickling the throat with the finger, will be sufficient, if the patient drinks rapidly all he can. Try this first.

Arsenic.—Excite vomiting as soon as possible, by any of the above measures, also give warm greasy water, warm milk, cream, equal parts of sweet oil or melted lard and lime-water, or the white of eggs. Either of the above articles, or two or three of them, should be given as soon as possible, in connection with the measures to excite vomiting, and should be repeated occasionally afterward.

Corrosive Sublimate.—Excite vomiting as soon as possible, and at the same time let the patient immediately drink freely of eggs stirred up in water. If eggs are not at hand, give milk, and if that cannot readily be obtained, give flour and water.

Copper or Verdigris.—Give warm water freely, and also milk and water, and eggs stirred up in water.

Lunar Caustic (Nitrate of Silver).—Give common salt in water, afterward flaxseed tea or gum-arabic water.

Oxalic Acid.—Give powdered chalk mixed with water, or the carbonate of magnesia, and excite vomiting by drinking freely of warm water. Do not give saleratus or potash in any form. A mixture of lime-water and sweet oil is good.

Oil of Vitriol (Sulphuric Acid), Nitric Acid, and Muriatic Acid.—In case of poisoning from either of these acids, give immediately soapsuds, wood ashes mixed with water, carbonate of magnesia, chalk, or lime-water, and let the patient drink freely of water or milk-and-water. Oil is also useful.

Iodine and Iodide of Potassium.—Give starch or wheat flour, mixed with water.

Sugar of Lead.—Excite vomiting and give epsom-salts or diluted sulphuric acid. Castor oil is good; also give milk freely.

Saltpetre (Nitre).—Cause vomiting by giving tepid water, and give flaxseed tea or gum-water.

Antimonial Wine and Tartar Emetic.—Give freely of warm water, tea, milk, warm water and butter or grease, or a tea made of oak bark or of Peruvian bark.

Shell Fish.—Clams, muscles, &c., are sometimes poisonous. Excite vomiting, give powdered charcoal or strong coffee without milk or sugar.

Alkaline Substances, Strong Lye, &c.—Give vinegar diluted with water.

Phosphorus.—Excite vomiting and give gum-water or flaxseed tea. Avoid all oily substances and drinks.

Prussic Acid.—Shower the head and spine with cold water, and let the patient smell of camphor or of ammonia.

Opium.—If a stomach pump is at hand, the stomach should be thoroughly rinsed out; but if one cannot be obtained immediately, excite vomiting as soon as possible, by any of the measures named near the commencement of this section. Pour cold water over the head, spine, and chest; if the patient is a child, plunge the body into warm water and suddenly remove it into the cold air occasionally. Do not let the patient fall asleep, keep him walking, slap his hands, feet, and body. Do not give vinegar, but you may give coffee or tea. Electricity is sometimes useful.

In cases of poisoning from Nux vomica, Strychnine, Hyoscyamus (Monk's hood) Belladonna, Stramonium, Cicuta, or Hemlock, or any other vegetable substance, excite vomiting as soon as possible, by the use of any of the means named near the commencement of this section, or use the stomach pump. Do not use cold water as directed in cases of poisoning by opium or morphine. You may give drop doses of *Camphor*, often repeated, also strong *Coffee*, and for convulsions, if they are severe and persist, let the patient breathe *Chloroform* during them, omitting it as soon as the convulsions abate.

Alcohol.—The effects of poisonous doses of alcohol may be counteracted by showering the head and body with cold water, when the body is hot. Also cause vomiting as soon as possible, or use the stomach pump.

If inflammation or other forms of disease result from the action of poisons, consult the section on such disease in this work, and follow the directions there found, only always avoid the use of the article which has caused the symptoms, and select some other remedy.

CHAPTER XII.

EMERGENCIES,

AND DISEASES AND SYMPTOMS NOT ALREADY NOTICED.

THERE are times when prompt action is requisite to rescue individuals from immediate danger and death. At such critical moments it is all-important that the right thing should be done on the spot, and it is perhaps equally essential that improper measures be avoided. The aim in this chapter is simply to point out separately what should be done *first*, and then to refer the reader to the page where he will find full directions for further treatment.

BLEEDING (HEMORRHAGE).

If from a wound the blood flows in jets, press directly one or more fingers into the wound on to the end of the bleeding vessel or vessels. If from a wound on the inner part of the thigh or leg, press in the wound, and also with one thumb press firmly on the artery as it passes from the abdomen over the bone into the groin.

For further directions, see page 385.

Bleeding from the lungs, if alarming: Place the patient halfway between a sitting and lying position, unfasten the garments about the neck, chest, and waist, and apply cold water to the chest. The patient should not speak. If you have at hand, give *Aconite* alternately with *Ipecac* fifteen minutes apart. If you have no remedies, dissolve a teaspoonful of salt in half a glass of water and give a teaspoonful of the solution every ten minutes.

For further directions, see page 161.

BURNS AND SCALDS (IF EXTENSIVE).

Protect the surface from the air by applying dry cotton, or cotton moistened with sweet oil, or dust the parts repeatedly with wheat flour; or if at hand, apply cloth moistened with a liniment of sweet oil and lime-water. For further directions, see page 383.

FREEZING, AND FROST-BITTEN PARTS.

Keep the patient away from the fire; apply snow, ice-water, or cold water. For further directions, see page 384.

FITS, CONVULSIONS, &c.

If a patient falls in a fit, and is convulsed, or has twitchings of the face or extremities, with or without frothing at the mouth, let him remain in the horizontal position, with the head and shoulders raised; remove everything tight from around the neck and chest; apply cold water to the head, and for further directions, see pages 318 and 321.

If the patient is motionless, with blowing out of lips, elevate the head and shoulders, and if the head is hot and the face flushed, apply cold water to the head. For further directions, consult the section on apoplexy, page 304.

FAINTING FITS—SWOONING.

The face is deathly pale, and the lips colorless, the patient is unconscious, respiration and circulation are apparently nearly or quite suspended. Place the patient *immediately* in the horizontal position, with the head and shoulders as low or lower than the body; admit fresh air, and dash cold water over the face and chest. If relief does not soon follow, resort to artificial respiration, as directed on page 388, in cases of drowning. Also see page 179.

APPARENT DEATH (ASPHYXIA),

FROM DROWNING, HANGING, CHOKING, OR SMOTHERING.

If from drowning, remove all wet garments. In all cases of apparent death from either of the above causes, place the patient in a horizontal position, and apply dry warm flannel to the surface of the body, and warm bricks and bottles of warm water to the extremities and sides. In cases from smothering, choking, or hanging, dash a little cold water over the face and chest two or three times, and wipe dry afterward. In all cases resort immediately to artificial respiration as directed on page 388.

APPARENT DEATH FROM GASES AND LIGHTNING.

Place the body in a current of cool, fresh air, and dash cold water repeatedly over the face, neck, and body, and resort to artificial respiration as directed in cases of apparent death from drowning, on page 388. If the body becomes cold, apply artificial warmth as directed in cases of drowning. For further directions, see page 389.

Apparent death from a fall, resort to artificial respiration and warmth. See page 389.

POISONS AND THEIR ANTIDOTES

In all cases, if a poison has been taken into the stomach, excite vomiting as soon as possible, by giving freely of tepid water, and by tickling the throat with the finger or a feather. For further directions, see pages 390, 391, and 392.

SIGNS OF DEATH.

It may be thought an easy matter to say whether an individual is dead or alive, but it is sometimes extremely difficult to determine with certainty, and yet very important to decide correctly; for severe cases of fainting, and of asphyxia, not unfrequently terminate fatally, through a neglect of proper restorative measures.

All apparent respiration and circulation may cease for hours, possibly for days, and yet the patient be alive, and finally recover.

There is but one sure sign of absolute death, and that is the beginning of decomposition, which is indicated by the smell, and by the greenish, or bluish discoloration of parts of the body. The darkish discolorations of the skin which are generally witnessed soon after or even before apparent death on dependent portions of the body, are not signs of decomposition.

There is but one certain sign that an individual is dying, and that, in cases where there is no organic change to render recovery absolutely impossible, restorative efforts are useless, and that is the *rigidity* or stiffness of the muscular system which usually follows within a few hours after apparent death, and continues from a few hours to four or five days in different cases. The limbs and body are stiff, and if forcibly bent, the part does not return to its former place, but remains where the force applied has left it. "This curious phenomenon is regarded by John Hunter as the last act of the vital principle," and by Nystern, as a "concentration of the remaining vital powers in the muscular system, preparatory to its final extinction." After this rigidity or stiffness has passed off, the body again becomes limber, and decomposition follows.

In cases of apparent death from drowning, asphyxia, fainting, and the like, we should not give up our efforts to restore the patient until this rigidity or stiffness makes its appearance.

In England, it is customary not to bury the dead until the commencement of decomposition, and this is as it should be. We should never think of interring a corpse till either decomposition has commenced, or rigidity makes it manifest recovery is impossible.

VARIOUS SYMPTOMS NOT ALREADY NOTICED.

For habitual cold feet and coldness of the lower extremities, give *Rhus tox.* in the morning and *Silicea* at night. Washing in cold water is of service. In such cases, patients should shun hot water, stoves, and fires, for they increase the difficulty.

For perspiration of the feet, give *Sulphur* every night for one week, and *Carbo veg.*, the next, and so continue. For an offensive cold perspiration, give *Silicea* every night.

For burning in the feet, give *Pulsatilla* every night and *Calcarea carb.*, every morning, and wash with warm water.

For numbness of the lower extremities, give *Nux vomica* every night and *Silicea* every morning.

For numbness of the upper extremities, give *Nux vomica* at night and *Belladonna* in the morning, and in all cases of numbness consult the sections on Paralysis and Apoplexy.

For a bad or offensive breath, if from bad teeth, consult a dentist, and wash the teeth and mouth frequently with water. In all cases, give *Nux vomica* at night and *Sulphur* in the morning, and if improvement does not follow within a month, give *Pulsatilla* instead of *Nux vomica* at night.

INDEX.

THE AVOIDABLE CAUSES OF DISEASE,

MARRIAGE, &c.,

(THE TWO VOLUMES IN ONE.)

BY JOHN ELLIS, M.D.

AND FOR SALE BY BOOKSELLERS GENERALLY THROUGHOUT THE COUNTRY.

TABLE OF CONTENTS:

CHAPTER IV.—Violation of the Conditions requisite for Physical Development and Preservation. *Water.* *Air*—Impure Air—Ventilation—Poisonous Gases—Hot Air—Dry Air—Moist Air—Breathing—How we should Breathe. *Sunlight*—Its Effects on Vegetable Development—On Animal Development—Deformity and Disease result where Light is excluded. *Exercise*—Mental and Physical—Exercise of the Intellectual Faculties—Effects—Physical Exercise—Its Influence on Development—On Health—Results which follow the Neglect of Exercise—Labor—Active Amusements—Outdoor Sports—Calisthenics and Gymnastic Exercises—Their Importance in Schools, Cities, and Villages—Exercise as a Curative Agency.

CHAPTER V.—Children and the Causes of their Diseases—Hereditary Predisposition to Disease and its Causes—Delicate Organization and its Causes—Wants of Very Young Children—Nursing and Obstacles to Nursing—Wet Nurses—Bringing up Children by Hand, and Proper Food—Dosing Infants—Crying—Frequency of Nursing—Deficiency of Milk—Beer and Alcoholic Drinks—Cow's Milk—Weaning and Proper Food for Children after Weaning—Exercise, Air, and Light—Playgrounds for Young Children—Moral Management of Children—Dress—Shoes—Flannel.

CHAPTER VI.—Education—Our Imperfect System of Education among the Causes of Disease, Insanity, and Deformity.

Neglect of Moral Education—Consequences—Insanity—The Education of the Affections more important than Intellectual Education—Importance of Physical Education—Its almost Total Neglect and the Consequences which result—Too Lengthy Confinement in School—Proposed Change in our Schools—Neglect of Elocution and Oratory in our Schools and Colleges—Clergymen's Throat-ail—Its Causes—Prevention and Cure.

In this and in the preceding chapter, comprising eighty-seven pages, will be found more useful and practical information in regard to the proper and improper management and education of children, than can be found in any other volume in the English language.

CHAPTER VII.—Fashions and Habits of the Ladies—Health of American Women—Excessive Confinement in Schools while Young—Dark Parlors and Rooms—Consequences.

CHAPTER VIII.—Neglect of Amusements—Motives which should prompt and restrain in seeking Amusements—Improper Amusements—Those which are Proper—Dancing—Abuse of Amusements.

CHAPTER IX.—Improper Use of Poisons—Signs by which Poisons can be recognized—Opium: Its Effects—Tobacco: Its Effects—As a Poison—Symptoms caused by its Habitual Use.

CHAPTER X—Alcoholic and Fermented Drinks—Physiological Testimony—Natural and Unnatural Stimulants—Effects of Unnatural Stimulants—Drunkenness—Wine—Beer.

CHAPTER XI.—Excessive Labor—Mental and Physical Labor—Clergymen—Physicians—Lawyers—Teachers—Farmers—Bad Positions of the Body.

MARRIAGE, &c.

EQUALITY OF THE SEXES.—Mental and Physical Characteristics of the two Sexes—Man is Superior as Man, and Woman as Woman—What Constitutes a True Marriage—Marriage of Similars or "Congenials," Mentally and Physically, and the Consequences which result to the Parties and their Offspring, both as to Mind and Body—Marriage of Opposites and the Results—The only True Foundation for Happiness in Married Life—Want of Congeniality or Affinity—The True Remedy—Licentiousness—Vice.

Of the Avoidable Causes of Disease, the New York *Independent* says:

"In the above book, Dr. Ellis, whom we personally know to be abundantly qualified for the work he has undertaken, attacks with a vigorous and fearless pen the evils of society, as it is at present constituted, revealing startling facts, the result of years of careful observation as to the physical *degeneration* of the American people, with the manifold causes which tend to produce this result Giving no quarter to the prevailing habits of rearing children from the cradle to the completion of their school education, the author follows them into the workshop and counting-room, dissecting out with a skilful hand the groundwork of ill health and premature decay, and laying bare the faulty manner of life with uncompromising fidelity. In this busy age attention must be *repeatedly* called to the habits of life which engender disease, before people will heed the warning; hence we are glad to recognize in the above work, one that we can cordially recommend and indeed urge upon our readers, as a book every way worthy their careful study."

If you would like the above work, call on the nearest bookseller, and if he has not got it, request him to send for it, and he will be able to furnish it to you at the New York price.

www.ingramcontent.com/pod-product-compliance
Lightning Source LLC
La Vergne TN
LVHW020104110826
845151LV00001B/56
* 9 7 8 1 4 2 5 5 4 3 9 3 8 *